Bloodline of Nitinol Stents

Iosif Rabkin • Dmitry J. Rabkin

Bloodline of Nitinol Stents

Springer

Iosif Rabkin
Malden, MA, USA

Dmitry J. Rabkin
Newton, MA, USA

ISBN 978-3-032-25696-6 ISBN 978-3-032-25697-3 (eBook)
https://doi.org/10.1007/978-3-032-25697-3

This Springer imprint is published by the registered company Springer Nature Switzerland AG
The registered company address is: Gewerbestrasse 11, 6330 Cham, Switzerland

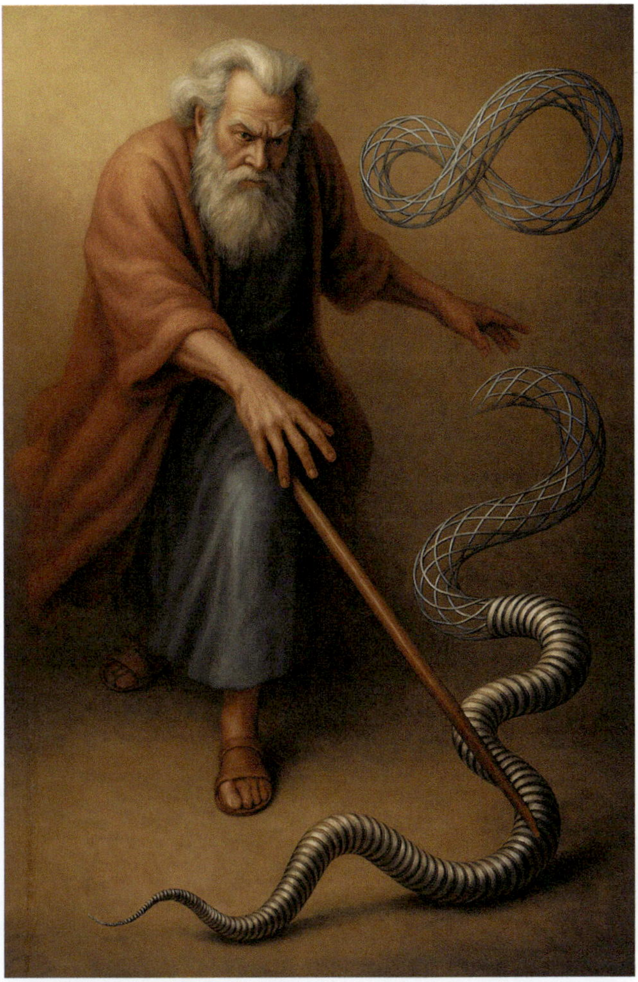

Annotation for the Book Front Illustration

There is a fanciful belief that Nitinol was known even in biblical times, and that the rod of Moses itself was fashioned from this extraordinary alloy. Warmed by the heat of his hand, the rod remained straight and rigid, obedient to its trained form. Yet when cast upon the cold ground, it softened and yielded, losing its rigidity and flowing into a sinuous, serpentine shape. In this imagined union of ancient wonder and modern science, the miracle is recast not as defiance of nature, but as a profound intuition of its hidden laws—an alloy responding faithfully to temperature, transforming stiffness into motion, and metal into lifelike form.

Acknowledgment

Writing this book has been a profound privilege, and I am deeply indebted to the many individuals who made this work possible. Foremost, I am grateful to my father and co-author, whose pioneering vision, intellectual rigor, and lifelong dedication to the field have been an enduring and incomparable source of inspiration.

I extend my heartfelt gratitude to my wife and children for their constant love, patience, and encouragement. Their unwavering support sustained me throughout my career and provided the strength and balance essential to my professional life.

I am also deeply thankful to my collaborators, colleagues, mentors, and peers, whose insight, guidance, and generous sharing of knowledge helped shape my understanding, refine the ideas presented here, and broaden the scope of my work. Their contributions have enriched my career as a whole.

Finally, I wish to acknowledge the readers of this book. It is for you that these pages were written, and it is my sincere hope that this work informs, inspires, and contributes meaningfully to the advancement of the specialty.

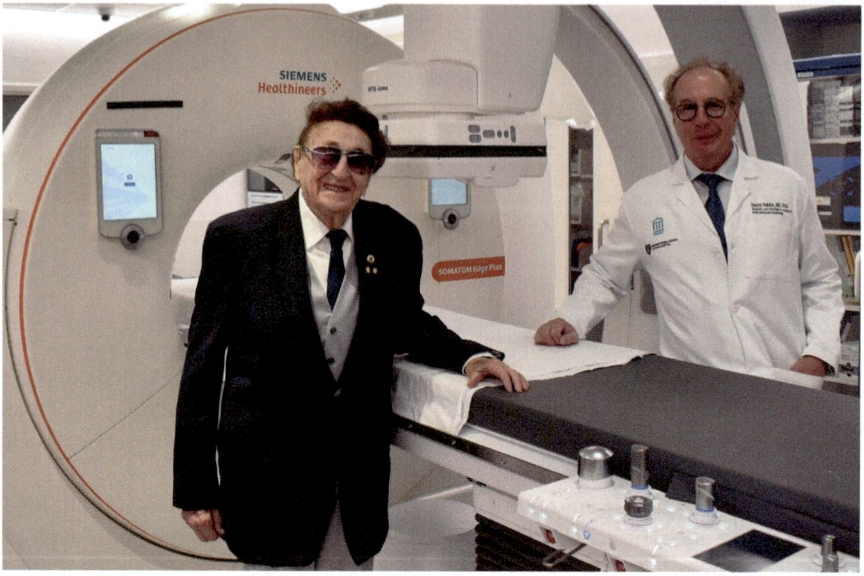

Dmitry Rabkin

Competing Interests The authors have no competing interests to declare that are relevant to the content of this manuscript.

Contents

Genetic Material

1

NITINOL has gained continuous increased popularity among the manufacturers of endoluminal devices. At the same time, most interventional radiologists know little about its unique properties. A thorough understanding of the physical properties of Nitinol, however, is important for optimizing selection and deployment of endoluminal devices in a given clinical scenario. This chapter reviews the unique physical characteristics of Nitinol, which make it the best suitable material for interventional devices, intended for introduction through small openings and expanding inside the body to its intended size and shape [1].

Discovery of Shape Memory Effect and Nitinol

Nitinol is an alloy comprised of approximately 50% nickel and 50% titanium. Nitinol has properties of superelasticity and shape memory. Superelasticity refers to the enhanced ability of a material to be deformed without irreversible change in shape. Shape memory is the ability of a material to regain its shape after plastic deformation at a lower temperature. These physical properties of Nitinol allow complex device configurations and high expansion ratios enabling percutaneous delivery through low-profile access systems. The discovery of superelasticity and shape memory dates back to as early as 1932 [2, 3]. Swedish physicist and metal expert Dr. Olander experimented with an alloy of gold and cadmium. He was the first to observe and report this alloy's "rubber-like behavior," which we now call superelasticity. Olander, however, could not explain the physical basis of his observation. In 1948, the Russian scientist Kurdiumov predicted and, in the following year together with his colleague Khandros, experimentally proved the mechanism of the internal transformations in alloys responsible for superelasticity [4]. Two years later, in 1951, American scientists Chan and Read found that the gold–cadmium alloy, which is now known as the alloy of Olander, possesses not only superelasticity, but also shape memory. At the International Exhibition in Brussels in 1958, a simple

I. Rabkin, D. J. Rabkin, *Bloodline of Nitinol Stents*,
https://doi.org/10.1007/978-3-032-25697-3_1

"engine" with shape memory capabilities was displayed to demonstrate potential applications of the new effect. (The "engine" was a vertically suspended shaped string of alloy that would contract during heating and lift an attached weight). These studies were ignored until 1963, when Buehler and his colleagues at the United States Naval Ordnance Laboratory attempted to develop a material with high resistance to corrosion, and created an alloy of approximately equal amounts of nickel and titanium [5]. Besides having very high anticorrosive properties, this alloy unexpectedly demonstrated remarkable capabilities of shape memory and superelasticity. This alloy was much cheaper than the alloy of Olander, which contains approximately 50% gold. The new alloy was named Nitinol, where Ni and Ti are the symbols for nickel and titanium, and NOL stands for the Naval Ordnance Laboratory.

Nitinol Properties for Interventional Devices

Structural Basics

Superelasticity and shape memory are based on the ability of Nitinol to exist in several crystal forms or phases. Phase transitions between liquid and solid phases are commonly known phenomena, such as water freezing to ice or solid metal melting into liquid. What makes Nitinol unique is its ability to exist in two distinctly different, reversible crystal phases in its solid state at clinically useful temperatures. The alignment of crystals at higher temperature is called austenite (A) phase, the alignment of crystals at the lower temperature is called martensite (M) phase. In between is a temperature interval of gradual transition between the A and M phases. Under external force, the shape of a Nitinol device can be greatly deformed without irreversible damage. Depending on the temperature at which this external force is applied, superelastic or shape memory effects prevail. In close vicinity to or above the temperature-defining transition into the full A state, superelasticity results as soon as the deforming force is released, the device immediately assumes its original shape (Fig. 1.1a). When Nitinol is deformed at or below the lower temperature of the complete M transition, the shape memory effect can be exploited. The device retains its deformed shape even after the external force is removed as long as the temperature of the environment stays below the temperature of transition into A phase, only during heating does the device resume its original shape (Fig. 1.1b). Nitinol memory can be compared with human memory and divided into three stages: imprint, storage, and recall. The first stage requires the imprint of a particular shape. This is achieved by winding Nitinol wire on a special jig into the shape of the desired device (Fig. 1.2), restraining the wire on the jig, and annealing the assembly in a furnace at 500 °C for 1 hour. The jig is then cooled to room temperature and the wire is removed. This configuration now represents the austenite state of the device. For the second stage, storage, one can straighten a device relying solely on its superelastic features by exerting constant force and restraint to keep it straight. For the shape memory effect to be utilized, the device can be gradually straightened and loaded at or below the temperature of the M transformation. The

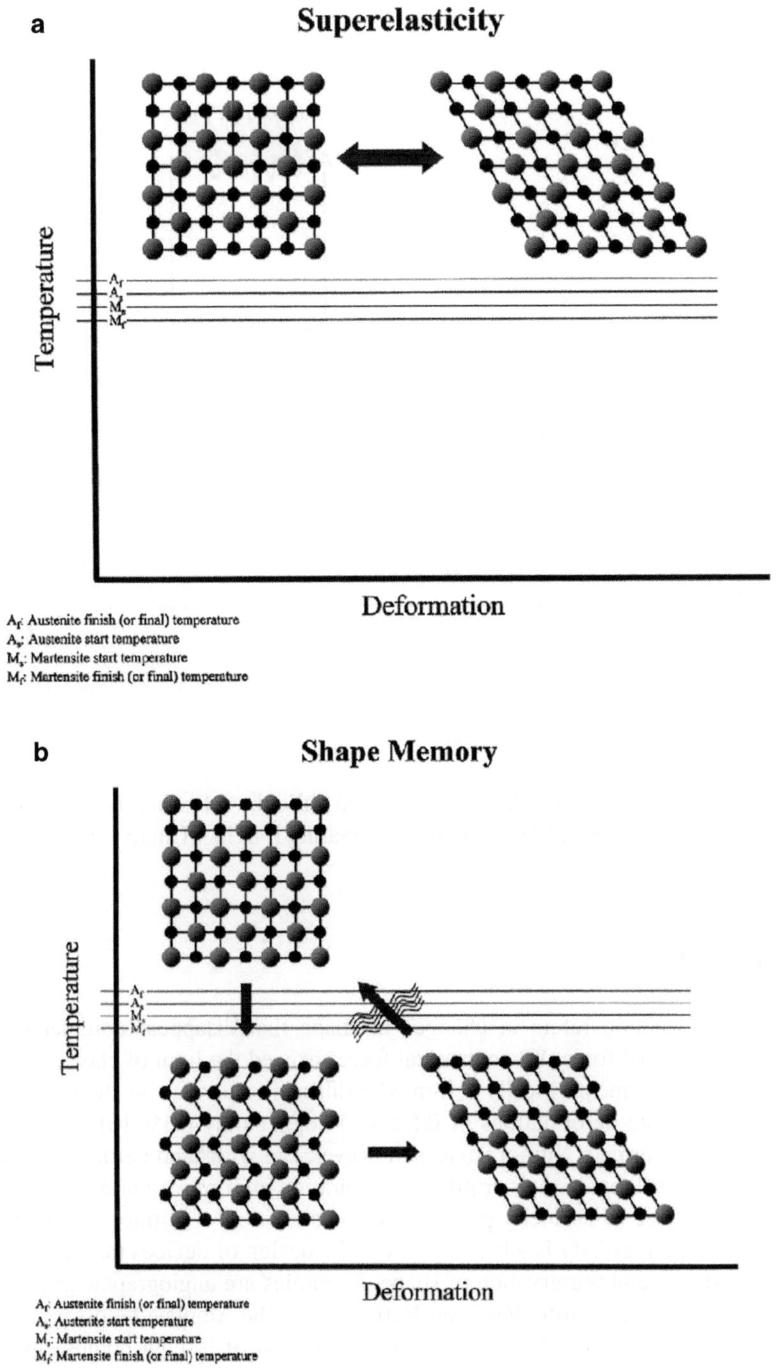

Fig. 1.1 Crystal model of Nitinol deformations. (**a**) Superelastic effects are leveraged by external force above the temperature of transformation, transformations between the states are "two way" and are limited to only two states. (**b**) Shape memory effects are exploited by temperature change. Note that transformations between the states are "one way" and include three states

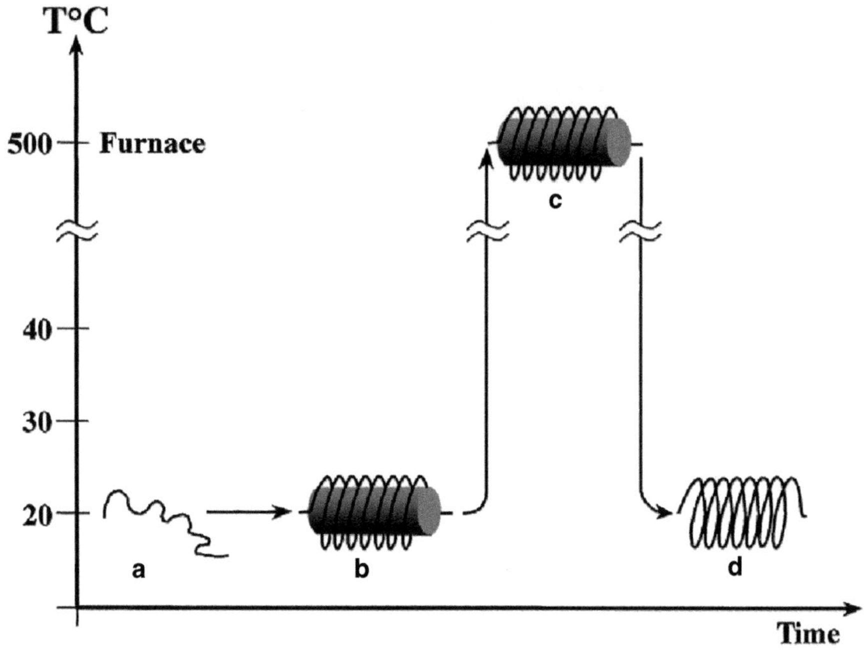

Fig. 1.2 Schematic diagram of imprinting process for manufacturing of Nitinol devices: (a) Nitinol wire, (b) modeling of wire around the jig, (c) annealing in a furnace, and (d) imprinted product removed from the jig after cooling

third stage, recall or retrieval, can be achieved either by releasing the external force from a device in its superelastic state or by heating it in its M state to activate shape memory (Fig. 1.3).

Superelasticity

Elastic deformation refers to changes in shape that disappear completely after release of external force. When external forces exceed the limit of elastic deformation, devices become plastically deformed resulting in a permanent change of shape. Steel can tolerate deformations of 0.5% and copper only 0.1% before becoming irreversibly deformed. Nitinol devices, however, can withstand deformations up to 10–12% and still regain their original configuration after release of external forces. This high degree of elasticity prompted the designation of Nitinol as superelastic material. Superelasticity is advantageous in the design of devices that require high kink resistance and preservation of shape. Examples are angiographic guide wires (Terumo; Boston Scientific Vascular, Natick, MA), the Amplatz Goose-neck snare (Microvena, White Bear Lake, MN) for the retrieval of foreign bodies, and orthodontic arch wires ("braces").

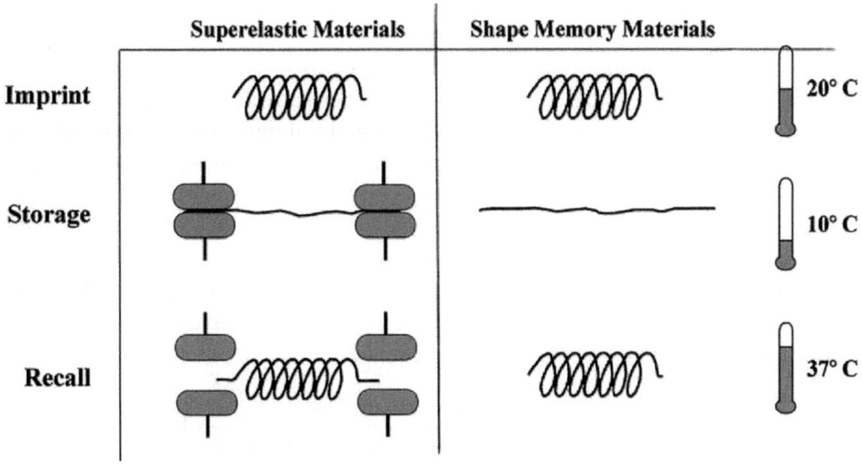

Fig. 1.3 Comparison of superelasticity and shape memory effects. Superelastic materials require external restraint for storage of a device in a deformed configuration, shape memory materials require cool temperatures to store the deformed shape

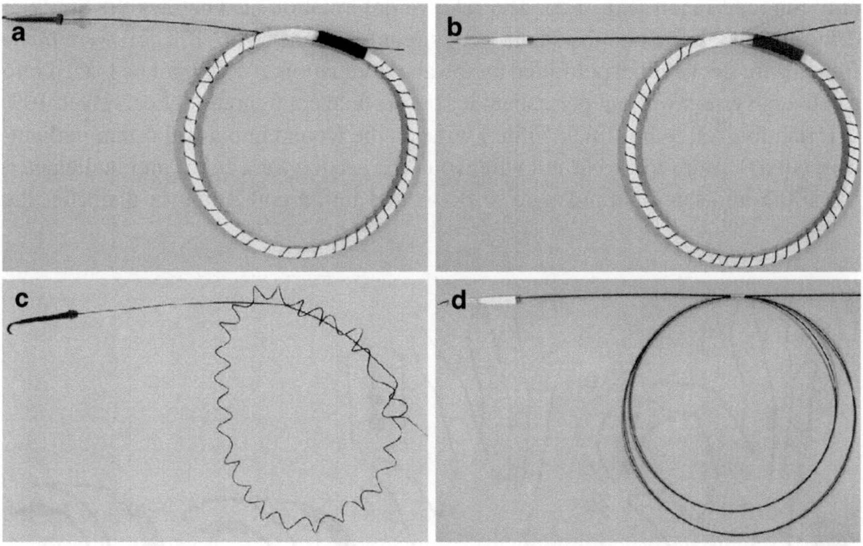

Fig. 1.4 (**a**) A regular 0.035-inch guide wire wound around a plastic housing. (**b**) A Nitinol 0.035-inch guide wire wound around a plastic housing. (**c**) Markedly deformed regular guide wire after removal from the plastic housing. (**d**) No residual deformation of the Nitinol guide wire after removal from the plastic housing

To demonstrate the superelastic effect of Nitinol and the difference between the metals, we wound a regular guide wire with a stainless steel core and a Glidewire with a Nitinol core around their plastic housings (Fig. 1.4a, b). After removal, the regular wire became markedly deformed and permanently damaged, while the Nitinol guide wire returned to its perfectly straight alignment (Fig. 1.4c, d). The degree of deformation was 12% for both guide wires; 12% is significantly higher than what stainless steel can accommodate (0.5%), thus resulting in permanent damage. On the other hand, 12% is within the elastic deformation limit for Nitinol, thus permitting total recovery.

The elastic properties of a device depend on the inherent elasticity and the thickness of the material from which it is constructed. The relative deformation of a device can be calculated by the following equation:

$$\text{Relative deformation} = \frac{\text{Thickness of the material}}{\text{Radius of deformation} \times 2} \times 100\%$$

According to this equation, thinner material allows greater deformation and thus greater flexibility. For example, a razor blade can be deformed into a semicircle, and still regain its original shape after it is released, whereas a thicker plate of the same material deformed to a semicircle of the same radius would remain deformed with only minimal recoil (Fig. 1.5). The relative deformation also defines the limits of device design. For example, smaller coils require thinner wire. If a coil were made from a wire thicker than permitted by the above equation, it could not be loaded into a delivery system without permanent loss of its final configuration. For a given 10% deformation, a 0.5-mm-thick Nitinol wire can be wound into a coil 5 mm in diameter, but a 0.2-mm-thick Nitinol wire would be needed for a coil 2 mm in diameter. If the 0.5-mm-thick Nitinol wire to be wound into a coil 2 mm in diameter, the

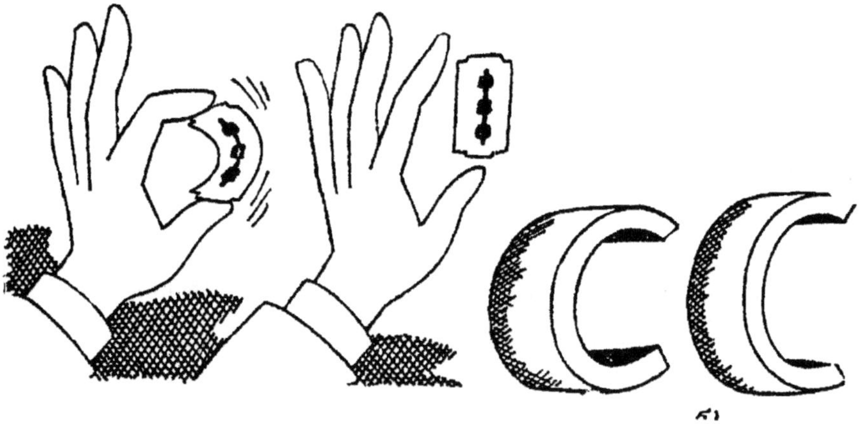

Fig. 1.5 Dependence of thickness of the material on the elastic properties, the thin razor returns to its imprint configuration after the deforming force is released, while the thicker metal remains in "c" deformity after release of the deforming pressure (Courtesy of Zaimovsky and Kolupaeva [3])

deformation would be 25%—above the permissible limit—and irreparable damage would occur.

Shape Memory

Shape memory is the capability of a plastically deformed material to restore its original shape with heating. Recovery of the imprinted shape of Nitinol devices occurs within a temperature range. For example, the coil in Fig. 1.6 recovers its shape completely at the body temperature of 37 °C (transition into the A phase), but starts its transformation at 34 °C. The range of this temperature interval can be varied by adjusting the alloy composition and the manufacturing conditions. The temperature of the final transformation (in this example 37 °C) can be moved up or down the temperature scale by changing alloy content. Lower nickel concentration is associated with a higher transition temperature to the final shape recovery. Examples of interventional devices that demonstrate shape memory effect are self-expanding stents, filters for the inferior vena cava, devices for closure of atrial septal defects, and heat-sensitive Harrington rods for spinal fusion [6, 7].

Knowledge of the transition temperature is important for the interventional radiologist because it affects implantation. If shape recovery occurs above body temperature, devices have to be heated after release into the body. Dotter used this heating technique in his original work with the Nitinol coil stents in animals [8]. If shape recovery occurs below body temperature, the device should be cooled during the delivery to prevent expansion inside the delivery catheter. This was

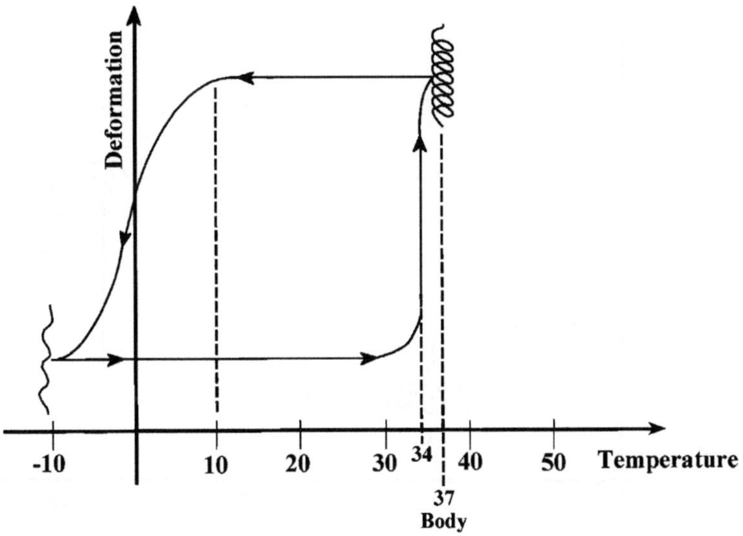

Fig. 1.6 Schematic presentation of Nitinol transformations showing the range of shape recovery between 34 and 37 °C

recommended for the delivery of the original Simon Nitinol filter (C.R. Bard). If shape recovery occurs at body temperature, no heating or cooling is necessary during the delivery and implantation, provided delivery is relatively speedy. If, however, tortuous iliac anatomy or other interferences delay prompt deployment of a Nitinol filter or aortic stent graft with these characteristics, premature warming to body temperature could cause expansion in the delivery sheath, increase friction, and interfere with delivery. In this instance, flushing with a cool solution may be helpful. When loading a Nitinol device that recovers at body or room temperature, it is helpful to do so in an ice water basin; the device becomes soft and pliable and can be easily straightened for introduction through the delivery system (Fig. 1.7). The ice water basin test is also useful when the interventionist receives the sample of a new device and it is unknown whether delivery is based on superelasticity or shape memory. If a Nitinol stent cannot be flattened in ice water, it has no shape memory in the clinical range.

Shape recovery of Nitinol devices at body temperature may not be desirable for all stent applications. The transition temperature to the A phase probably should be lower for tracheobronchial stents than for intravascular devices to prevent varying temperatures of inhaled air changing the mechanical forces and characteristics of the device.

Complete shape recovery of a Nitinol device in vivo depends on the absolute temperature at which the A transition is completed, the temperature range of M-A transition, and the time required for implantation. When delivery is protracted, the device is exposed to body temperature inside the delivery system. As pointed out

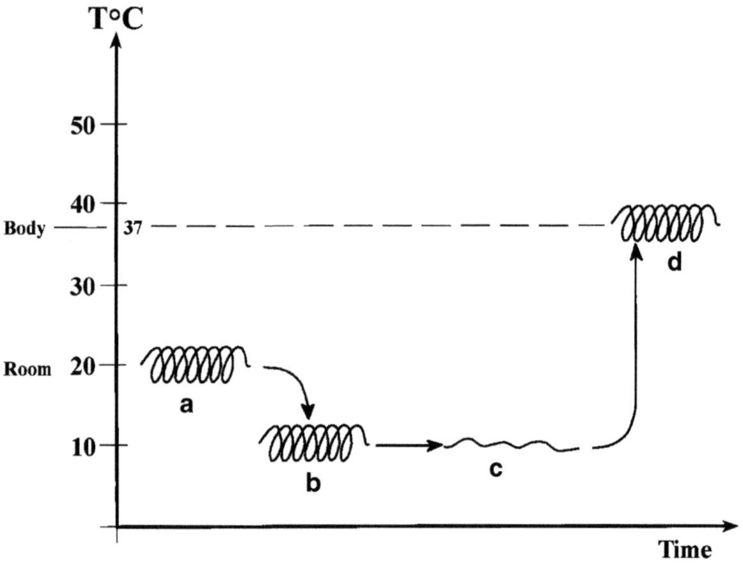

Fig. 1.7 Schematic presentation of transformations of Nitinol coil before and during delivery into the body. (a) expanded at room temperature, (b, c) cooled to allow easier placement within delivery housing, and (d) shape recall after deployment at body temperature

previously, the release process can then become more difficult, the device may open abruptly after being freed from the delivery system and may "jump" beyond its target.

Familiarity with shape recovery is important when exact deployment against the forces of the blood stream is required. The rapidity by which large aortic stent grafts open into their final configuration may dictate whether a reduction in arterial flow (by balloon or decrease in blood pressure) is necessary during deployment. A too slow opening risks folding of the device and its distal migration by the blood stream, too rapid opening may result in a jump proximal to target.

In situations in which shape recovery is not critical, but superelastic properties are paramount, the alloy composition is chosen such that the transition temperature is far below body and even room temperature (e.g., for guide wires or foreign body retrieval snares).

Biocompatibility

Nitinol is a highly biocompatible and nontoxic material [9, 10], although Nitinol alloys contain approximately 50% nickel, which is considered toxic. However, assessment of nickel metabolism in humans indicates that the body burden on nickel in normal adult averages 0.5 mg (7 μg per kg for a 70-kg adult person). The maximum recommended permissible amount of nickel administered to a human as a contaminant in intravenous fluids should not exceed 0.5 μg per kg per day (35 μg per day for a 70-kg adult) [11]. The average weight of a Nitinol IVC Filter is under 300 mg and the weight of the 8-mm-diameter/23-mm-length stent is around 100 mg. Considering that there is approximately 50% nickel in Nitinol, if this particular stent released into the blood stream more than 35 μg of nickel per day, it would have turned into pure titanium in less than 3.5 years, which is completely unrealistic. Experimental studies on animals showed that there is no significant change in total weight of the interventional devices years after their implantation (less than 1% loss of mass was detected in Simon Nitinol filters 4 years after insertion into the experimental animals) [12]. The relatively small weight of the available interventional Nitinol devices and marked stability of the alloy make exposure to nickel almost negligible. The bonding forces of nickel and titanium in Nitinol are very strong and prevent release of nickel ions into the body in large amounts. Moreover, as Nitinol oxidizes after proper surface treatment, it forms a titanium oxide layer with no nickel present at the surface, allowing only minimal diffusion of the nickel ions from the deeper layers through the surface [13]. Evaluation of the possible nickel release from Nitinol implants has shown that the expected nickel concentration in the biological liquids of the body will be less than natural nickel levels in the human blood serum [14]. Extensive laboratory testing of Nitinol demonstrated its higher chemical stability and more prominent anticorrosive properties than stainless steel.

Animal and human experience showed high biocompatibility of Nitinol and, thus, suitability as an implant material. Putters et al. compared different materials and quantified toxicity of implantable devices by evaluation of inhibition of mitosis in human fibroblasts exposed to nickel, titanium, and Nitinol [15]. In this study, nickel significantly inhibited mitosis in human fibroblasts, whereas titanium and Nitinol lacked such effect. These findings provided the basis for acceptance of Nitinol as a surgical implant material.

Nitinol-based medical devices have been used in humans since the mid-1970s. Besides interventional implantable devices (such as vascular, tracheobronchial, esophageal, intestinal, and biliary stents and inferior vena cava filters), a rod for correction of scoliosis, compression staples, artificial hip sockets, bone plates, aneurysm clips, and various orthodontic devices and implants (all made of Nitinol) have been used in humans. To our knowledge, there are no documented reports of toxicity, adverse effects, or biologic incompatibility of Nitinol in vivo.

General Considerations

Nitinol devices can generate tremendous force (up to 80 kg/mm^2) if they meet resistance during their recovery. Varying the thickness of the Nitinol wire, the overall shape of the device, and the spatial arrangement of the Nitinol wire within this shape can regulate the force. These design features, as well as the characteristics of the Nitinol alloy used, should be taken into account when designing, selecting, and deploying interventional devices for specific clinical applications.

Self-expanding Nitinol devices with shape memory capabilities, such as stents, stent-grafts, and filters are typically oversized in respect to the target organ by 10–20%, and continue to apply a sustained expansion force as they attempt to return to their unconstrained diameter. Thus, the final device diameter may be larger than the one obtained at the end of a procedure, such as stent placement in a bronchus or bile duct encased by a tumor. In such an instance, a follow-up film may be more reflective of the final shape of the device. This feature may also make it superfluous to balloon dilation after deployment and thus minimize tissue injury. On the other hand, a Nitinol device will not expand beyond its nominal diameter, even if dilated by a larger-sized balloon. The patient is, therefore, not exposed to the risks of overexpansion.

Although a self-expanding Nitinol device cannot generate the expansion force of an angioplasty balloon, more than enough force can be generated to prevent vessel recoil and contraction [16]. Some investigators have suggested that the continuous pressure exerted by a self-expanding Nitinol device on the vessel wall may induce increased intimal hyperplasia over time [17]. Clinical evidence suggests, however, that this application of force actually helps ensure an open lumen [18, 19].

Further studies in animal models have demonstrated that the design geometry of intravascular endoprostheses can significantly influence the rate of stenosis in normal vessels, underscoring the importance of wire thickness, spatial configuration, and device oversizing [20].

Nitinol is a nonferromagnetic material and has lower magnetic susceptibility than stainless steel, which produces less artifacts during MR imaging. This feature of Nitinol is important when follow-up studies are planned to evaluate position and patency of the implanted devices, or when imaging is performed for unrelated indications.

Nitinol produces a fluoroscopic image comparable to stainless steel, provided the mass and dimensions of the devices are equal. Although sufficient in many cases, an improvement would be beneficial in certain clinical situations, particularly in obese patients. Radiopacity of Nitinol endoluminal implants can be enhanced by application of small radiopaque gold markers at the ends of the devices, which do not interfere or alter the properties and behavior of Nitinol construction. This technique is now utilized by nearly all manufacturers of Nitinol stents.

Conclusion

The features of superelasticity and shape memory make Nitinol an excellent material for interventional devices. These physical characteristics permit manufacture of complex shapes of devices and introduction through low-profile delivery systems. Familiarity with the characteristics of Nitinol aids in selecting the most suitable device for a specific clinical indication.

References

1. Rabkin D, Lang E, Brophy D. Nitinol properties affecting uses in interventional radiology. J Vasc Interv Radiol. 2000;11:343–50.
2. Schetky LM. Shape memory alloys. Sci Am. 1979;241:74–83.
3. Zaimovsky VA, Kolupaeva TL. Unusual properties of usual metals [in Russian]. Moscow: Science; 1984. p. 111–3.
4. Kurdiumov GV, Khandros LG. About a thermoelastic balance in martensite transformations. [in Russian]. Dokl Akad Nauk SSSR. 1949;66(2):211–5.
5. Buehler WJ, Wang FE. A summary of recent research on the nitinol alloys and their potential application in ocean engineering. Ocean Eng. 1968;1:105–20.
6. Shmerling MA, Wilkov MA, Sanders AE, Woosley JE. Using the shape recovery of nitinol in the Harrington rod treatment of scoliosis. J Biomed Mater Res. 1976;10:879–92.
7. Wayman CM. Some applications of shape memory alloys. J Met. 1980;32:129–37.
8. Dotter CT, Buschman RW, McKinney MK, Rosch J. Transluminal expandable nitinol coil stent grafting. Radiology. 1983;147:259–60.
9. Castleman LS, Motzkin SM. Biocompatibility of nitinol. In: Williams DF, editor. Biocompatibility of clinical implant materials. Boca Raton: CRC Press; 1981. p. 129–54.
10. Oshida Y, Miyazaki S. Corrosion and biocompatibility of shape memory alloys. Corros Eng. 1991;40:1009–25.
11. Sunderman FW. Potential toxicity from nickel contamination of intravenous fluids. Ann Clin Lab Sci. 1983;13:1–4.
12. Prince MR, Salzman EW, Schoen FJ, Palestrant AM, Simon M. Local intravascular effects of the nitinol wire blood clot filter. Investig Radiol. 1988;23:294–300.
13. Rabkin DJ. Experimental basis of endovascular stenting. PhD thesis. Moscow: Moscow Institute of Radiology; 1987. Russian.
14. Shabalovskaya SA. On the nature of the biocompatibility and on medical applications of NiTi shape memory and superelastic alloys. Biomed Mater Eng. 1996;6:267–89.

15. Putters JL, Kaulesar Sukul DM, De Zeeuw GR, Bijma A, Besselink PA. Comparative cell culture effects of shape memory metal (Nitinol), nickel and titanium: a biocompatibility estimation. Eur Surg Res. 1992;24:378–82.
16. Kleshinski SJ, Harry JD. Medical stenting: a synthesis of design principles. In: Proceedings of the international conference on shape memory and superelastic technologies; 1997. p. 561–6.
17. Froelich JJ, Alfke H, Wilke A, et al. Effects of nitinol Strecker stent placement on vascular response in normal and stenotic porcine iliac arteries. J Vasc Interv Radiol. 1999;10:329–38.
18. Mangell P, Malina M, Vogt K, et al. Are self-expanding stents superior to balloon-expanded in dilating aortas? An experimental study in pigs. Eur J Vasc Endovasc Surg. 1996;12:287–94.
19. Ozaki Y, Violaris AG, Hamburger J, et al. Short- and long-term clinical and quantitative angiographic results with the new, less shortening Wallstent for vessel reconstruction in chronic total occlusion: a quantitative angiographic study. J Am Coll Cardiol. 1996;28:354–60.
20. Tominaga R, Kambic H, Emoto H, Harasaki H, Sutton C, Hollman J. Effects of design geometry of intravascular endoprostheses on stenosis rate in normal rabbits. Am Heart J. 1992;123:21–8.

Conception 2

Pre-clinical Proof of Concept of Endovascular Nitinol Stenting

Prior Art

The first attempts of placing vascular stents through the catheters in order to dilate the vessel and provide support precluding restenosis in the diseased zone were made in the late 1960s–early 1970s [1–3]. Unsatisfactory clinical experience gained from the use of angioplasty and recanalization made the scientists led by Ch. Dotter, the founder of this method, find new technical means which could be used for setting up a supporting framework in the vessel to maintain the dilated lumen and to preclude restenosis in the diseased vessel.

The experimental technique of nonoperative transluminal introduction of the stent was described by Ch. Dotter for the first time in 1969. The 1.0–3.5 mm in diameter tubular cylindrical prostheses were made of polyethylene, polyamide, plastic, and teflon and introduced through the catheters into femoral and popliteal arteries in dogs. The stents were patent for no longer than 24 hours after implantation and became totally thrombosed, which was proven angiographically and morphologically [1].

Spiral tubular prostheses made of silicon-coated stainless steel wire showed more promise. Charles Dotter performed experiments in six dogs, placing the stents into the femoral arteries. They were patent for a longer period of time, owing to the fact that the metallic coils of the stents were rapidly covered by a neointima. The angiographic studies performed within 2.5 years after implantation had proved patency of the reinforced arteries [1].

Despite these promising results, however, the suggested method failed to find wide recognition in clinical practice due to the following disadvantages:

1. Significant narrowing of the blood vessel lumen due to intimal hyperplasia over the metallic wire.

I. Rabkin, D. J. Rabkin, *Bloodline of Nitinol Stents*, https://doi.org/10.1007/978-3-032-25697-3_2

2. Injury of the vessels at the entry site of a large guiding catheter.

The object of intravascular stenting consists in that the prosthesis introduced through the angiographic catheter into the vessel maintains its luminal size resisting the internal and external compression forces. Thus, the vessel lumen is preserved for free flow of blood [1].

The progress in the development of intravascular stenting depends on solution of two problems, that is, biological implantation of prostheses (compatibility, toxicology, corrosion-resistance, and other problems) and development of the method and device for delivery of an intravascular stent. From these problems, two major tasks follow, that is, to find materials best suited for stenting from the biological point of view and to develop a reasonably effective device for delivery of a stent [1].

In June 1972, R. Alfidi, C. Falls, and B. Gross claimed in the USA a device which was essentially a framework made of a memory metal comprising nickel and titanium in a ratio of 52–56% and 44–48%, respectively [4]. The device was designed for implantation in an animal vessel. The framework had a shape of a cylinder open at both ends, which shape could be restored in an animal vessel by means of a controllable device. The framework shape could be changed at a temperature lower than the shape-restoration temperature. Before introduction into the animal vessel this framework was deformed to a structure of smaller diameter. The device comprised an elongated tool, which could be disengaged from the expanding framework, and a special electric heater [4].

The first application of Nitinol for endovascular purposes goes back to 1977, when it was used for manufacture of an Inferior Vena Cava (IVC) Filter to prevent pulmonary embolism by mechanically trapping the blood clots, traveling from the lower extremities due to deep vein thrombosis [5]. A construction was made from the Nitinol wires, which were straightened and introduced into the Inferior Vena Cava through a catheter, inserted from the femoral or jugular vein access. After being released into the IVC and heated to a blood temperature, the wires assumed their original shape of crossed loops which filtered emboli out of blood.

In April 1983, two independent research groups of American radiologists, led by Ch. Dotter and A. Cragg (Fig. 2.1) reported on an experimental model of a spiral intravascular stent made from a shape memory alloy Nitinol [6–9]. Being designed for structural support of stenotic or collapsed vessels, these constructions were intended for transformation and subsequent introduction into the vessels through angiographic catheters. Once the stents were released from the catheter, they expanded assuming the form of a cylinder inside vessels.

The devices designed by these two groups were similar in appearance, but substantially differed in the method of their introduction. The stents comprised spiral coils from a Nitinol wire. The coils were straightened and delivered through the catheters into the blood vessels. After deployment the straight wires restored their original spiral shape, thereby expanding the vessel lumen and providing internal support for it. The purpose of such stents was to expand the narrow lumen of a vessel and maintain its patency. Also, in certain conditions the stents can protect the

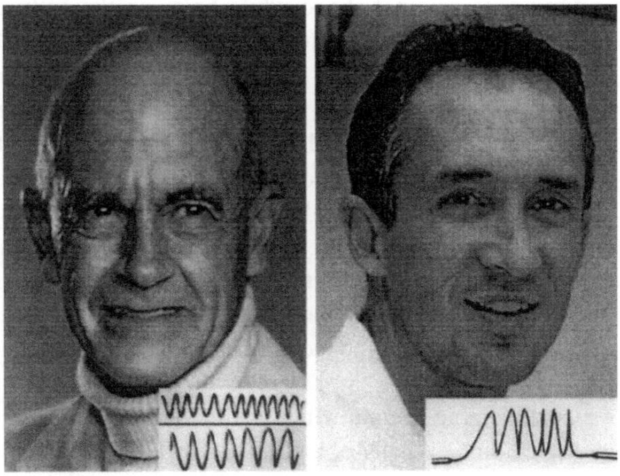

Fig. 2.1 Charles Dotter and Andrew Cragg and their prototypes of Nitinol spiral stents

vessel from compression by surrounding tissues and provide unobstructed flow of blood.

The construction proposed by A. Gragg comprised of 5–11 mm in diameter and 1–6 cm long Nitinol spirals with the turns either tightly pressed against one another or spaced apart to a distance of up to 1 cm. The 0.045 cm straight Nitinol wire was pushed through a catheter until it extended beyond the distal end thereof and the spiral was formed in the vessel as it was heated by the blood. As soon as the Nitinol wire emerged outside the catheter, a newly formed spiral was accurately fixed by introducing a guide wire into the vessel (dog aorta). The spiral was disengaged from the guide wire by unscrewing the latter from the spiral adapter. The authors implanted ten intravascular stents in the dog aortas ranging from 0.5 to 1.0 cm in diameter [6–8].

A similar device was patented by J. James in 1987 [10].

The use of this technique, however, is complicated by the property of Nitinol to restore its original shape not at a certain temperature, but during temperature variations within a certain range. Normally, this range, termed A_s–A_f covers about 10 °C for the existing alloys. Owing to this fact, the straightened Nitinol wire which is to become a spiral at a body temperature (A_f = 33 °C) begins changing its shape just in a warm room (A_s = 25 °C). Besides, the Nitinol alloy which completely restores the original shape at body temperature is pliable only at a temperature close to a freezing point. Therefore, to make the spiral a straight wire before placing the stent into the angiographic catheter, substantial cooling is required (e.g., placing it in sterile ice-cold water) [6, 7].

Hence, it becomes apparent that as the wire moves along the catheter in warm blood, the risk of premature restoration of spiral form is substantially high. Also, when Nitinol starts "recalling" its shape (though this process may be impeded inside the cannula or delivery tube) "dislocating" plastic deformation takes place in the alloy and when it emerges from the catheter, the restoration of the desired original form is made difficult and sometimes even impossible. In order to prevent wire from assuming its original shape while being in the catheter, the authors permanently injected therein a cold isotonic solution of sodium chloride (10 °C). Besides, the Cragg's technique used for forcing the stent out of the catheter makes it difficult to accurately deploy it within the desired portion of the vessel.

All stents implanted in the animals remained patent for 7–150 days. However, in a week after implantation of the stent the artery caliber decreased in the place of stent implantation; especially in case when the spirals were tightly coiled, due to deposition of fibrin on the turns of, which was proven by macroscopic and histologic examinations. Despite this fact, later examinations did not reveal further decrease in the lumen of the artery [8].

The limitations of the techniques and device include:

- Considerable trauma which is inflicted to the vessel in the place of puncture by the guiding catheter of a comparably large diameter;
- Possible risk that the spiral will begin to recall the shape long before its delivery to the place of deployment as the straight wire will be moved in the catheter in warm blood since the transition temperature range for the wire in use starts at 25 °C.

Besides, the fact that this process is restricted by the guiding catheter, it may lead to deformation which adversely affects the shape restoration capabilities.

Quite another solution was proposed by Ch. Dotter et al. Their spiral was introduced in the form of a small diameter spring. Such "spiral" was fitted to the end portion of the inner delivery catheter having a blind end and a plurality of side openings uniformly distributed according to the spiral rings.

This spring was then transformed to a shorter spiral having a larger diameter. The decisive factor in that case was that the Dotter spring did not change its dimensions at a body temperature and restores its original shape only after infusion of 20–30 ml of a heated isotonic solution of sodium chloride. The hot isotonic solution of sodium chloride forced through the side openings of the catheter caused rapid heating and expansion of the spiral (US Patent No. 4.503.569 as of March *V*, 1985).

The transition temperature may be changed by slightly varying the alloy composition and production process. The authors used a transition temperature ranging from 54 to 60 °C. Such temperature was selected based on the fact that in their opinion it provided a stability phase required for production, storage, and placement of the Nitinol framework. Besides, it was well endured during those few seconds which were required to restore the original shape of the spiral. Thus, the Nitinol spiral with a smaller diameter could easily be installed in a stenotic artery segment where it could then assume the original shape and its diameter increased nearly to a diameter of the adjacent intact segments of the vessel. Due to expansion of the spiral, it was fixed in the zone of slightly extended but in all other respects intact vessel [9].

Experiments in animals involving injection of a physiologic solution heated to 80 °C in a blood vessel have revealed no signs of thrombogenesis and other unwanted effects and showed that the vascular tissue and blood are not adversely affected in case of short-time temperature rise [9] (Fig. 2.2).

The experimental results on the use of a 5 mm in diameter Nitinol stents in dogs have been published. For dogs weighing 25–30 kg the stents were made 5 mm for placement in an iliac artery. The spiral was easily coiled at a room temperature around the distal end of the guiding catheter. The capability of alloy to memorize shape was activated by heating it up to 40–50 °C. The stents were delivered by means of a seven French catheter and its diameter before introduction was 2.2 mm. After the stents had been introduced, 10 ml of a physiologic solution heated up to 60–65 °C were injected in the desired segment of the artery; therefore, the stents rapidly increased its diameter to an initial size of 5 mm.

Angiography was made 1–6 to 12–24 months after implantation of the stents. All 12 stents were patent with autopsy coming in 12–24 months. However, angiographic examination had found that one of the endoprostheses was occluded a month after implantation. At 1 and 2 years it was found that the stents had completely grown into the artery wall. Its inner surface was coated with neointima. No enlargement or fibrosis of the vessel wall was revealed [11]. According to the information of the US National Heart, Lung and Blood Institute, vessel response to intravascular stents is

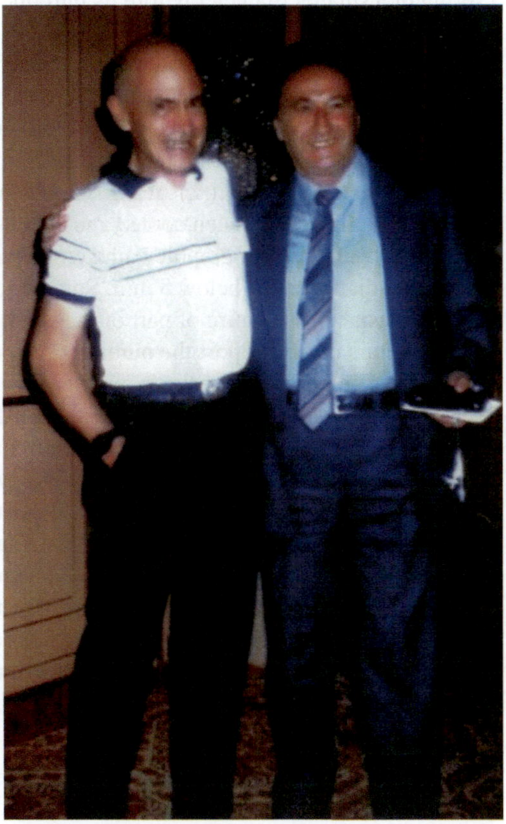

Fig. 2.2 Charles Dotter and Iosif Rabkin at RSNA meeting in Chicago in 1985

governed by the surface characteristics, properties of the material and its capabilities to cause thrombogenesis, or to impede formation of endothelium. The research work done by Ch. Sutton et al. did not reveal such reactions [11].

However, the method proposed by Ch. Dotter has some limitations. For example, the size of the catheter required to accommodate the Nitinol spring and to ensure infusion of a hot physiological solution is excessively large to pass through peripheral vessels. Such catheter with a comparably large diameter has poor bending properties and cannot be percutaneously introduced in a tortuous vessel. This substantially limits the use of Nitinol spirals to large arteries and veins where the vessel portion following the place of catheter introduction must be straight [12]. Besides, it was discovered that owing to blood flow a hot physiological solution rapidly cooled. To preclude such cooling of the solution and heating of the Nitinol spring until it assumes its original form, a larger amount of liquid heated to higher temperatures should be injected. Attempts were made to use special balloon catheters to block blood flow so as to enhance efficiency of a hot physiological solution. But even though the method was so modified, its application remained limited. In the peripheral vessels, blood flow can easily be blocked but this technique is of course unacceptable for an aorta and other main arteries [12].

The most difficult problem was presented by the necessity of coiling the spiral to a spring of a smaller diameter before its introduction into the catheter. For example, coiling a 6 mm in diameter spiral to a 3 mm in diameter spiral degraded memory effect. When such stent was heated, it failed to fully restore its original shape. The stress raised by coiling, even carefully performed in ice cold water, increased the A_s–A_f, restoration range by 10–20 °C on the average and limited the final diameter of the spiral to 80% of the desired magnitude. For example, if a Nitinol wire restored its shape at a temperature (A_f) of 40 °C and the final diameter of the spiral was 10 mm, then, after it had been cooled and coiled to a smaller diameter spiral before introduction into an angiographic catheter, the value of A increased to 60 °C while the original diameter fell below 8 mm. Sometimes, the coiling process caused complete “amnesia” of the entire of part of the spiral.

The authors did not report the number of experiments and number of implanted stents. It was noted, however, that a month after implantation of the Nitinol stents in the vessels, the caliber of femoral arteries in places of spiral implantation sharply decreased (by more than 50%) as compared to their original luminal size [7].

In April 1983, an application filed by Kogyo Gijutsu Intio was published in Japan, entitled to the benefits of priority under the International Convention as of March 15, 1980 [13]. This application claimed a tube made of special alloy which was capable of restoring its original shape. The tube was intended for restoration of stenotic portions of blood vessels. The alloy components were not specified in the application. The tube of a desired diameter was cast at a temperature higher than the point of phase transformation. Then the tube diameter was decreased by flattening it and folding about the longitudinal axis thereof. The folded tube was implanted in a stenotic portion of the blood vessel [13].

As apparent from the specification, the Kogyo's tube, even folded, is still less suitable for implantation in the vessel than a spiral stenting frame coiled to a small spring and will inevitably traumatize the vessel in the place of puncture.

Thus, the analysis of patent literature and experimental research pertaining to percutaneous transluminal implantation of Nitinol endoprostheses has revealed significant difficulties experienced in their delivery and implantation. Also, the long-term results cause concern since the luminal size of the dilated vessel sharply narrows due to massive intimal formations. Owing to this fact the authors refused from this method for treatment of stenotic lesions of vessels in a clinical setting. No more reports on experimental works and especially on clinical applications of the intravascular stents in arterial vessels were found by the authors in the literature. The first experimental works conducted by Ch. Dotter and A. Cragg were not continued and the problem remained unsolved.

For example, the components of Nitinol alloy were not exactly matched to ensure production of stents with optimal characteristics for catheter-based introduction and accurate placement in the vessel. These first Nitinol stents did not meet medical and technical requirements for their clinical applications. Besides, no technique was developed for application of intravascular stents in a clinical setting.

How We Did It

The experiments on practical use of the Nitinol coils for endovascular stenting have been started in the National Research Center of Surgery of the USSR Academy of Medical Sciences since October 1983. Technical support required for solution of this problem was provided by a creative group of physicians headed by B.V. Petrovsky (Fig. 2.3) and metallurgists (members of the Moscow Institute of Steel and Alloys) including P.I. Polukhin, M.L. Bernshtein, V.A. Zaymovsky, V.A. Khasyanov, I.Y. Khmelevsky, A.I. Kadnikov, and B. Khasenov [14–16]. The idea resided in the installation of the intravascular stent by implanting it through an angiographic catheter introduced percutaneously. The object was to create a prosthesis which could be introduced through a narrow space (2–3 mm) of the angiographic catheter and which later could assume the form of the vessel. The purposes of the intravascular stent were to maintain the caliber of the dilated vessel, precluding restenosis, and opposing the external compression force exerted by the surrounding tissue. Thus, the intravascular stent served to maintain the luminal size of the vessel and ensure free flow of blood.

Why was the nickel–titanium alloy (Nitinol) chosen out of a wide variety of metals? The research conducted together with the metallurgists had shown that Nitinol possessed the super properties which were absent in the other metals. These properties included [15–17]:

1. Supernatural memory
2. Superelasticity
3. Superstrength
4. Superplasticity

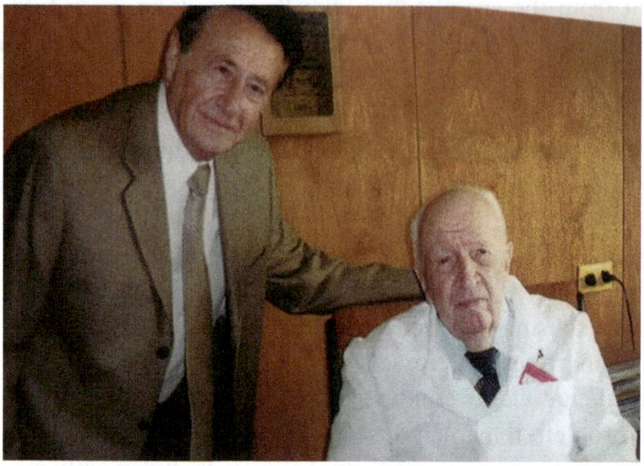

Fig. 2.3 Boris Petrovsky, Soviet and Russian surgeon, scientist and clinician, Director of the All-Union Scientific Center of Surgery of the USSR Academy of Medical Sciences, Academician of the Russian Academy of Science, and Iosif Rabkin, who was the Head of Radiology Department at the same institution and close collaborator and friend of B. Petrovsky

To solve the problem faced by the group, the following medical and technical requirements for intravascular stents were developed:

1. Biocompatibility with living organism tissue, hemocompatibility;
2. Delivery through an angiographic catheter in the form of uncoiled stretched filament;
3. Accurate placement of the intravascular stent in the vessel monitored through an X-ray Fluoroscopy;
4. Restoration of the original shape of the stent due to coiling to the spiral under the effect of natural heating to a blood temperature;
5. Adjustable pressure to the vessel due to plastic expansion of the stent, with the pressure not adversely affecting the vessel wall;
6. Reliable self-fixation in the desired portion of the vessel;
7. Incompressibility under the action of external force [16].

With this aim in view, we have partnered and collaborated with the metallo-physicists of the Moscow Institute of Steel and Alloys in developing a new modification of the alloy based on nickel and titanium, that is, medical Nitinol specially intended for intravascular stents and restoring its original shape at a temperature of 37 °C (Fig. 2.4). The temperature range within which the alloy restored its shape covered 3 °C, that is, the restoration process began after heating to 34 °C [17].

A unique intravascular stenting framework (Inventor's Certificate No. 1237201, convention priority as of April 4, 1985) and a special introducer for its delivery and implantation were developed and manufactured. Also, a radically new technique was developed to introduce the stent through an angiographic catheter and

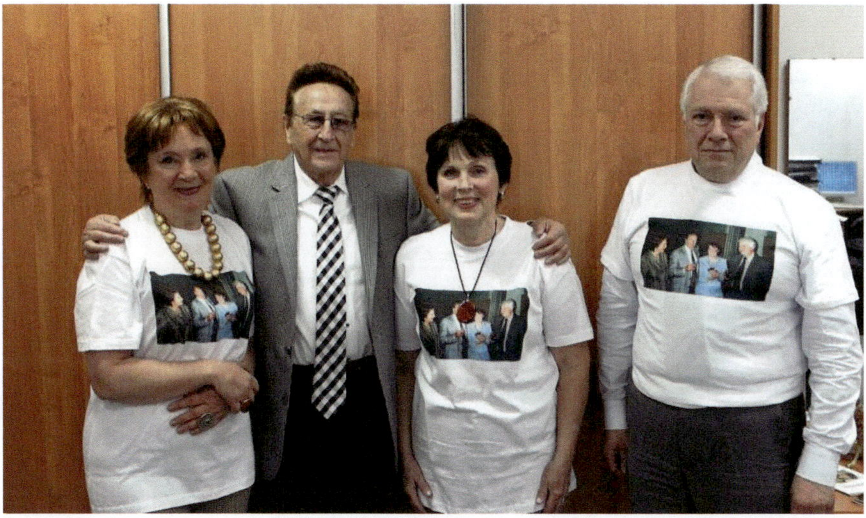

Fig. 2.4 Close inter-disciplinary collaborators: Iosif Rabkin with metallo-physicists Elena Ryklina, Irina Khmelevskaya, and Sergei Prokoshkin

accurately place it in the desired portion of the vessel (Inventors Certificate No. 1342511, convention priority as of May 20, 1985) (Fig. 2.5).

The intravascular stents were made of a Nitinol wire having a diameter of 0.2–0.5 mm. The stents were made to have various lengths and diameters. The length of coiled spirals varied from 1.5 to 6.0 cm and their diameter from 4 to 16 mm. Besides, the turns of springs were differently spaced—from intimate mating to a distance of 3–7 mm. A special silicon coating was applied to each stent [16, 18].

The spiral stent has a special lug externally disposed at the distal end thereof was secured in the lock of a special introducer (Fig. 2.6). Then, it was cooled, stretched, and delivered by means of the introducer through the guiding catheter to the desired location. After the stent had assumed its original spiral shape due to heating to a body temperature in the vessel, the introducer lock was released, the spiral end was freed, and the introducer was removed from the vessel (Fig. 2.7) [18–20]. A unique memory effect intrinsic in the Nitinol wire made it possible to deliver the transformed spiral through a small caliber angiographic catheter percutaneously introduced into the vessel [18, 21].

We have also developed a second way of delivering and deploying the spiral stent by introducing it through the delivery catheter not as a straight wire, but as a coil of much smaller diameter. With this technique the coil is fixed on the delivery system at both proximal and distal ends. By spinning the proximal fixation lock, the coil is reduced in size under cooling conditions into a spiral of a much smaller diameter, so it "hugs" the delivery introducer, allowing to minimize the profile of the system with the loaded stent. When the stent is delivered to the desired location, both proximal and distal locks are released and the originally restrained coil expands from its

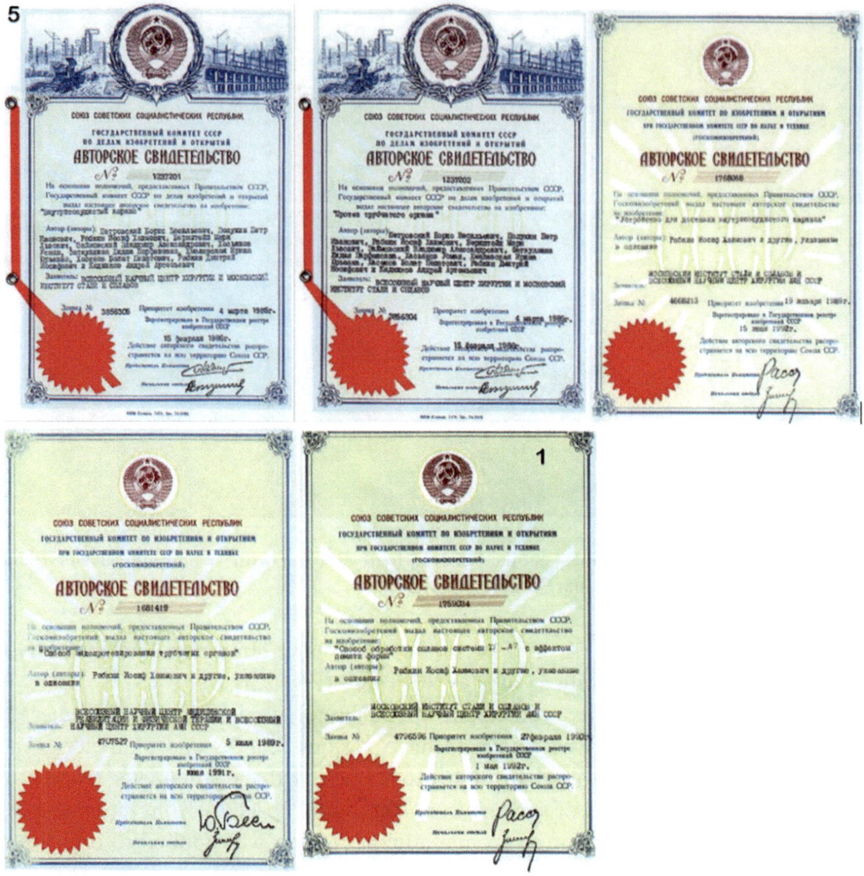

Fig. 2.5 Multiple Inventor's Certificates have been issued in the Russian Federation for innovative unique design of the Nitinol Spiral Endoprosthesis and the methods and mechanisms for their delivery and deployment

restrained diameter to its final intended size (Fig. 2.8). With the expansion of the coil there is some shortening of the stent, but overall, this method makes the positioning and deployment more precise and less traumatic than the transformation of the coil stent from the straight wire, although the delivery system has to be slightly higher profile.

Bio- and Hemocompatibility on Nitinol Stents

Toxicological studies performed during experiments in vitro and on biological test objects showed that the Nitinol wire had good compatibility with living tissue, caused no anatomic abnormalities, and facilitated formation of neointima.

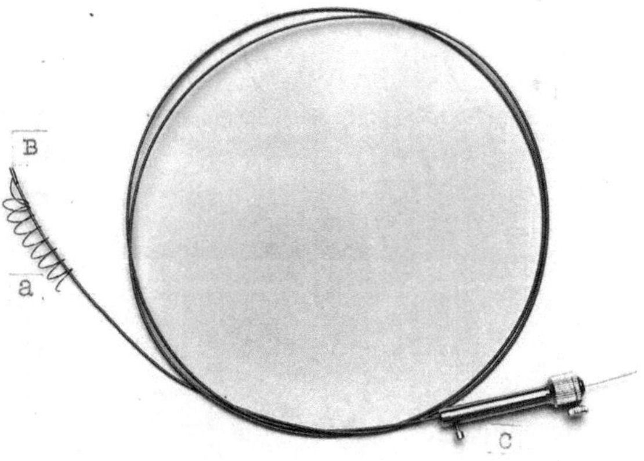

Fig. 2.6 Nitinol spiral stent is locked on an introducer in preparation for delivery

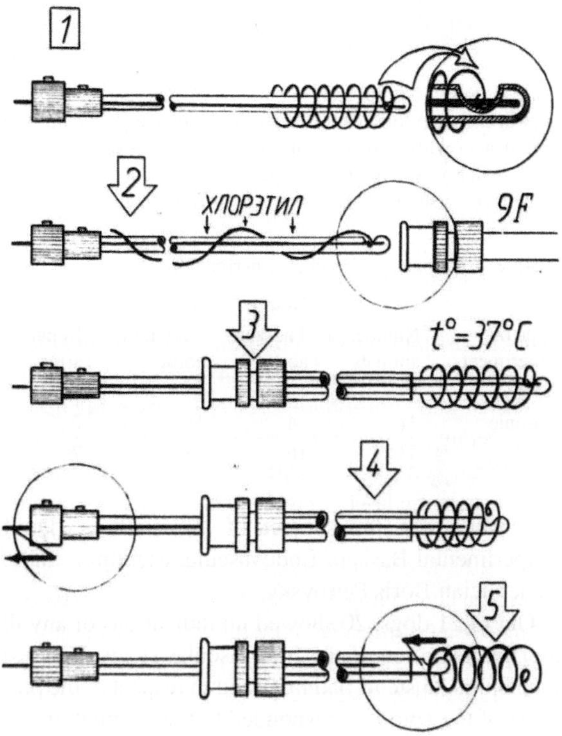

Fig. 2.7 Steps of fixation, delivery, and deployment of Nitinol spiral stent

Then, the experiments were conducted in 53 mongrel dogs. Of these dogs 32 were subject to acute experiment and 21 were left for dynamic observation and investigation at different follow-up time after the implantation of stents from 12 hours to 15 months. Total 85 intravascular spiral Nitinol stents were implanted (Table 2.1), including 16 in a thoracic aorta, 37 in an abdominal aorta, 7 in renal arteries, 17 in iliac arteries, and 8 in femoral arteries (Figs. 2.9 and 2.10) [18, 24].

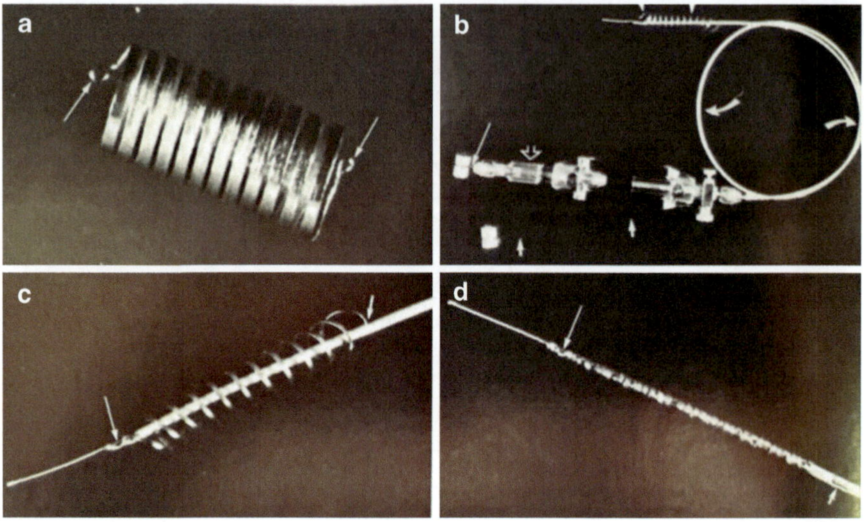

Fig. 2.8 Spiral Nitinol stent with flat wire and its delivery system. (**a**) Rabkin Nitinol stent with loops at each end for secure fixation on the delivery system. (**b**) Delivery system with loaded spiral Nitinol stent with its fixation at both ends. (**c**) Close-up view of the spiral stent fixed at both ends on the delivery system. (**d**) The spiral stent is reduced in size to a minimal diameter and secured on the delivery system in preparation for its introduction

Table 2.1 Summary of animal experiments

Type of experiments	Number of animals	Number of stented vessels					Total number of stents
		Thoracic aorta	Abdominal aorta	Renal artery	Iliac artery	Femoral artery	
Acute	32	12	21	5	10	3	51
Chronic	21	4	16	2	7	5	34
Total	53	16	37	7	17	8	85

This work was the subject of the author's (Dmitry Rabkin) PhD thesis on "Experimental Basis of Endovascular Stenting," under the scientific supervision of academician Boris Petrovsky.

Out of 21 dogs, 20 showed no indications of any illness, fever, or abnormal gait after implantation of the intravascular stents. The X-ray test studies revealed that none of the 34 stents had migrated in respect to the place of initial implantation. The shape of the spiral corresponded to the original one. Angiography of 21 dogs, performed in different periods after stent implantation, showed no signs of thrombogenesis and vascular occlusion at the sites of implantation in 19 dogs (Fig. 2.11).

The experiments revealed that in the early period after implantation, the silicon-coated stents exhibited pronounced thromboresistant properties even in such zones complex in hemodynamic respect as vascular bifurcations and trifurcation, as well as the levels at which smaller branches were originating from the main vascular trunk. Besides, at a later period after implantation, the Nitinol spirals caused no growth of intima without narrowing of the vascular lumen [18, 22]. It became

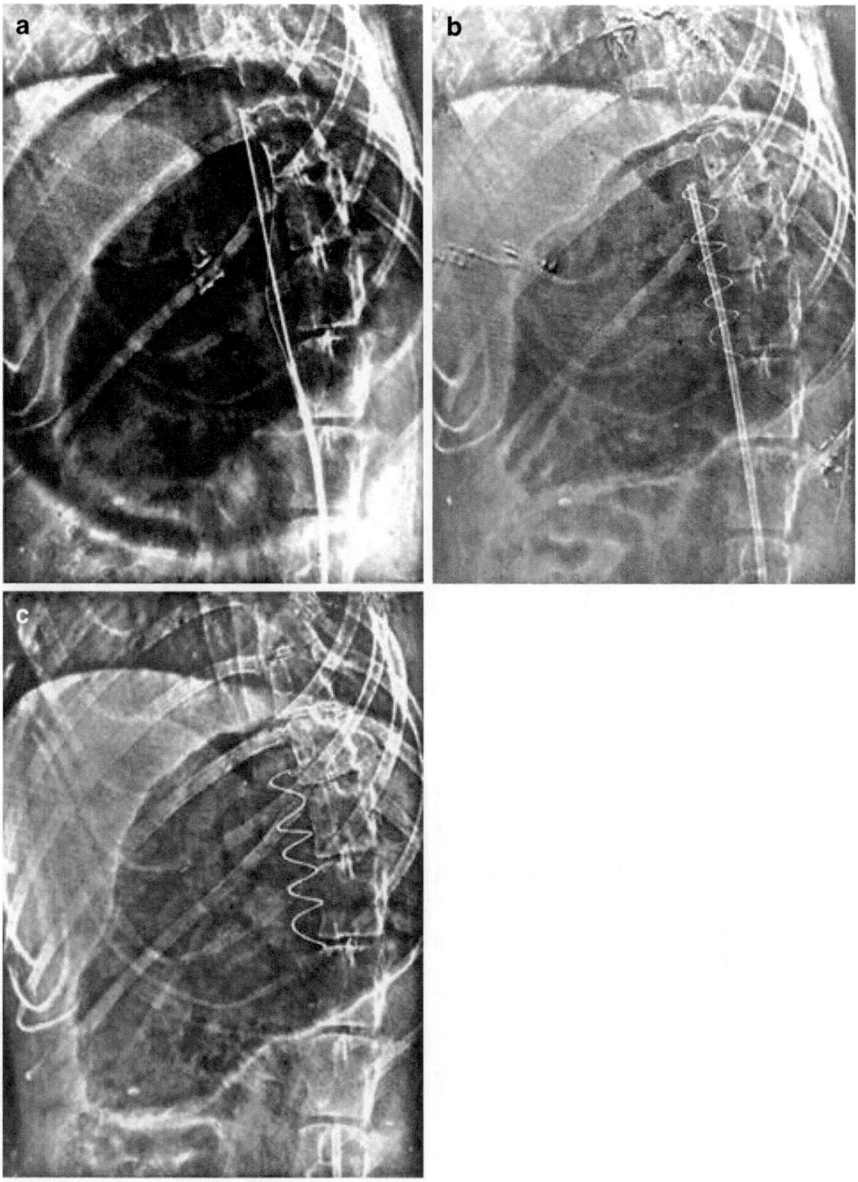

Fig. 2.9 Steps of implantation of Nitinol spiral stent into an abdominal aorta: (**a**) Straightened stent locked at an introduced delivered to abdominal aorta; (**b**) Stents assumes spiral shape, while still attached to introducer; (**c**) Stent detached from introducer and fully deployed.

obvious that the Nitinol stents themselves could not be responsible for thrombogenesis in the places of their implantation. No relationship was discovered between thrombosis of the stents and their length, location, thickness of a wire, and frequency of a spiral turns [23].

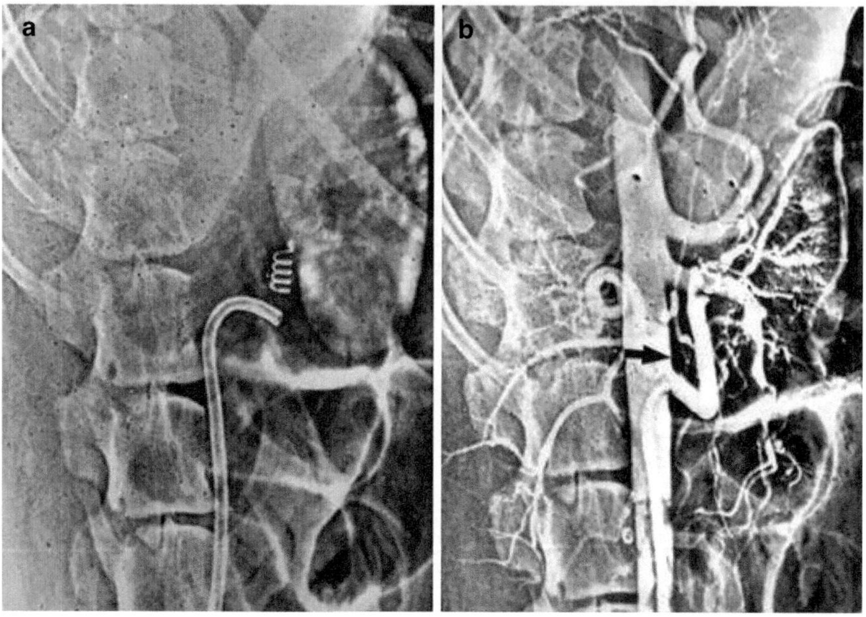

Fig. 2.10 Implantation of the Nitinol spiral stent into the tortuous left renal: (**a**) Spiral stent deployed into left renal artery; (**b**) Angiogram after stent implantation demonstrates wide patency of the stented left renal artery

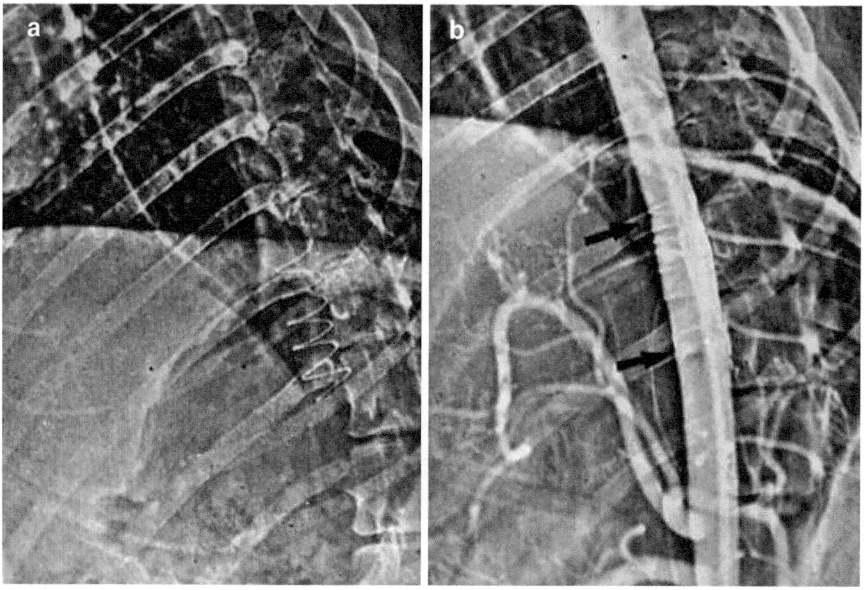

Fig. 2.11 Nitinol spiral stent remains in the site of original placement (**a**) and widely patent (**b**) 15 months after its implantation

Complications with thrombosis of the stented segments of the vessels was observed in two animals. One of these dogs died 12 hours after the implantation of three stents without silicon coating into the abdominal aorta. The reason was that the second stent touched the distal turns of the already-placed spiral thereby causing their twisting and subsequent injury of the vessel.

Morphologic and histologic examinations of 23 stented vascular segments of 15 dogs were conducted in 1–15 months. It was disclosed that the endoprosthesis turns are first coated with a light film of albumin precipitated from blood flow. In the places, where the spiral turns contacted the internal layer of the artery, impressions in the vessel wall were found (Fig. 2.12). Three to five days later, fibroblasts grew through an albumin coat and immature granular connective tissue was formed encircling the stent turns. Bands of newly formed capillaries oriented around the spiral were found. Regenerative processes developed mainly due to formation of granular connective tissue surrounding metal parts of the spiral (Fig. 2.13).

Further, the maturing granular tissue showed a trend of its fibrillar structures to formation of fibrosis in the form of a sleeve around each individual turn of the stent. The fibrotic ring so formed protruded into the vascular lumen by no more than 0.03–0.05 mm. The bridge of connective tissue provided smooth transition from the artery wall to the spiral turns, improving hemodynamic conditions (Fig. 2.14). On the side of the unchanged part of the arterial intima, marked proliferation of endothelium and cells of a subendothelial layer toward the spiral turns was found (Fig. 2.15) [18, 22, 24]. The authors have concluded that they had succeeded in the establishment of basic principles of implantation and angiogenesis of the intravascular stents. Owing to biological inertness of such stents, a new vascular bed is formed on top of them providing a laminar blood flow function. Thus, by the end of the second week the implanted intravascular spiral is no longer exposed to the direct contact with blood flow and blood cells. However, 2 or 3 weeks more are obviously required for final incorporation of the Nitinol stents into the vessel wall [17, 18].

At the same time, intravascular stenting of intact vessels cannot be regarded as an ideal model for the study of morphogenesis since in a clinical setting

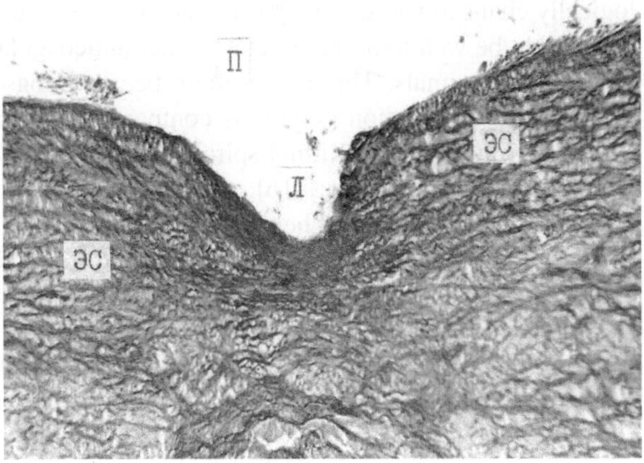

Fig. 2.12 Fragment of the abdominal aorta 24 hours after the implantation of the Nitinol spiral stent demonstrates indentation in the vessel wall with increased density of the elastic fibers from the pressure of the stent

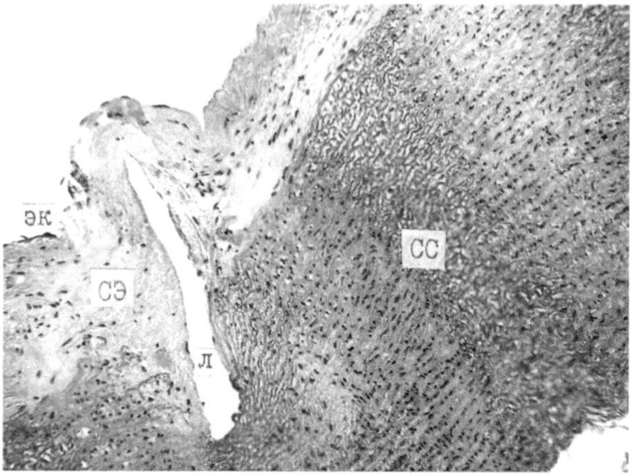

Fig. 2.13 Fragment of the abdominal aortic wall 14 days after implantation of Nitinol spiral stent demonstrates formation of a neointima, covering the stent strut on the side of a vessel lumen

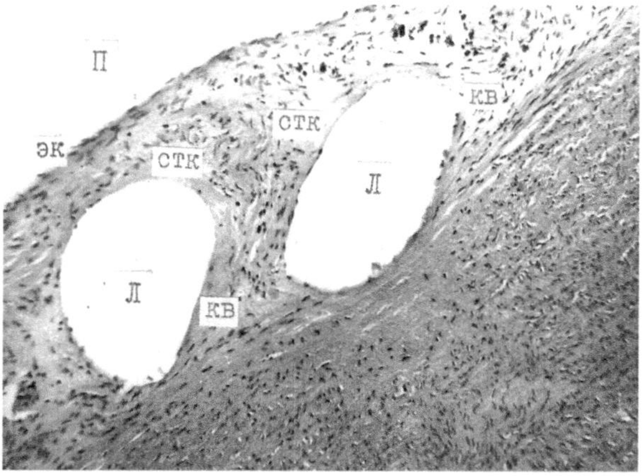

Fig. 2.14 Fragment of the abdominal aortic wall 9 months after implantation of Nitinol spiral stent demonstrates complete coverage of each stent struts with a thin layer of neointima, which consisted predominantly of collagen fibers

intravascular stents are intended for implantation in obliterated by atherosclerotic plaque or extrinsically compressed vessels and the response of a normal and pathologically changed vascular wall is not always the same [24].

It might be well to point out that neither anticoagulants nor antiaggregants were given to the animals. This is important because dogs are known to have a more active blood coagulation system as compared to humans. Therefore, a long-term patency of intravascular Nitinol spiral stents implanted in humans is also possible and was regarded promising [16].

To reveal the behavior of hemocoagulation, hemostasis factors were investigated in ten dogs during implantation of intravascular stents. The analysis of experimental data obtained from comparing the results of different samples taken from the peripheral artery (I), place of contemplated placement of the stent in the vessel (II), and from the lumen of the intravascular stent immediately after its implantation (III) had shown a trend toward the increase in the hypercoagulation potential of blood. Statistically reliable in this case were shortened time indexes of thrombelastography,

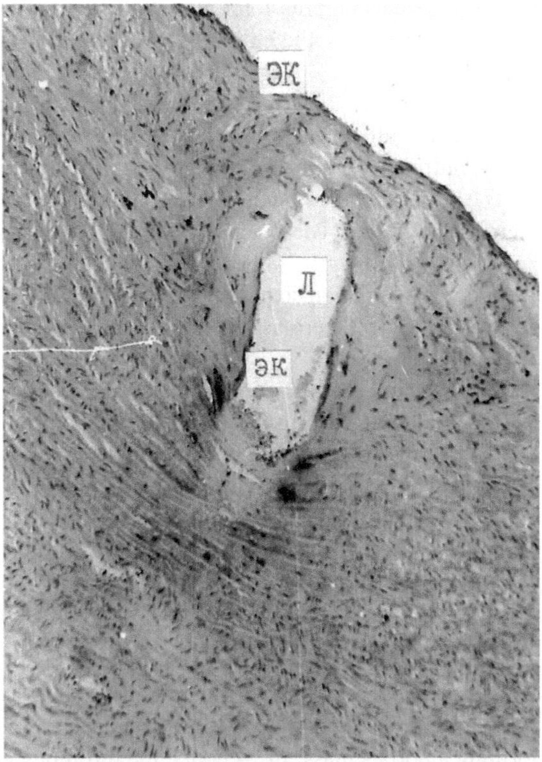

Fig. 2.15 Fragment of the abdominal aortic wall 15 months after implantation of Nitinol spiral stent demonstrates that neointima over the stent strut is covered with a vascular endothelium for its entire length on the luminal side

prothrombin time, increased rate of thrombocyte aggregation, and decrease in the level of antithrombin III. In this case, the main substrate of blood coagulation, fibrinogen, and fibrin-stabilizing factor (fibrinase) remain stable during the entire manipulation.

For the first lime the fact was established that thrombogenic properties of Nitinol are intimately related to its absorptive selectivity with respect to albumin rather than fibrinogen or gamma-globulin which stimulate adhesion of thrombocytes. This was proved by means of electrophoresis of blood plasma protein of samples II and III. It appeared that it was just albumin that was adsorbed on the surface of the intravascular stents, which promotes inhibition process of blood coagulation and adhesion of thrombocytes, thereby preventing thrombogenesis and intimal overgrowth [25].

To our knowledge this is the first most comprehensive experimental analysis of bio- and hemocompatibility of endovascular Nitinol stents, demonstrating stages of vessel wall reaction and neointima formation after the implantation of these devices.

Thus, it may be concluded that the Nitinol intravascular stents possess a substantially high hemocompatibility and are suitable for intravascular stenting in a clinical setting [16, 25]. The acute and chronic experiments proved the possibility of intravascular delivery and accurate placement of a spiral stent through a catheter. Also, the experiments proved that the stent was not dislocated in the vessel and exerted adjustable pressure on the wall of the vessel, not impairing it and protecting it against external compression force. With continuous observations during long-term chronic experiments, the Nitinol spiral stents experienced no change [20, 24].

According to I.Kh. Rabkin et al., it should be concluded that the silicon-treated Nitinol spiral stents behave like porous bypasses, allowing exchange of ions between the vessel wall and lumen and acts as a frame for endothelium and newly grown intima.

The experimental studies allowed the authors to formulate main advantages of their Nitinol stents. These advantages are:

I. From implantation standpoint:
   (a) Biological inertness
   (b) Nontoxicity
II. From technical standpoint [16, 20, 50]:
   (a) Capability of Nitinol to "recall" its shape at a temperature of 34 °C
   (b) Corrosion resistance
   (c) Self-fixation
   (d) Elasticity
   (e) Incompressibility
   (f) Functional mobility
   (g) Adjustable nondestructive pressure on the wall of the vessel

As was reported by J. Palmaz and H. Rousseau [26–30], a metal mesh placed in the artery blood environment was rapidly coated with a soft thrombus. The thrombus was composed mainly of red blood cells which adhered to the metal, thereby forming a porous mass. In 24 hours, the thrombus was replaced by a compact layer of fibrin with the fibers oriented along the blood flow. After staining by silver nitrate, it was clearly visible how endothelial cells grew on the fibrin-coated metal framework 72 hours after its deployment. The experiments performed a week later in rabbits revealed that the stent was completely coated with endothelium. In dogs, pigs, and baboons, this process took 1.5–3 weeks [27, 31–33]. In humans, neointima developed during 6–8 weeks [20, 34–36]. The stents implanted in the veins of dogs had 80% of their inner surface coated with neointima after 4 weeks and 100% after 6 months [20, 24].

The primary source of thrombogenesis after stenting is the metal itself, which comes into contact with circulating blood and blood cells. Therefore, to preclude occlusion of the stented segment, special care should be exercised until the end of endothelialization process. After the endothelial bed has been formed, it provides a reasonably good protection against thrombosis that usually accompanies a decrease in the blood flow velocity. The thrombogenesis process should closely be controlled, but not completely prevented since a light thrombotic coat is required for endothelium growth [37]. The study of thrombogenesis, using platelets labeled by indium-III has revealed that thrombogenesis intensity is inversely proportional to the quantity of anticoagulants and antiaggregants, which are given to the animal before stenting. Quantitatively estimated thrombogenic capability has shown the absence of relation between the increasing diameter of the framework and formation of a thrombus, provided the thrombus perception area remains constant. Artificially restricted blood flow facilitates thrombogenesis that progresses to complete occlusion. Such process can be slowed and even precluded by means of anticoagulants [18, 19, 38]. At the same time endothelium cannot grow on a metal surface. Such growth becomes possible only after fibrin and small thrombi have settled on the inner surface of the intravascular stent. Protein absorption is higher on such metals as silver, copper, and platinum [17, 39]. Thrombogenesis is directly related to thickness of the wire and porosity of the endoprosthesis [40]. The type Gianturco-Roubin and Palmaz stents are made of a 0.015 mm dia wire, whereas the type Wallstent endoprosthesis is made of a 0.08 mm wire. Probably owing to this difference, 13 animals out of 43 in which the Wallstents were implanted had partial or full thrombosis [41]. For Palmaz stents, thrombosis was encountered more rarely while for the Gianturco stents it was practically absent except for the cases when they were implanted in 3 mm arteries and when no sufficiently long antiaggregant therapy was prescribed for the animals [42–45]. In addition to anticoagulant therapy, thrombogenicity of the stainless steel stents can be reduced by polishing filaments or introducing dextran intraoperative, whereby attraction of platelets (having negative electric charge) to the metal (having positive electric charge) is reduced [46, 47]. Thrombogenicity of the Nitinol stents is lower as compared with steel [8]. Long-term biocompatibility depends on such factors as oxidation of the stent surface, corrosion, and repeated flexions of flexible intravascular stents due to contraction of the artery wall [48]. At that time, I.Kh. Rabkin et al. were the only physicians reporting a long-term (5.5 years) experience in observation of stents biocompatibility [49, 50]. The possibility of biodegradation of the stents is still under consideration as well [51, 52].

A major threat to intravascular stenting is presented by thrombosis. The frequency and quality of thrombotic complications as well as the degree of intimal hyperplasia regulate short-term and long-term patency of the stented vessels.

The study of thrombogenesis in dogs after implantation of stainless steel endoprostheses without silicon coat proved the leading role of anticoagulant therapy for obtaining positive results in stenting of arteries [53, 54]. This is in contradiction to the chronic experience gained from dog studies performed by J. Palmaz et al. Though anticoagulants were not used, the authors had found that after 35 weeks of observation 77% of the stented vessels were fully patent (when the vessel diameter was less than 5 mm, patency decreased to 40%) [7].

References

1. Dotter CT. Transluminal angioplasty: a long view. Radiology. 1980;135(3):561–4.
2. Dotter CT, Judkins MP. Transluminal treatment of arteriosclerotic obstruction: description of a new technique and preliminary report. Circulation. 1964;30:654–70.
3. Dotter CT, Rösch J, Judkins MP. Transluminal dilatation of atherosclerotic stenoses. Surg Gynecol Obstet. 1968;127:794–6.
4. Alfidi R, Falls C, Cross W. Vessel implantable appliance and method of implanting it. US Patent 3,868,956; 1975 Mar 4.

5. Simon G, Borrelly J, Gazel P, et al. Endoscopic treatment of postintubation subglottic stenosis. Ann Chir. 1981;35(8):622–4. French.
6. Cragg A. Percutaneous arterial grafting: experimental results. In: XIII World Congress of the International Union of Angiology. Abstracts. Rochester, MN; 1983 Sept 11–16.
7. Cragg A, Gunnar L, Rysavy J, et al. Nonsurgical placement of arterial endoprostheses: a new technique using nitinol wire. Radiology. 1983;147(1):261–3.
8. Cragg A, Lund JA, Rysavy JA. Percutaneous arterial grafting. Radiology. 1984;150:45–9.
9. Dotter CT, Buschmann RW, McKinney MK, et al. Transluminal expandable nitinol coil stent grafting. Radiology. 1983;147(1):259–60.
10. Jervis J. Medical devices incorporating SIM alloy elements. US Patent 4,665,906; 1987.
11. Sutton C, Oku T, Harasaki H, et al. Titanium-nickel intravascular endoprosthesis: 2-year study in dogs. AJR. 1988;151:597–601.
12. McKinney D. Nitinol devices for interventional radiology: report. Oregon Health Sciences University, Department of Diagnostic Radiology; 1983. 10 p.
13. Kogyo Gijutsu Intio. Japan Patent Application; No. 58-17615; 1983.
14. Bernshtein ML, Prokoshkin SD. Nature of shape "memory" effect in alloys. In: New technologies in roentgenosurgery. Moscow; 1989. p. 23–36. Russian.
15. Petrovski BV, Polukhin PI, Rabkin IK, et al. Endovascular (catheter) therapy. In: Endovascular surgery. Theses of the all-union symposium, No. 7. Moscow; 1985. p. 5–7. Russian.
16. Rabkin IK, Zaymovsky VA, Khmelevskaya IY, et al. Experimental basis and early experience in intravascular stenting of vessels. Vestn Rentgenol Radiol. 1984;(4):57–61. Russian.
17. Rabkin IK, Zaymovsky VA, Khmelevskaya IY, et al. Intravascular stenting of vessels. In: Interventional radiology. Theses of the all-union symposium, 7th; 1985. p. 16–8. Russian.
18. Rabkin DI. Experimental substantiation of endovascular stenting. Abstract of the candidate's dissertation. Moscow; 1987. 25 p. Russian.
19. Rabkin IK. Endovascular stenting. Khirurgiia (Mosk). 1988;(6):137–41. Russian.
20. Rabkin IK, Matevosov AL, Gotman LI. Interventional radiology. Moscow: Meditsina; 1987. Russian.
21. Koroleva NS, Samokhin AY, Zenger VG. Selection of treatment method for cicatricial stenoses of trachea. In: 31st All-union congress of surgeons. Theses of reports. Tashkent: Meditsina; 1986. p. 401–2. Russian.
22. Minkina SM, Rabkin DI. Experimental morphological studies on the dynamics of "implantation" of endovascular prostheses in the vessel wall. In: Endovascular revascularization. Theses of the all-union symposium, No. 8. Moscow–Yerevan; 1987. p. 19–20. Russian.
23. Rabkin DI. Endovascular stenting of arterial vessels in experimental use. In: Endovascular revascularization. Theses of the all-union symposium, No. 8. Moscow–Yerevan; 1987. p. 9–13. Russian.
24. Rabkin DI, Minkina SM, Kadnikov AA, Khasenov BP. Experimental and morphological substantiation of endovascular stenting of vessels. Med Radiol (Mosk). 1986;(10):55–63. Russian.
25. Smirnova LA, Rabkin DI. Hemocoagulation system changes in intravascular stenting: experimental data. In: Endovascular revascularization. Theses of the all-union symposium, 8th. Moscow–Yerevan: AMS USSR, National Research Center of Surgery; 1987. p. 14–5. Russian.
26. Palmaz JC, Richter G, Noeldge G, et al. Balloon-expandable intraluminal stenting of iliac artery stenosis or occlusion: multicenter trial. In: 17th international congress of radiology; 1989 July 1–8. Paris. p. 418.
27. Palmaz JC, Kopp DT, Hayashi H, et al. Normal and stenotic renal arteries: experimental balloon-expandable stenting. Radiology. 1987;164:705–8.
28. Palmaz JC, Garcia OJ, Copp DT, et al. Anticoagulation and balloon-expandable intra-arterial stents. Circulation. 1987;76(Suppl IV):IV–45. Abstract.
29. Palmaz JC, Richter GM, Noeldge G, et al. Intraluminal stents in atherosclerotic iliac artery stenosis: preliminary multicenter report. Radiology. 1988;168:721–31.
30. Palmaz JC, Tio FO, Schatz RA, et al. Early endothelialization of balloon-expandable stents: experimental observations. J Intervent Radiol. 1988;3:119–24.

31. Maass D, Zollikotek C, Vangiader F, et al. Radiological follow-up of transluminally inserted vascular endoprostheses: expanding spirals in animals. Radiology. 1984;152:659–63.
32. Maassen W, Greschuchna D, Vogt-Moykopf I, et al. Tracheal resection—state of the art. Thorac Cardiovasc Surg. 1985;33(1):2–7.
33. Sigwart U, Kaufmann U, Goy J, et al. Prevention of coronary restenosis by stenting. Eur Heart J. 1988;9:C31–7.
34. Zubairov FS, Kochkin VV, Gunter VE, et al. Titanium nickelide device for treatment of congenital dislocation of the hip. In: Superelasticity, shape memory effect and their use in new equipment. Tomsk; 1985. p. 156. Russian.
35. Rabkin IK. Endovascular surgery (achievements and development prospects). In: Endovascular surgery. Theses of the all-union symposium, No. 6. Moscow; 1982. p. 5–11. Russian.
36. Rabkin IK, Germashev VG. Five-year experience in intravascular stenting of main arteries. In: New technologies in interventional radiology. Moscow; 1989. p. 14–8. Russian.
37. Dotter CT, Krippaehne WW, Judkins MP. Transluminal recanalization and dilatation in femoropopliteal obstruction. Am Surg. 1965;35:453–9.
38. Palmaz JC, Sibbitt RR, Reuter SR, et al. Expandable intraluminal graft: a preliminary study. Radiology. 1985;156:73–7.
39. Williams DF, Skill IN, Smith R. Protein adsorption and desorption on metal surfaces. J Biomed Mater Res. 1985;19:313–20.
40. Zeitler W, Richter EJ, Roth FJ, et al. Results of percutaneous transluminal angioplasty. Radiology. 1983;145(1):57–60.
41. Rousseau H, Puel J, Joffre F, et al. Self-expanding endovascular prostheses: an experimental study. Radiology. 1987;164:709–24.
42. Duprat J, Wright KC, Charnsangavej C, et al. Flexible balloon-expanded stent for small vessels. Radiology. 1987;162:276–8.
43. Duprat G, Wright KC, Charnsangavej C, et al. Self-expanding metallic stents for small vessels: an experimental evaluation. Radiology. 1987;162:469–72.
44. Rollin N, Wright KC, Charnsangavej C, et al. Self-expanding metallic stents: preliminary evaluation in atherosclerotic model. Radiology. 1987;163:739–42.
45. Roubin GS, Robinson KA, King SB, et al. Intracoronary arterial stenting after angioplasty: early and late results. Circulation. 1987;6:891–7.
46. Palmaz JC. Balloon-expandable intravascular stent. AJR. 1988;150:1263–9.
47. Palmaz JC, Richter GM, Noeldge G. Intraluminale Stent-Implantation nach Palmaz: erste klinische Erfahrung. Radiologe. 1987;27:560–3. German.
48. Ratner BD, Johnston AB, Lenk TJ. Biomaterial surfaces. J Biomed Mater Res. 1987;21:59–90.
49. Rabkin IK. Discussing the four-year Russian experience with stents. In: Laser and stent therapy in vascular disease. International congress II. Scottsdale, AZ: The Phoenician Resort; 1989. p. 365.
50. Rabkin IK, Germashev VG. Five-year experience in intravascular stenting of main arteries by shape-memory stents. In: Shape memory and superelasticity effects and their employment for medical purposes. Tomsk; 1989. p. 115–6. Russian.
51. Ellis S, Topol E. Intracoronary stents: will they fulfill their promise as adjunct to angioplasty? J Am Coll Cardiol. 1989;13(6):1425–30.
52. Ellis SG, Topol EJ, Gallison L, et al. Predictors of success for coronary angioplasty performed for acute myocardial infarction. J Am Coll Cardiol. 1988;12:1407–15.
53. Noeldge G, Richter GM, Palmaz JC, et al. Thrombogenicity of balloon-expandable intraluminal stents with varying outflow obstruction. In: International congress; 1988 Feb; Toulouse, France. Abstract.
54. Noeldge G, Richter GM, Palmaz JC. Balloon-expandable stents in iliac arteries: first long-term results. In: International congress; 1988 Feb; Toulouse, France. Abstract.

Firstborn

3

Clinical Applications of Spiral Nitinol Stents

Endovascular Stenting with Spiral Nitinol Stents

Launch of the Clinical Application

Positive experimental results allowed the authors (I.Kh. Rabkin) to perform intravascular stenting for the first time in the clinical practice using a Nitinol stent of his own design. In March 1984, the stent was successfully implanted in the left external iliac artery of a 56-year-old patient, who had ischemia of the lower extremity (stage III) with trophic changes in the great toe of the left foot [1]. In 2.5 years, however, stenosis of the right common iliac artery developed. A stent was implanted on the right side. Thus, bifurcation stenting was performed with good long-term results (5.5 years on the left side and 3 years on the right side) [1–3] (Fig. 3.1).

Intravascular stenting was performed based on an inventive technique and utilizing specially designed mechanism of stent delivery through an angiographic catheter to the stenotic section of an artery, after balloon angioplasty or, in case of an occlusion, after recanalization followed by balloon dilatation. The entire intervention procedure including recanalization, angiography, and stenting usually took about 45 min. Drug therapy was performed before and after implantation and its results were monitored with reference to coagulograms, thrombelastograms, and variations in aggregation of thrombocytes. Intravenous Reopolyglucin-40 (Dextran) was most often given once daily for 5–7 days before and 3–5 days after the intervention in combination with the solutions of Dipyridamole, Trental, and Complamin (Xanthinol) in a dosage corresponding to the age and degree of disease. High aggregation of thrombocytes was decreased by aspirin (75–125 mg daily) and Ticlid (Clopidogrel equivalent), the doses being selected on an individual basis depending on variations in the aggregation of thrombocytes. Disaggregating preparations and indirect anticoagulants were given for a longer time period (up to 6–8 months) on

I. Rabkin, D. J. Rabkin, *Bloodline of Nitinol Stents*,
https://doi.org/10.1007/978-3-032-25697-3_3

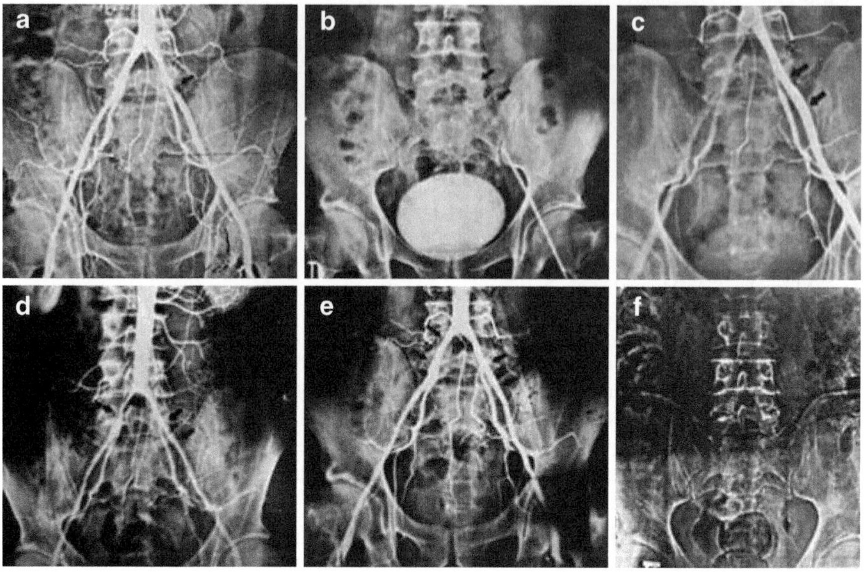

Fig. 3.1 Fifty-six-year-old man with intermittent claudication. (**a**) Initial pelvic arteriogram demonstrates focal left external iliac artery stenosis. (**b**) X-ray after deployment of the spiral Nitinol stent (double arrows). (**c**) Control angiogram after balloon angioplasty and spiral Nitinol stent deployment demonstrates good angiographic result. (**d**) Pelvic arteriogram of the same patient 2 years later performed for right lower extremity claudication, demonstrates right common iliac artery stenosis (single arrow). The previously stented left external iliac artery remains widely patent (double arrow). (**e**) Pelvic angiogram after the deployment of the spiral Nitinol stent into the right common iliac artery demonstrates restoration of the lumen and flow, and persistent patency of the previously stented left external iliac artery (arrows). (**f**) Plain radiograph of the pelvis shows a spiral Nitinol stent in the right common iliac artery and left external iliac artery

an outpatient basis when a trend toward increase of blood prothrombin was indicated. Also, an antisclerotic vessel dilating therapy was done [4].

In 1987, I.Kh. Rabkin et al. published their general experience gained during the first 4 years of intravascular stenting—a radically new and leading direction of medicine in this country. As was noted by the authors, though the period was not long, still it was quite sufficient to sum up the first results. A 2-year intensive research work done by the authors in cooperation with Interventional Radiologists, metallophysicists, surgeons, hematologists, and morphologists made it possible to implement the idea from the experiment into a clinical practice [1, 5, 6] (Fig. 3.2).

At that time this group of authors was holding a leading position in the world not only in the number of implanted intravascular stents, but also in the scope in which this problem has been studied. By 1989 the authors have gained an experience from intravascular stenting in 208 patients with diseased subclavian, renal, iliac, femoral, and popliteal arteries, including 11 patients who underwent multiple stenting in the same zone [2, 3] (Table 3.1).

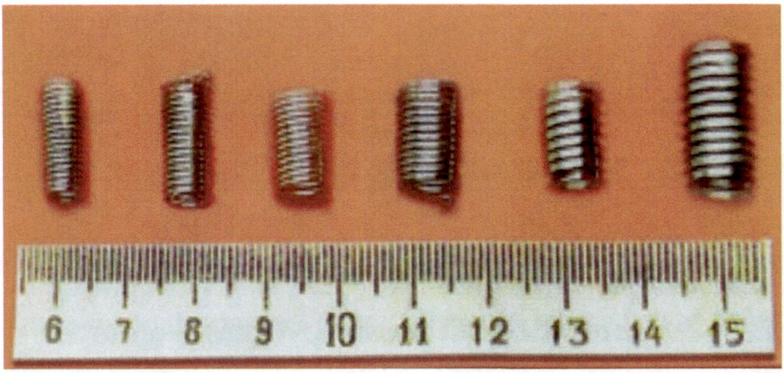

Fig. 3.2 Rabkin Nitinol spiral arterial stents of different diameter, length, and coil pitch

Table 3.1 Localization and the Number of Intravascular Stents

Location	Number of patients	Type of stenting		Total of implanted stents
		Single	Multiple	
Common iliac	57	55	2	59
External iliac	48	45	3	51
Superficial femoral	66	60	6	72
Popliteal	19	19	–	19
Subclavian	9	9	–	9
Renal	9	9	–	9
Total	208	197	11	219

Implanted in the National Research Center of Surgery of the USSR Academy of Medical Sciences (1989)

The age of patients ranged from 21 to 73 years. Of them, 86.7% suffered from atherosclerosis, 9.8% from aortoarteritis, and 3.6% from fibromuscular dysplasia [2, 3, 7] (Figs. 3.3 and 3.4).

No other clinic in the world had such clinical experience at that time. Among the above-mentioned patients 76.6% had such accompanying serious medical conditions, as post-myocardial infarction cardiosclerosis (23.7%), serious diabetes, including that with accompanying angiopathy and retinopathy (20.4%), disturbance of cerebral circulation (12.9%) including patients with hemiparesis, other pathology (19.6%). These data once again emphasize the utmost importance of intravascular interventions and intravascular stenting in particular for treating various vascular diseases, as many of these patients were not surgical candidates due to their serious comorbidities [3].

The indications for intravascular stenting are as follows:

1. Prevention of restenosis in case of atherosclerosis after balloon dilation;
2. Maintaining a hemodynamically effective channel in case of fibromuscular dysplasia, aorto-arteritis, extrinsic compression;
3. Extensive vascular calcifications unresponsive to balloon angioplasty;

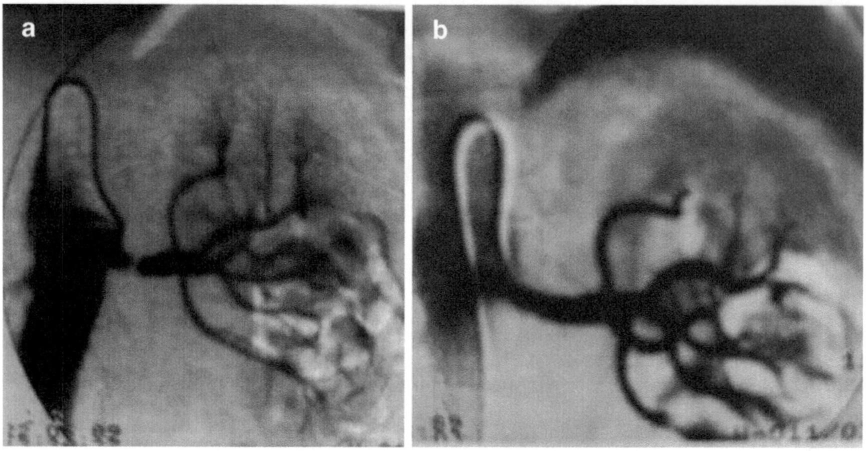

Fig. 3.3 (**a**) Angiogram demonstrates tight stenosis of the left renal artery. (**b**) Angiogram after implantation of the Nitinol spiral stent demonstrates wide patency of the left renal artery without evidence of a residual stenosis

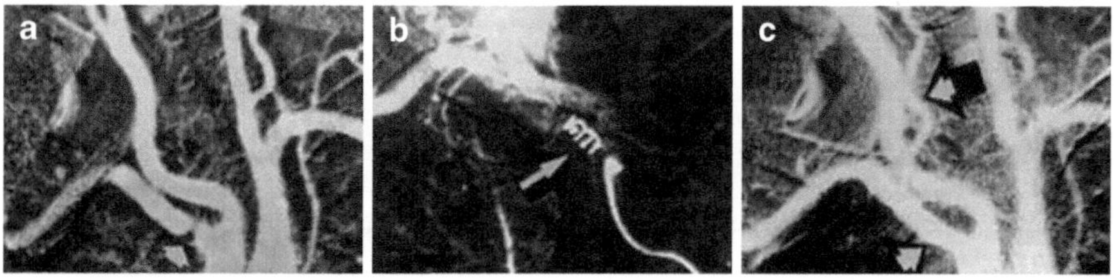

Fig. 3.4 (**a**) Thoracic aortogram demonstrates high-grade stenosis of the proximal right subclavian artery. (**b**) Implanted spiral Nitinol stent into the area of subclavian artery stenosis. (**c**) Thoracic aortogram after stenting of the right subclavian artery with a spiral Nitinol stent demonstrates no residual stenosis and wide patency of the subclavian artery

4. Stenoses of bypass anastomoses;
5. Pathological tortuosity of the vessels [8].

For the purpose of answering a question whether intravascular stenting in case of vascular atherosclerosis is indicated, the authors deeply investigated the mechanism of angioplasty and intravascular stenting, demonstrating that dilatation causes atherosclerotic plaque compression, plaque fluid extrusion, plaque flattening, and plaque destruction. Also, it leads to rupture of intima and media followed by organization and partial regeneration of the vessel wall. At the same time, dilatation leaves the basis for a relapse of atherosclerotic process, that is, rejection of the plaque proper, adhesive surface, small thrombosis, and turbulent blood flow [1, 9].

What intravascular stenting is intended for? The implanted intravascular stent confines compressed atherosclerotic masses to the vascular wall, precluding their separation from intima. The implanted Nitinol spiral exerts uniform pressure on the vessel baroceptors, facilitates rapid regeneration of the vessel, and formation of neointima even at 2 weeks after stent implantation. Such endothelium-coated neointima provides smooth no-adhesive and no-thrombogenic surface, providing laminar blood flow. The author stresses that the study of the problem of intimal hyperplasia which sometimes takes place after intravascular stenting lies ahead. Probably this phenomenon maybe attributed to improper selection of the diameter of the stent which in this case exerts excessive pressure on the vessel wall. Of paramount importance is the fact that since the beginning of the process after intravascular stenting filaments of albumin rather than fibrin are deposited on the stent turns. They are compacted, form a smooth surface, which is indicative of rearrangement of the internal layer during the first days. What is clear is that the intravascular stent provides a "working area," while the blood cells and connective tissue are used as a building material to form neointima. It is essentially the implantation of an artificial prosthesis in the vessel wall [8].

Intravascular stenting may also be used when direct surgery is either limited or contraindicated [10–12].

It is important that 96.2% of patients underwent intravascular stenting without complications and regained their working abilities soon after stenting had been performed (this post-implantation period took only 15 h) [2, 3, 13]. In six patients, thrombosis developed.

Of some interest is one of the above instances when mismatching between the diameters of the vessel and the spiral, as well as the stenosis in the flexure of the iliac artery caused implantation of the Nitinol stent in the dilated segment with spontaneous coiling of the spiral in the proximally intact, but moderately expanded portion of the vessel, whereby the vessel lumen was closed. A basket for removal of foreign bodies was introduced through the catheter into the artery lumen; the spiral was caught and removed through the telescopic catheter.

The publication describing the removal of a large foreign body from the artery was presented [5].

A 2-year follow-up of 86 patients (85.4%) showed that only 12 (14%) of them had aggravation of symptoms (Table 3.2). Similarly, worsening was observed in

Table 3.2 Long-term Results of Intravascular Stenting of Main Arteries

	Follow-up (3 years or longer)			
		Results		
Artery	Number of patients	Good	Satisfactory	Poor
Common iliac	10	10 (100%)	–	–
Internal iliac	12	11 (90.1%)	1 (9.9%)	–
Common femoral	1	1 (100%)	–	–
SFA	14	7 (50%)	2 (14%)	5 (36%)
Popliteal	4	1 (25%)	1 (25%)	2 (50%)
Subclavian	2	2 (100%)	–	–
Brachiocephalic	1	1 (100%)	–	–
Rena	3	3 (100%)	–	–
Total	47	35	4	7

seven patients (15%) out of 47 (46.6%) at 3 years after stent implantation. By aggravation we meant manifestation of clinical symptoms of the main underlying condition, thrombosis of the intravascular stent zone, which necessitated direct reconstruction interventions. It should be noted that exacerbation of symptoms took place only in cases when the stents were implanted in the vessels of comparatively small diameter (femoral and popliteal arteries). In all other cases the stenting results were good or satisfactory [2, 3] (Fig. 3.5). Thus, intravascular stenting by means of Nitinol prostheses proved to be an original, new, low-traumatic, organ-saving, and painless method of revascularization. Implantation of a stent is reasonably simple, requires local anesthesia, and offers a good means of salvage in patients for whom surgery is contraindicated [14–16].

The authors are well aware of the fact that their method had certain limitations, for example, as poorly visible process of stent transformation from a straight filament to a spiral as it is displayed on the screen and complications pertaining to implantation of spiral stents in tortuous vessels. The latter is caused by the fact that the linear portion of the wire, one end of which is secured to the introducer, gradually assumes a spiral shape and traverses a long path as a partially shaped structure inside the vessel, thereby inflicting trauma to its walls and the more tortuous is the vessel the heavier is the potential trauma that may be inflicted [17]. The author is now concerned with the work aimed at obviating these disadvantages. New type of less traumatic and more effective intravascular stents and means of their delivery have been developed and used in a clinical setting, whereby the field of application of the Nitinol spirals has been substantially expanded [18–22]. Clinical experience has been gained thus far in the implantation of such new stents in trachea, esophagus, biliary ducts (this experience is described in the following section), and in the neck of the uterus and urethra. It can be asserted that future clinical experience,

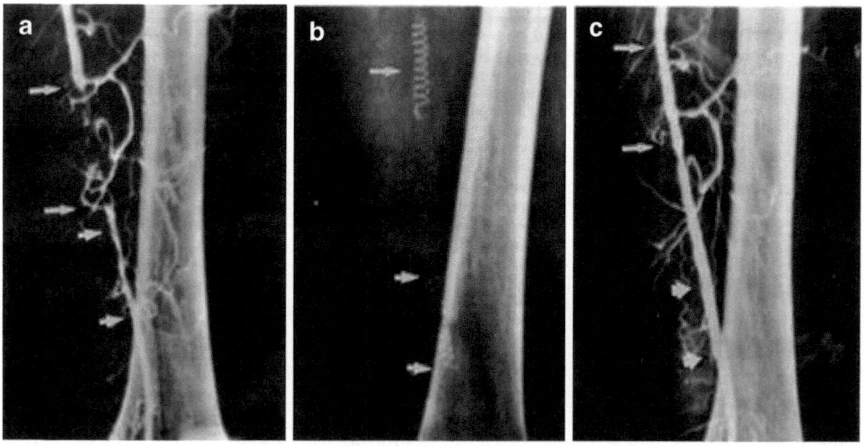

Fig. 3.5 (**a**) Leg angiogram demonstrates occlusion of the mid-superficial femoral artery. (**b**) Two spiral Nitinol stents were implanted into the SFA. (**c**) Angiogram post-stent implantation demonstrates wide patency of the superficial femoral artery

study of the long-term results, morphologic, and hemodynamic examinations will assist in a more objective estimation of this new and promising line of vessel-saving treatment [2, 3, 10–12]. Much promise is undoubtedly offered by a clinically new, combined, and single-step technique of sequential application of laser angioplasty, dilatation, and stenting with the aid of Nitinol spirals [23]. Based on the clinical experience gained from the independent use of laser angioplasty and intravascular stenting, the authors working in the National Research Center of Surgery of the USSR Academy of Medical Sciences combined these two techniques and utilized them in a sequential manner for single-step treatment of segmental occlusion of the external iliac artery. The patient underwent laser recanalization of the occluded segment of the left external iliac artery, balloon dilatation of this zone, and implantation of the Nitinol framework. Angioplasty was done by means of a laser. Recanalization of occlusion required an energy of 193 J and was accomplished with the aid of a sapphire end piece having a diameter of 2.2 mm. The test angiogram showed a nearly 2.5 mm in diameter channel. A tunnel was created and a balloon dilatation catheter was introduced therein. The 4 cm long balloon had a diameter of 6 mm and inflation was performed sequentially three times. Follow-up angiography revealed complete restoration of the artery caliber. To preclude restenosis of the revascularized zone, a 6.6 mm in diameter Nitinol framework was implanted in compliance with the method developed in the clinic. Subsequent angiography proved good patency of the recanalized, dilated, and stented segment of the external iliac artery. Immediately after intervention, palpable pulse appeared in the popliteal artery and foot arteries [23].

By September 1, 1989, I.Kh. Rabkin, Z.G. Natsvlishvili, Z.A. Bubanashvili, and A.M. Kavteladze have accumulated a unique experience of intravascular stenting with the use of a Nitinol prosthesis after laser⁻ and rotor recanalization. Total 17 intravascular stents were implanted in iliac [6], femoral [10], and renal [1] arteries after laser recanalization and 12 intravascular stents were implanted after rotor recanalization. This research work is very important and proves wide possibilities of revascularization in the instances when balloon angioplasty is limited by occlusion in the vessel [7, 23].

Thus, a new technique of intravascular stenting performed after balloon dilatation, laser, and rotor recanalization allows the authors to offer intravascular interventions as an alternative treatment to the bypass surgery [18].

Endobiliary Stenting with Spiral Nitinol Stents

Background

Among the diseases of the biliary system, strictures of bile ducts present the most serious difficulties for treatment. The strictures of bile ducts may be caused by operative injuries comprising up to 60% of all strictures [14, 24]. Sometimes, their appearance is caused by tumorous lesion of ducts (in 16% of oncological patients) and by compression of metastatic nodes from outside. Encountered more rarely are inflammatory strictures and strictures caused by sclerosing cholangitis.

The strictures of bile ducts are usually treated by surgical intervention. The operation is aimed at restoration of bile passage along its normal path, which can be managed extremely rarely, or it is directed to creation of bypass biliodigestive anastomoses [15, 16]. However, under such pathological conditions the operations present a serious problem because of clearly defined changes in topological relationships between the organs and due to the presence of coarse cicatricial changes in the region of portal fissure. Recurrent strictures after operations make up 5.3–53% [14, 25–27]. Complications related to the operations for strictures may comprise 47%. In 25–35% of patients repeated operations are required [28–33]. Mortality after such operations comes to 4–13% and even to 18.4% [34], which is usually associated with the serious general condition of patients, caused by a long-term jaundice, cholangitis, external biliary fistulas, portal hypertension, disturbance of coagulation of blood system, hepatic insufficiency. There is a large group of patients for whom operative treatment is contraindicated due to serious general condition or technically impossible. This applies in an even greater degree to the patients with malignant tumors [35–38].

Deficiencies of operative treatment of bile duct strictures and obstruction of ducts by tumors require searching for more sparing methods of treatment of these patients. This served as an impetus for development of endobiliary manipulations for the treatment of this disease. Balloon dilatation of bile duct strictures adopted in the last few decades gives 24–58% of relapses, its application in patients with tumorous injuries of bile ducts is not possible [27]. Decompression of biliary tree by external or internal–external drainage also has a number of serious shortcomings, such as loss of bile and associated with it loss of protein and electrolyte, dislocation of drain from the stricture zone, incrustation of drain tube by the salts of bile, and psychological discomfort experienced by patients who have to wear a drain tube and bile collection bag [15].

Nonoperative methods providing decompression and patency of bile ducts especially when they are obturated by tumors present an essential alternative of surgical interventions [39–44]. In the opinion of authors, nonoperative decompression should be considered as the main method of treatment of this disease due to a short life expectancy of patients with obstruction of bile ducts caused by inoperable carcinoma of pancreas.

To restore the patency of bile ducts in case of mechanical obstruction, caused by neglected advanced tumorous process, has been already made for many years with a great selection of palliative surgical interventions providing, for the implantation of endoprostheses in the obstructed region [29, 40–53]. However, there were no clearly enough defined optimal capabilities of various decompression methods, such as endoscopic, transcutaneous (interventional) and surgical, when used separately or in a combination. There was no comparative study of various methods, including the evaluation of technical capabilities and assessment of the rate of possible success. There was no study of physiological changes in the bile production and secretion. For instance, it is unclear why the concentration of bilirubin in such patients remains high despite establishing an adequate outflow of bile and problems connected with immediate and early mortality, rate of complications, recurrent occlusions, and average survival rate of patients, belonging to different groups.

A polyethylene endoprosthesis was used for palliative purpose to stop jaundice accompanied by pruritus and threat of cholangitis in 277 patients with carcinoma of pancreas to give success in 89% of cases. Some 18% of patients died within 30 days after application of drainage, but endoscopic implantation of stent proper never caused a need for surgical intervention or was responsible for lethal outcome. Complications were reported in 21% of cases. The authors, having made an analysis of own data and published by other scientists, came to a conclusion that biliary drain placed endoscopically has certain advantages over percutaneous drain and both are in disadvantage related to palliative surgical interventions, as far as patients with inoperable carcinoma of pancreas are concerned [44]. The same viewpoint in relation to endostenting of bile ducts in case of inoperable carcinoma of pancreas is held by other authors [33, 54–57].

There are data confirming that percutaneous drainage of bile ducts normally used in patients with compression of bile ducts due to tumors may fail in providing normalization of bilirubin level in blood. Mortality of such patients within 30 days after operation, involving preliminary use of drainage, comprises up to 90% [46, 51]. However, this opinion is not shared by all authors. R. Gibson et al. [28] note that percutaneous transhepatic stenting in patients with inoperable cholangiocarcinoma provides sometimes the only accessible and executable palliative methods. In 28 out of 30 patients, percutaneous transhepatic implantation of endoprosthesis (PBN–Plastics) has been used to advantage. The authors believe that percutaneous transhepatic stenting may improve the quality of life of these patients and serves as a very useful palliative therapeutic means in case of cholangiocarcinoma of porta hepatis even under the conditions of very advanced process.

Percutaneous method of insertion of endoprosthesis made under fluoroscopy offers certain advantages over its implantation through the endoscope, especially in case of portal fissure tumors. First, because with such tumors it is rather difficult to manipulate through the endoscope (only 42–75% of positive results), as compared with 90% of successful attempts in case of tumors of more distal localizations [32, 33, 58]. Percutaneous transhepatic insertion of endoprosthesis gives from 75–80% to 100% of positive results. Besides, percutaneous manipulation allows selection of the most suitable segment of liver for access and insertion of drain. This viewpoint, in particular, is held by H. Ahlstrom et al. [59], who used percutaneous transhepatic insertion of endoprosthesis in 68 patients with obstruction of bile ducts by inoperable tumors of various origins. Of them, normalization of bilirubinemia was obtained in 45 patients and reduction of bilirubinemia, in 10 patients. Thirteen patients received two to three endoprostheses, four of these patients had portal fissure tumor, in six patients restenting was necessary because of dislocation of the first endoprosthesis, and in three patients, because of tumor growth.

Stenting of bile ducts with various synthetic tubes [45, 60, 61] has a number of disadvantages, such as dislocation of prostheses from its place, occlusion of stent due to its incrustation by the salts of bile acid, need for replacement of tube every 2–3 months, need for the use of large diameter delivery catheters to pass the prosthesis to the region of implantation, which is complicated with subsequent bile outflow into the abdominal cavity. An attempt to use a polyurethane prosthesis bent on both ends for percutaneous transhepatic insertion in patients with inoperable tumors produced a clinical effect and prevented displacement of prosthesis, but it did not clear some other negative aspects of application of tubes made from synthetic materials [61]. Application of autovein has not gained acceptance because of frequent rejection of transplant and development of sclerosis in the plasty region [25].

Use of silicon prostheses mainly for dilatation of bile ducts obstructed by malignant tumors, as suggested in 1977 by B. Kron [35] may be considered as a definite stage in the development of endobiliary interventions. About 600 such cases were described in the literature [36–38, 62–64].

B. Kron and J. Reynier [38] analyzed 500 cases of application of such prostheses for tumorous obstructions of bile ducts described in the literature and their own experience (33 cases) and came to a conclusion that the mortality in such cases made up 6%. Among the complications they pointed was biliary fistulas in 8% of patients, the number of fistulas decreased in the subsequent years after adoption of non-absorbable sutural materials and fixation of prosthesis in the region of implantation by means of purse-string sutures. After implantation of prostheses, jaundice has left in 5% of patients. One reason for retention of jaundice are twists in prostheses or their displacement. Ascending cholangitis in the long-term period took place in 3% of patients. Migration of prosthesis was observed in 1% of patients.

In 1989, there was offered a new modification of prosthesis made from specially treated silicon (which does not adhere to the tissues). On its external surfaces are provided hooks (to prevent migration), and in the upper portion, multiple perforations ensuring better outflow of bile. The endoprosthesis is sufficiently flexible. The material of endoprosthesis is radiopaque. The endoprosthesis comes in various diameters [65]. In the comment to this work, J. Braasch from the Lahey Clinic Medical Center points out that in many patients endoprosthesis was obstructed by bile plaster or encrustations, which is not the case with the patients who received bypass anastomoses. The survival rate was the same as in the group of patients with biliodigestive anastomoses, therefore, it is recommended to apply endoprostheses only in patients for whom the use of biliodigestive anastomoses is contraindicated [66].

Some authors even believe that in case of sutural stenoses of bile ducts it is preferable to restore stenosed bile ducts by means of a transplant made of jejunum wall [67–70]. A new case of application of vascularized jejunal patch to restore patency of bile duct is described by Th. Junginger et al. [69]. In their description the authors note that 10 months after operation the ducts of the patient remained patent and in the region of jejunal patch there was only a light nonprogressing diverticulum. Similar diverticula in the region of implanted jejunal patch are also described in other publications [67]. The authors came to the conclusion that plastic surgery on the common bile duct wall by the use of a jejunal patch is one of the methods for the restoration of patency of extrahepatic bile ducts, especially if stricture is localized in the upper portion of hepatic duct. The majority of modern specialists believe, however, that insertion of endoprostheses in case of strictures of bile ducts and during palliative operations when the ducts arc obturated by tumors is a reliable procedure [20–22, 30, 43, 44, 71–76].

In order to improve long-term results for the patients with mechanical jaundice, most authors first perform percutaneous transhepatic or nasobiliary drainage for providing outflow of bile and, after the improvement of patients' condition, insert the endoprosthesis into the bile ducts. In all cases, they attempt first to insert the prosthesis endoscopically and, if this fails, they immediately perform percutaneous transhepatic insertion. In their opinion, the first procedure is indicated in case of obstruction of ducts by malignant tumor [77].

For patients with mechanical jaundice where bile ducts are obstructed due to the growth of malignant tumors, R. Passarello [78] inserts endoprostheses for palliative purpose either percutaneously or endoscopically. The selection of method depends on localization of tumor: for obstructed proximal portions of ducts, he uses percutaneous drainage, in other cases he prefers endoscopic drainage.

With the type Miller (French Miller Double Mushroom) prosthesis used, the longest time during which the prosthesis remained patent made up usually 11 months; however, one patient lived for 2 years (with endoprosthesis patency retained). Repeated mechanical jaundice developed almost in all patients who received prostheses by this technique. The cause of repeated jaundice was obstruction of endoprosthesis as a result of tumorous growth or accumulation of bile plaster in the endoprosthesis lumen. The endoprosthesis, as a rule, migrated (upward or downward). In three patients the endoprostheses disintegrated after 6 months [79]. In order to permit performance of cholangiography of endoprosthesis, as well as to open up an obstruction (when the endoprosthesis becomes obstructed), an attempt was made to use a special endoprosthesis connected to a small closed reservoir placed in the subcutaneous fat. If indicated, the above-mentioned reservoir, in the opinion of authors, can be punctured and cholangiography can be carried out and bile ducts washed out [80].

Launch of the Clinical Application

In 1983, I.Kh. Rabkin introduced a fundamentally new high priority method of treating bile duct strictures, which entails that a spiral shaped Nitinol prosthesis is implanted in the region of stricture after dilatation, thus producing an internal stent providing for free flow of bile and preventing compression of bile duct from outside. He also validated the application of Nitinol prosthesis for stenting bile ducts.

To enable endobiliary stenting, the author created a prosthesis that is inserted into bile ducts in a constrained state, then is expanded and self-locked. The prosthesis has no adhesive properties. A Nitinol alloy having a shape memory, described in detail in the section which covers endovascular stenting, served as a material for manufacturing stents required for restoration of patency of suture-related post-operative strictures and recanalization of tumorous strictures. A specific feature of this prosthesis is the fact that this stent having the shape of the required size spiral can be reshaped, after cooling, into the coil of smaller diameter, which permits its passage through a delivery catheter into the strictured area. After being heated to an intermediate temperature ($t = +37$ °C), the spiral regains its original shape [20].

The temperature interval within which the original shape being restored is only few degrees; by changing the composition of alloy and manufacturing stent treatment conditions, it is possible to shift this interval over the temperature scale. Owing to its physical and mechanical properties, Nitinol device is capable of exerting high stress pressure up to 700 MPa while restoring its original shape within the bile stricture. It means that in the process of recovering of the preset size and configuration, the Nitinol prosthesis will overcome circumferential elastic resistance of tissues, it will exert on them a very high pressure, depending on the construction of prosthesis [81, 82].

The technology of manufacturing wire endovascular prostheses is described by D.I. Rabkin [6] and is also presented above. The same technology is used for manufacturing spiral endobiliary prostheses, but in the latter case two fixing loops are made instead of one, and instead of straightening the coil for delivery, the spiral is made into a smaller in diameter coil and fixed with locking mechanisms on both ends. To recanalize tumorous strictures, Nitinol tape (flat ribbon coil rather than round wire coil) endoprostheses is also being used [20–22]. When it expands to its final size, such stent creates essentially a flexible metallic cylinder, exerting high radial force and preventing ingrowth of tumorous tissues inside the lumen.

To verify application of endobiliary Nitinol spiral stents, an experimental study has been carried out for investigation of the effect of Nitinol spiral stents on the bile duct wall and lithogenicity of bile in 15 dogs. Laparotomy under general anesthesia was performed with dissection of common bile duct (CBD), then a restrained Nitinol prosthesis was inserted into the proximal portion of CBD, allowed to expand with the diameter of prosthesis after restoration of its shape exceeding the diameter of the dog's common bile duct by 1–1.5 mm (to prevent displacement of prosthesis). The wall of bile duct was closed, using absorbable atraumatic suture with a magnifying device [19].

Histological investigation of the common bile duct wall at the site of implanted Nitinol spiral stent showed that after 6 days and at 1 month post-stenting, coil-shaped impressions in the mucosa were seen from the wire imprints. Within the first week after stenting the inflammation is practically absent. After 3 months the mucosa in the impressions from the prosthesis becomes atrophied and hyperplastic growth develops between the prosthesis struts. Separate macrophages, white blood cells, lymphocytes are detected under the epithelium. In the spaces between the coils, the mucosa protrudes into the common bile duct, the crypts get opened, deformed, and the lumens of alveolar glands of the wall become larger. After 6 months the stent coils grow into the mucosa. They rest either in the layer of connective tissue or in the mucosa. Papillary growth of mucosa is observed against the background of moderately expressed inflammatory infiltration of stroma of lymphohistiocytic character and, as a rule, by the fourth to sixth month it ends with sclerosis. Complete isolation of spiral is accompanied with the formation of a channel made of connective tissue and coated with prismatic epithelium [21, 22].

The study was carried out 6 days, 14 days, and 2.5 months after the implantation of spiral stents; in 9 dogs the spirals were left for further investigations after 6, 9, and 12 months. In all cases the endoprostheses remained patent, no lithogenic activity was noted, the spiral retained its smooth surface and original shine. On the sixth day, the internal surface of the common bile duct had traversed impressions left by the spiral coils. Histological study did not show any inflammatory changes in the CBD wall. In the places where the spiral exerts pressure on the wall the elements of connective tissue are brought closer together, the epithelium of mucosa in the early term period is not present. After 2.5 months, these areas are already lined with epithelium. Beyond the pressure area from the coil turns there was hyperplasia of mucous glands, microcystic expansion of their lumen, and accumulation of mucous secretion. The stroma of bile duct in the spiral projection area showed loosely defined with intermittent macrophage reaction.

Experimental studies confirmed the possibility of placing a stent in the bile duct so that the stent does not displace and provides free outflow of bile. The obtained results are indicative of biological inertness of Nitinol stent with respect to bile and choledochal wall. The conducted experiment made it possible to refine the mechanism of action of Nitinol stent on the bile duct wall and possible ways of passage of prosthesis into the biliary tree. The results of experiment allowed proceeding with clinical investigations [19].

A specific feature of the tape-type prosthesis from flat Nitinol ribbon is that tumorous tissue cannot grow into the prosthesis lumen. No signs of immersion of tape-type stent into the submucous layer were detected [22].

Clinical application of Nitinol endoprosthesis was started after experimental and toxicological studies. Fluoroscopically guided controlled endobiliary stenting by use of Nitinol prosthesis was made in 11 patients with anastomotic and tumorous strictures of bile ducts. Percutaneous transhepatic implantation was made in four patients, and intraoperative endostenting, in seven patients. The follow-up observation continued for 1 year. To perform endobiliary implantation under fluoroscopy, the most complicated patients were taken, who have had a number of operations for anastomotic strictures and had a propagated tumorous growth and for whom it was impossible or dangerous to perform any further invasive treatments other than endobiliary stenting under fluoroscopy.

On the basis of experience on the use of fluoroscopically guided endobiliary stenting of bile duct strictures with Nitinol prosthesis, an algorithm of treatment of patients with anastomotic and tumorous strictures of bile ducts was worked out [10, 11, 17, 20–22]. Anastomotic strictures of bile ducts were recanalized by wire Nitinol endoprostheses, and tumorous strictures, by tape-type endoprostheses [20, 21].

Implantation of endoprostheses was made after balloon dilatation of stricture region. In cases when due to rigidity of stricture it was not possible to pass the delivery catheter or metal guide wire through the stricture zone, intraoperative endobiliary stenting was made under fluoroscopy. In this case, the stricture area was recanalized with Doliotti probe that was passed in a retrograde fashion through the created opening of the common bile duct. The prosthesis was also implanted by means of delivery catheter inserted through CBD puncture. An important thing for implantation is proper selection of prosthesis diameter. Reliable placement of prosthesis is achieved when the prosthesis diameter is 2 mm larger than that of the duct (Fig. 3.6).

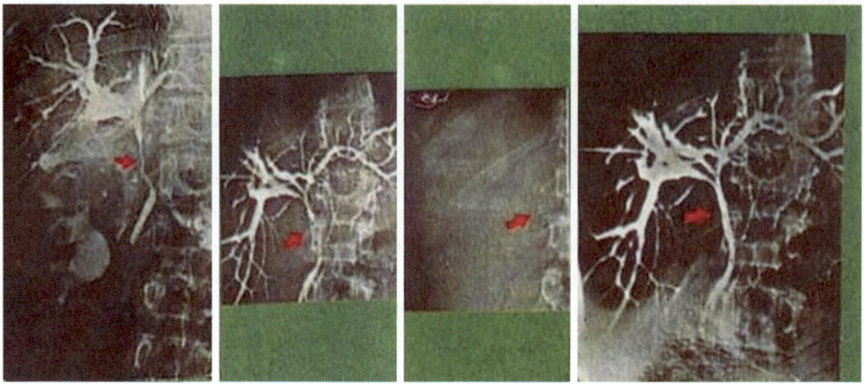

Fig. 3.6 Transhepatic cholangiogram before and after endobiliary spiral Nitinol stent placement into a tight stricture of the common duct with good result

In performing fluoroscopically guided endobiliary implantation, the prosthesis in one case could not restore its original shape because of improperly chosen diameter. The day after it was removed through the delivery catheter and sometime later the patient received a prosthesis that fully complied with the diameter of duct. In another case, the length of smaller radius of stent coiled into spiral exceeded the length of extrahepatic bile ducts. This suggested that in stenting of long strictures it is better to use a number of endoprostheses, placing them one after another. The experience of fluoroscopically guided endobiliary stenting of bile duct strictures by means of Nitinol prosthesis shows that this technique permits improving the condition of patients for whom operative treatment is impossible or associated with a high degree of risk for patient's life [20–22].

Endotracheal/Bronchial Spiral Nitinol Stents

Background

Treatment of stenotic diseases of trachea remains a complicated and actual problem of the modern thoracal surgery [83, 84]. In the last 20–25 years, reconstructive and corrective tracheal surgery in our country and abroad was progressing rapidly [84–90]. A numerous group of patients for whom the intervention on the trachea is indicated represents patients with chronic non-oncologic, mainly acquired stenoses. Usually, they are caused by tracheostomy and long-term artificial pulmonary ventilation. The rate of occurrence of stenoses, according to statistics, varies widely from 0 to 20% and makes up on the average 3–4% [84, 86, 91–94]. New surgical means, such as cryogenic surgery and laser, can also badly injure airway and cause stenosis if used improperly [95].

Post-intubation and post-tracheostomal stenoses are mainly attributable to the pressure exerted by inflated cuff or tube end pressure on the trachea wall, to the injury of mucosa caused by the movement of tube along the trachea and due to infections. The pressure exerted by intubation tube on the cuff balloon may cause erosion of tracheal mucosa, exposure of cartilages, their fragmentation with subsequent tracheomalacia. Contamination of ischemic cartilages results in necrosis and gradual replacement by granulation tissue and then to the development of fibrosis and stenosis. Most commonly found in practice is a combination of corrosive stenosis of trachea and chondromalacia of trachea rings which are adjacent to the place of location of corrosive stenosis [86].

Treatment of chronic stenoses is aimed at restoration of normal functioning of trachea, correction of stenosis, and creation of permanent adequate patency of trachea. In order to achieve it, conservative, endoscopic and surgical methods of treatment were developed and frequently used in their combination.

Conservative treatment is effective, as a rule, only for fresh corrosive stenoses of trachea when structural tissue is not yet formed and there is only a narrowing due to immature granulation and fibrous tissue and infiltration and inflammation changes in the tracheal wall [93]. Considered as an optimal method of treatment is a surgical intervention, that is, resection of diseased segment of trachea with end-to-end anastomosis [86, 96–98]. However, most surgeons consider as an indication for this operation only such stenoses the length of which does not exceed 2 cm. For longer stenoses of trachea, dilatation with the use of T-shaped silicon tubes is undertaken [99]. For stenoses in the intrathoracic portion of trachea, endoscopic intervention (bouginage, laser photocoagulation, and cryodestruction) is usually carried out, the lumen of trachea is restored and split intubation tube is inserted through a stoma of caudal narrowing [86, 96, 97, 99]. Loss of supporting function by damaged tracheal cartilages is often the cause of failure both of endoscopic and surgical treatment of cicatricial stenoses of trachea [100–102].

In the literature many reports dwell on complications occurring after performance of reconstructive/restorative operations on trachea [89, 103, 104]. This fact possibly explains a common trend for application of endoscopic means when treating nonmalignant strictures of trachea. However, modern methods of treatment of extended post-intubation and post-tracheostomic stenoses with domination of tracheomalacia suffer from serious disadvantages. In such cases, the surgeons usually insert various provisional tubes into the trachea for a long period of time, counting on a gradual consolidation of softened tracheal wail and development of rigid lumen [86, 105]. The main disadvantages of these methods are failure of implantation of the tube in the trachea tissues, absence of epithelization of internal surface of the tube, and subsequent disturbance of evacuation of tracheobronchial secretion, long-term impairment of quality of life and disability of patient, and often failure to restore sufficient rigidity of tracheal wall despite a year-long wear of prosthesis.

Such disadvantages are also inherent in the "Swiss roll" prosthesis made of silastic [106] that was used for a long time as a stent for treatment of children. A sheet of silastic foil is rolled into a tube and then inserted into the cavity of larynx and trachea. To fix the stent in the subcutaneous fat, a polyethylene tube was placed at the front surface of trachea and the stent was attached to this tube by means of a few stitches. The sheet of silastic rolled into a tube has a tendency to expand, thus exerting a light pressure on the mucosa and preventing formation of dead spaces between the stent and the larynx and trachea wall. The cigar-shaped "Aboulker" stent retained its value from the 1960th [105], but it did not solve the problem. Sometimes, the softened wall of the chest portion of trachea is externally reinforced by different materials, such as polypropylene rings, segments of cartilage, and marlex gauze. This rather complicated and traumatic operation is not always possible and is met with numerous complications [107].

Therefore, loss of rigidity of tracheal wall presents an uneasy problem for the surgeon. On one hand, conservative and endoscopic methods of treatment are often ineffective in tracheomalacia; on the other hand, surgical intervention is either too risky, because of large area of softened tracheal segment subject to removal or it is inefficient. This difficulty can be obviated when tracheal endoprostheses are used. However, there is no "ideal" endoprosthesis that would fully satisfy all requirements: implantability in the recipient's tissues under the conditions of infected medium, epithelization on the side of cavity, absence of allergic reactions, tumoral growth or formation of granulomas, quick manufacture in the course of operation, sufficient rigidity and possibility of lateral and longitudinal movement [107].

Temporary endoprostheses, such as tracheostomatic cannulas, intubation tubes made of various plastics, straight and T-shaped tubes made of rubber, silicon, latex are used to create and retain the patency of trachea restored during operation and to provide adequate breathing [90, 96, 97, 108]. After various reconstructive operations on the larynx and trachea, provisional or permanent devices are used, but not implanted prostheses. Permanent prostheses are to be used as a palliative measure in the cases when restorative operations have no effect or there are intrathoracic tumors pressing on the trachea [109]. However, a presence of foreign material, even an inert one, with a potentially infected mucosa of airways remains an unsolvable biological problem [110].

One possible way of solving this problem would be development of implantable tracheal endoprostheses that might be coated with airway mucosa and serve as an artificial framework for trachea.

Metal constructions are being used for a long time for experimental and clinical studies aimed at searching for new methods of treatment of tracheal stenoses. As early as 1952, an attempt was made to implant a hollow cylinder made of cobalt–chromium alloy in the lumen of trachea to treat chronic scar stenosis of its upper part [111]. It was revealed that this results in a disappearance of cellular cilia, loss of surface layers of tracheal epithelium, and moderate inflammation in the area of contact of endoprosthesis and, besides, dry mucus accumulated in the lumen restricts the breathing. A case is described [112] when after a failed tracheal dilatation, a stainless steel spiral was implanted into the tracheal lumen of a female patient to support tracheal walls and to prevent renarrowing of trachea. Owing to a very quick proliferation of granulation tissue, the endoprosthesis and tantalum framework used in angioplasty of the trachea were removed. The patient was required to permanently wear a cannula.

In 1986, a report was given about the invention of an expandable metal endoprosthesis for treatment of tracheobronchial stenoses, tracheomalacia, and collapse of trachea after its reconstruction [113]. The prosthesis made from stainless steel wire had a cylindrical zigzag configuration with five to ten turns. The diameter of expanded endoprosthesis was 2 and 4 cm, and its length 2.5 cm. With the prosthesis implanted in the trachea and bronchi of dogs, it was revealed that in all cases there was an inflammatory reaction on the side of tracheal tree and sometimes migration of prosthesis was noted. Endoprostheses of this design were used for treatment of two oncological patients. In one patient the prosthesis served to dilate postoperative bronchial stenosis, and in the other patient, to mechanically support the replaced trachea. In both patients it was possible to expand the airway, but both of them died: one patient died 7 months and the other 3 weeks after stenting from cerebral metastases and intoxication. Despite the large diameter of expanded endoprosthesis which considerably exceeded the diameter of trachea, the stent has migrated. In our opinion, an excessively large diameter of expanded stent may cause serious complications in case of appearance of pressure sores and the expanding stent itself requires further development due to its inability of reliable self-fixation. The literature cites a report about the use of stainless steel wire spiral endoprosthesis in a woman patient to impart rigidity to the fully epithelized fibrous tube connecting cricoid cartilage to the remaining tracheal segment 2 months after disconnection of laryngotracheal anastomosis [114]. The operation provided for normal breathing for 18 months, although the formed lumen decreased to 50% as compared to the initial postoperative lumen, even without clinical symptoms.

Launch of the Clinical Application

A remarkable progress in various branches of medicine took place as result of discovery and study of properties of metal alloys having shape memory and superelasticity. Development and successful clinical use of endovascular stenting of stenosed vessels by the use of spiral Nitinol endoprosthesis with shape memory have led to an idea that studies on Nitinol spirals as implantable endotracheal prostheses hold much promise [107, 115].

The method consists of implantation of artificial intramural-supporting tracheal framework in place of diseased original segment. This is achieved by inserting a spiral Nitinol endoprosthesis having shape memory into the wall of the affected portion of trachea. When the endoprosthesis whose diameter exceeds that of the trachea lumen is implanted in the trachea, the Nitinol spiral, after being heated to the body temperature and after assuming the preset shape, embeds into the mucosa and gets into the thickness of tracheal wail, playing the part of an artificial supporting framework [107].

To reveal the response of trachea and lungs to the implantation of Nitinol spiral endoprosthesis into an intact and stenosed trachea, the authors carried out 82 experiments on 63 rabbits. In 23 animals (the first series of experiments), endoprostheses of different diameters were implanted in the intact trachea. On one end the endoprosthesis was provided with a special loop that served to attach it to the guide. The guide with attached endoprosthesis cooled down to 0 °C, was inserted into the tracheal lumen through a radio-opaque catheter placed in the tracheotomy hole or through an intubation tube. After the endoprosthesis was positioned at the required level, it was quickly heated by the body temperature and self-fixed due to the pressure of spiral coils on the tracheal wall. All manipulations connected with implantation of endoprosthesis into the trachea were performed under fluoroscopy.

In 40 rabbits (the second series of experiments) nonrigid stenosis of trachea was first formed. Experimental studies showed that the spiral Nitinol endoprosthesis being implanted both in an intact and stenosed trachea remained biologically inert with respect to the tracheal wall and did not exert an adverse effect on the lungs. Some abnormalities in the course of post-implantation period in the animals with stented trachea were revealed. Potential infectivity of intratracheal secretions and air led to the fact that implantation of endoprosthesis into the tracheal lumen caused in all animals in the very first few days inflammatory reaction of the tracheal wall as a response to the foreign body. Pathomorphological investigation of euthanatized animals showed that mucosa in the area of localization of endoprosthesis was hyperemic, there was considerable accumulation of mucus, especially at the caudal end of endoprosthesis. In some animals, growth of granulation tissue was revealed. Histological investigations of portions of the stented segment of trachea confirmed the presence of obvious inflammation of all layers of the tracheal wall. Some 3–4 weeks and later after implantation of endoprosthesis, the reaction of trachea depended on the level of position of endoprosthesis and on the ratio between its diameter and that of the tracheal lumen. Location of endoprosthesis (even partial) in the subglottic space of larynx was accompanied by a clearly expressed chondroperichondritis and growth of granulation into the organ lumen. If the endoprosthesis was arranged fully in the trachea, the success of stenting depended on the fact whether all coils of endoprosthesis imbedded in the tracheal wall or protruded into the tracheal lumen. The conduct of endoprosthesis coils with the infected medium of trachea lumen in conjunction with permanent mechanical irritation of mucosa contributed to maintenance of chronic inflammation that was retained for a long time (up to 1.5 years) and had no trend to stopping. In the cases when it was possible to manage quick and full "growth" of endoprosthesis coils into the tracheal wall with restoration of epithelial lining over the whole length, no macroscopic indications of inflammation in trachea were observed already 2 months after implantation of endoprosthesis and slowly going chronic inflammation in the vicinity of endoprosthesis coils, determined by histological methods, had no effect on the condition of animals. It should be noted that tracheal lumen in the stented segment was retained in a full measure, the endoprosthesis was embedded in the tracheal wall and on the macro specimen its coils were observed through smooth, lucid mucosa. This regularity was noted both in the group of rabbits with intact trachea and in the group with stenotic trachea. One of factors contributing to the successful stenting of trachea is minimum traumatization of mucosa during stenting and accurate placement of endoprosthesis during the first attempt.

Full "growth" of endoprosthesis coils into the tracheal wall was observed in those cases when the diameter of endoprosthesis was 2–3 mm larger than that of the tracheal lumen. A sleeve-like expansion of trachea at the level of location of endoprosthesis was never accompanied by perforation or formation of pressure sores on the adjacent organs. The coils of endoprosthesis embedded in the thracheal wall had no adverse effect on the esophagus. No dysphagia disturbances were noted in the animals, and during autopsy the stented portion of trachea could be easily separated from the esophagus [107].

Implantation of Nitinol spiral endoprosthesis into the trachea of rabbits did not require any special fixation. Due to a difference in the diameter of endoprosthesis and tracheal lumen, the pressure exerted by the coils on the tracheal wall enabled the endoprosthesis to remain in the original place, although in 9 out of 42 animals the endoprosthesis migrated with time in cranial [4] or caudal [5] directions. This was the case only when the endoprosthesis diameter was not large enough (less than 7.1 mm). When endoprostheses of larger diameter (from 7.2 to 7.7 mm) were used, it was possible to achieve reliable and stable fixation of endoprostheses implanted both in the intact and in the stenotic trachea of rabbits. So, in the experiments on tracheal stenting in rabbits it was revealed that correct selection of diameter of Nitinol spiral endoprosthesis is a factor of primary importance. To prevent migration of endoprosthesis during the postoperative period and to provide adequate lumen of the stenosed segment of trachea at which the endoprosthesis would be fully coated with tracheal mucosa and would effectively act as an intramural artificial supporting framework of trachea, the diameter of endoprosthesis should be 2–3 mm larger than that of the trachea segment being stented [107].

Positive results of experiments on implantation of Nitinol spiral endoprosthesis in the intact and stenosed trachea of rabbits enabled the authors to use it in six patients (three women and three men) with cicatricial stenosis of trachea, complicated by tracheomalacia in order to create an artificial intramural supporting framework for the trachea and to restore its patency. The patients were 22–48 years old. The etiology of tracheal stenosis were a long-term artificial pulmonary ventilation (APV) and use of tracheostomic cannula. If, apart from soft tracheomalacial stenosis, there was also rigid cicatricial stenosis, the first step was to remove cicatricial tissue, narrowing the lumen via the bronchoscope tube, using tongs or AIG—neodymium laser, followed by the expansion and reinforcement of softened segment of trachea. Then, the endoprosthesis cooled down to 0 °C was implanted through the bronchoscope tube under fluoroscopic control or directly by hand through the tracheostoma. In the trachea, the endoprosthesis was warmed up to the body temperature within a few minutes and allowed to assume a correct spiral shape of preset diameter. In all cases, the implantation of endoprosthesis was performed under anesthesia with APV by the injection method or with high frequency APV [2, 3, 107, 116].

Immediately before implantation, the endoprosthesis was cooled down 0 °C in ice water. The endoprosthesis was shaped into a correct spiral by its spontaneous natural warming to the body temperature and by spraying the prosthesis with hot physiological solution. Control over the location of endoprosthesis and condition of the internal surface of the trachea was accomplished under fluoroscopy, fluorography, tracheography, and bronchoscopy [107, 116].

The early experience of clinical application of Nitinol endoprosthesis for treatment of cicatricial stenoses of trachea with tracheomalacia has shown its efficiency. As a result of implantation of endoprosthesis in the softened segment of trachea, this diseased tracheal segment obtains the lost intramural framework that serves as a support for available rigid elements of the tracheal wall (fragments of cartilage, fibrous, and cicatricial tissue, etc.) and keeps the trachea from collapse. The new framework possesses sufficient elasticity and strength to resist the pressure exerted by the surrounding structures on the trachea and to prevent its mechanical narrowing. An adequate selection of endoprosthesis makes it possible in most of cases to avoid its additional fixation to the tracheal wall. Self-fixation of endoprostheses takes place due to elastic forces of endoprosthesis proper that exerts pressure on the tracheal wall with the result that the coils of endoprosthesis press into the mucosa and are kept by the latter firmly enough. In this case, the spiral coils cut the mucosa and get embedded in the tracheal wall, leaving on the mucosa linear spiral defect that heals with time [107, 117].

The experience suggests that in the conditions of infected intratracheal medium, especially in the presence of tracheostoma, there may be no smooth healing of tracheal mucosa after stenting. If the endoprosthesis has "grown in" only partially, the continuing inflammatory process in the trachea will cause a growth of granulation tissue into the trachea lumen, narrowing of airway that requires repeated endoscopic interventions. Combatting the growth of granulations in the presence of an endoprosthesis partially imbedded in the tracheal wall presents a serious problem that cannot be solved by endoscopic removal of granulation tissue, by the action of an AIG-neodymium laser or silver nitrate, combined with antibacterial therapy that give temporary improvements. In such a situation a need arises for insertion of protector tube (split intubation tube) for 4–6 months until all coils of endoprosthesis are fully imbedded in the tracheal wall and a layer of epithelium is formed on the tracheal mucosa over the endoprosthesis [2, 3, 107, 116, 117].

Having analyzed the causes of complications observed in the first patients, the authors changed the tactics of postoperative period. Immediately after implantation of endoprosthesis in the trachea and its deployment, they installed a protector tube (split intubation tube) into its lumen for the time required for complete "growth" of endoprosthesis into the tracheal wall and epithelialization of trachea over its entire length. This enabled them to reduce the time of full immersion of endoprosthesis into the tracheal wall and restoration of epithelial lining on trachea and to avoid repeated endoscopic interventions [2, 3, 107].

The authors considered as indications for the implantation of spiral Nitinol endoprosthesis in the trachea extended (more than 2–3 cm long) nonrigid stenoses of trachea, represented by tracheomalacia or combination of cicatricial stenosis of trachea with tracheomalacia, especially in case of localization of stenosis in the intrathoracic portion of trachea, as well as stenoses occurring after repeated unsuccessful surgical interventions. Considered as contraindications for implantation of spiral Nitinol endoprosthesis in the trachea are rigid cicatricial stenoses as well as tracheal stenoses extending as far as the subglottic space and the bifurcation of trachea.

By this means, experimental studies and the first experience of application of spiral Nitinol endoprosthesis in the treatment of six patients with cicatricial stenoses of trachea and tracheomalacia have shown a sufficiently high efficiency and safety of this method of treatment. Spiral Nitinol endoprostheses may successfully perform the function of an artificial supporting framework of trachea in the cases when tracheal cartilages are damaged [107].

Besides, the conducted experiments have shown that development of porous materials based on titanium nickelide with open through porosity of 40–75% looks promising for their application in the tracheobronchial surgery and for substitution of diseased segments of trachea. An implant made of plates of porous titanium nickelide can be easily shaped by hand during operation. A porous plate implanted into the muscular graft prevents the slippage of the neck soft tissue graft and firmly keeps the shape of the tracheal lumen. Endoscopic investigation made it possible to conclude that epithelization is completed in 7–10 days after operation [100, 101].

Endoesophageal Spiral Nitinol Stenting

Background

Elimination of strictures in the esophagus is one of the most complicated problems of gastroenteric surgery. The strictures are caused most frequently by malignant tumors or scarring process after burning of esophagus by corrosive agents. According to the summary statistical data [118], complications during intervention occurs in 39% of patients and the mortality alter such operations makes up to 29%. In the recent years there was a trend for widening of applications for palliative resections in esophageal carcinomas, but in case of neglected tumors palliative resection of esophagus can be undertaken in not more than 15–20% of patients [119]. According to D. Prochter, for 260 resections of esophagus (both radical and palliative) the postoperative mortality was 12% [120].

Mortality in one-stage plastic surgery for burn-induced esophageal strictures is 3.3% [121]. Bougienage and balloon dilation, when performed as part of a combination treatment for nonmalignant strictures, did not achieve the desired results in all cases, and in esophageal carcinoma, the efficiency of these measures was transitory. Gastrostomy placement causes a psychical trauma in patients and substantially worsens the quality of life. The patients agree with this intervention only in case of complete obstruction of esophagus, when the treatment has already limited promise and can cause a lethal outcome [121].

Attempts to use such methods of palliative approach as stenting for treatment of carcinoma of esophagus were made already in the last century. These interventions were mainly aimed at elimination of dysphagia which is met in 70–97.6% of patients with carcinoma of esophagus, whereas in 14.5–38.2% it has a clearly defined character [122]. To eliminate dysphagia in such patients, intubation of esophagus is carried out (after preliminary dilatation of tumorous stenosis). In the opinion of some authors, intubation should be performed as early as during the first endoscopy [120]. The prostheses are implanted either through surgical operation or by endoscopy. Endoscopic stenting has a number of advantages over other palliative interventions: it restores peroral nutrition and does not require special care for patients. The healing process was documented [122]. The following types of endoprostheses are used abroad: Celes-tin, Souttar, Mackler, Mousseau-Barbin, Atkinson,

Prochter-Livingston, Collis, Didcott, Holinger, Tytgat, Palmer, Goni, Stirnemann, Sachs, and Gottstcin. In the former USSR, tubes of G.K. Tkachenko, R.A. Toshchakov, and other constructions made of polymers found wide application. The same prostheses are also implanted for treatment of esophageal and tracheal fistulas, rupture of esophagus, as well as nonmalignant strictures.

D. Prochter (1980) collected information about intubation of esophagus, performed by 18 authors from different countries [120]. Mortality after insertion of the tube varied from zero with most authors and up to 32%. The authors personally carried out 2000 intubations of esophagus. Some 16.5% of patients died in the first 2 weeks after intubation. Other authors cite similar figures of mortality (from 2% to 25%) for the cases when the prosthesis was implanted endoscopically [31, 32, 123–125]. These figures are lower than the figures of mortality for the cases when the prosthesis was implanted intraoperatively (10–45%) [124].

The presence of tube in the esophagus does not preclude performing radiotherapy. After esophageal stenting, the condition of patients usually improves which, in turn, facilitates the conditions for the initiation of chemo- and radiotherapy [120]. The author believes that dilatation of tumorous stenoses does not increase the risk of tumor dissemination. Some of the patients showed only minor signs of mediastinitis that disappeared after a course of antibiotic therapy. After the courses of radio- and chemotherapy, reverse development of tumor was sometimes observed, which enabled removal of tubes in these patients.

Various complications were noted resulting from the use of all existing constructions of prostheses, such as perforation of esophagus, perforation of stomach by the distal end of tubes, gastric hemorrhage (in case of injury of gastric mucosa by the tube end), gastroesophageal reflux, obstruction of tube. Complications were associated with rigidity and narrow lumen of some stents (for example, Celestin). The number of complications decreased to some extent when more sophisticated stents, such as Prochtei-Livingston were used [120].

In 1976, R.A. Toshchakov and S.A. Volokitin have developed a bloodless method of esophageal stenting using a recanalization device, which comprises threaded plastic stents moving along the string provided with a spring-type guide [126]. The method made it possible to reduce the probability of esophageal perforation, to shorten the time of hospital stay of patients to 2–3 days since peroral nutrition became possible immediately after the operation. Later on, the authors have developed a new device for stenting of esophagus that lacks deficiencies of the previous one.

To intubate the esophagus, they used a threaded polyethylene prosthesis [122, 126].

Still more important is the choice of stenting procedure for fibrotic strictures of esophagus since the length of life of such patients is incomparably longer and the danger of complications in such cases increases. To prevent the gastroesophageal reflux, which often led to restenosis, these patients received an endoprosthesis provided with an anti-reflux valve. The authors report that after removal of endoprosthesis 1–1.5 years after its placement by using a rigid endoscope no inflammatory changes in the boundary portion of esophagus were observed in the patients [127].

Despite the fact that application of different synthetic stents produces relatively satisfactory results, no construction can be considered ideal or universal. All these constructions have disadvantages to a lesser or greater degree: considerable incidence of stent displacements, local complications (pressure sores, erosions, hemorrhages), a danger of esophageal perforation by the stent during its implantation, limitations of endoscopic interventions for implantation of some type of endoprostheses.

Attempts were made to find new ways in the development of endoprostheses. E. Frirmberger (1983) reported application of stainless steel spiral in ten patients suffering from the carcinoma of esophagus [128]. The spiral is tightly fitted on the endoscope tube; the tube is brought to the diseased segment and then the endoprosthesis is implanted. However, in this case one of the main requirements, that is, reliable self-fixation of endoprosthesis, is not always met. Displacement of the spiral is noted in three out of ten patients.

Launch of the Clinical Application

As it was mentioned above, in 1984 I.Kh. Rabkin for the first time in the world practice implanted a Nitinol prosthesis in the iliac artery of a patient [1]. Five-year experience on endovascular stenting and 3-year of endobiliary and endotracheal stenting with Nitinol spirals allowed proceeding to the development of endoesophageal stenting under fluoroscopy, based on the same principles of employment of Nitinol shape memory.

Under endoluminal stenting the authors understand implanting into a vessel or hollow organ special radiopaque metal alloy prosthesis having shape memory. In this case, the entire therapeutic manipulation is performed by the interventional radiologist under fluoroscopy control. The method is based on the shape memory of Nitinol: on cooling, the Nitinol spiral can be straightened into a linear element or shaped into a spiral of much lesser diameter and in such form it may be passed by means of special device to the required segment. Under the action of temperature of patient's body, the device memorizes the preset shape, expands, self-locks, and performs the function of internal framework [17, 129, 130].

The following problems were raised in the course of experiments: setting up a model of burn stricture of esophagus, which will be suitable for subsequent stenting; developing a procedure of endostenting of esophageal strictures with a Nitinol spiral under fluoroscopy; studying the influence on the mucosa, submucous and deep layers of esophagus [130, 131].

Experiments on simulating the burn strictures of esophagus began in April 1986, the first experiments on endoscopic stenting of esophagus under fluoroscopy started in January 1987. The endoprostheses were implanted under fluoroscopy in 20 rabbits with intact esophagus, in 5 rabbits with burn stricture, and in 7 rabbits with esophageal stricture caused by surgical intervention. All stented rabbits were intact. The follow-up after operation lasted from 1 to 98 days. Endoesophageal stenting under fluoroscopy in the animals was accomplished in an interventional operating room of specially organized section of National Research Center of Surgery under adequate anesthesia [130, 131].

In the course of experiments two procedures of endoesophageal stenting were developed. The first procedure involves fixing the spiral in the guide lock by means of an attachment ring, straightening it under the action of chlorethyl and inserting on the guide into the catheter. Then, according to the procedure, the end of catheter is brought to the lower end of stricture. The guide lock together with attached spiral is accommodated in the same place. The catheter is removed. The spiral starts assuming the preset shape under the action of temperature of animal's body. After deployment of the spiral, the guide is disconnected and taken out. According to the second procedure, the spiral is not straightened before implantation into the esophagus. It is twisted, by contrast, into the spiral of lesser diameter by cooling with chlorethyl and then is implanted in the required segment of esophagus. All stages of endostenting are controlled by fluoroscopy.

The experiments revealed that to avoid subsequent displacement the diameter of spiral should be 2–3 mm larger than that of esophageal stricture and 3–4 mm larger than the diameter of intact esophagus of rabbits. In the animals with an intact esophagus, the diameter of spiral should be 150% as large as the diameter of esophagus. Spirals for stenting were selected from the measurements on preceding esophagogram with oral contrast material [130].

Morphological investigation showed that tissues around the esophagus had not undergone macroscopic changes. In the early period the spiral coils are pressed 1–2 mm deep into the esophageal wall. After 2–3 months, the esophageal wall in the area of implantation of the spiral gets thickened, on macroscopic observation the mucosa looks fibrotic, its longitudinal folds are not seen. When observing the longitudinal section of esophagus, the spiral coils are embedded in the wall and they are surrounded by hard fibrotic tissue.

Histological investigation performed on the fifth day after stenting shows that the spiral coils are buried in the esophageal wall, forming funnel-like hollows, the bottom of which is lined with detritus and soft granulations. The underlying tissues are compacted, edematous, focally and diffusely infiltrated with round-shaped cells, where neutrophilic leukocytes are dominant. In the surface layers of the wall, the funnel-shaped hollows are lined with squamous epithelium. Beginning with the third week, channels start forming around the spiral coils. In the submucous layer they are lined with ripening granulations and soft fibrous tissue diffusely infiltrated with lymphocytes and histiocytes with insignificant admixture of neutrophilic leukocytes. The channels located in the surface layers of mucosa are lined with multilayer squamous epithelium. After 2 months the inflammatory infiltration around the spiral coils considerably decreases, the granulations ripen and turn into fibrous tissue. After 3 months the spiral is surrounded with multilayer squamous epithelium and fibrous tissue. Inflammatory infiltration around the spiral is expressed insignificantly. Single lymphocytes may also be encountered [130–132].

From these investigations, morphological studies show that Nitinol spiral-shaped endoprosthesis does not cause coarse changes in the esophageal wall and can be used in the clinical practice.

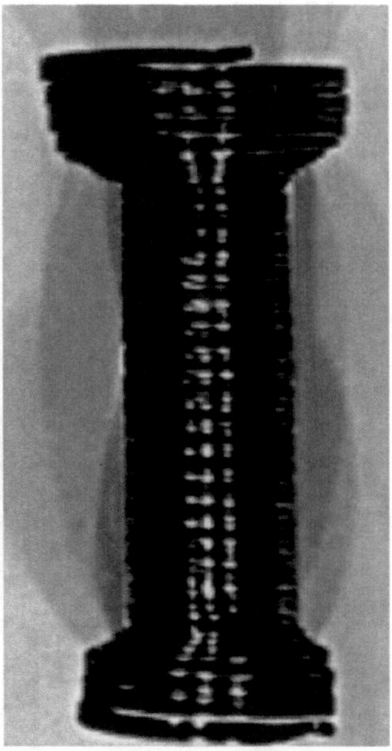

Fig. 3.7 Rabkin Nitinol spiral endoesophageal stent with flared ends for secure fixation

This enabled the authors to apply Nitinol endoprosthesis for the palliative treatment of carcinoma of esophagus [131, 132].

Endoesophageal stenting under fluoroscopy was performed in seven patients with carcinoma of esophagus (Fig. 3.7). The age of patients was from 44 to 78 years; the average age was 64.3 years. Among the patients were six men and one woman. All patients had accompanying diseases; six patients suffered from serious cardiovascular pathology. In five patients the tumoral process was localized in the middle third of esophagus, and in two patients, in the lower third of esophagus. Middle age of patients, serious comorbidities, clinical and radiologic signs of unresectable tumor made it impossible to perform radical surgery. Radiation therapy could not be carried out due to poor condition of patients. The patients have refused to gastrostomy placements.

Implantation of Nitinol spiral endoprosthesis did not require special preparation or anesthesia. Before the implantation the patients received 2.0 ml Valium and 0.5–1.0 ml Atropin. In six patients the esophageal lumen in the strictured area was dilated before implantation of Nitinol spiral endoprosthesis. In three patients, balloon dilatation was performed; in two patients the stricture was dilated with a bougie which was passed by a standard procedure along the guide wire. In one patient balloon dilatation was performed, followed by bougienage. The purpose of bougienage and balloon dilatation was to dilate the stricture of esophagus to a diameter of 7.5–8 mm so that the bougie with the spiral attached to it can easily enter the stricture.

During implantation no perforations or injuries to the esophageal wall were noted. Immediately after intervention the patients reported better passage of food

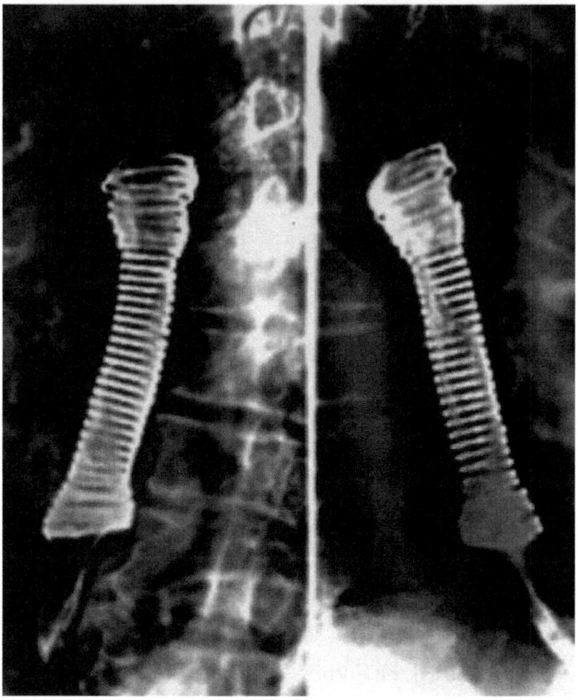

Fig. 3.8 Implantation of the endoesophageal Nitinol stent into a patient with inoperable esophageal cancer

through the esophagus that was evidenced by fluoroscopy. The first successful endoesophageal stenting under fluoroscopy was performed in February 1988 (Fig. 3.8). Clinical investigations allowed considerably improving Nitinol spiral endoprosthesis [131, 132].

In order to recanalize tumorous stricture of the cardia portion of esophagus since January 1988, we have developed a crown-shaped Nitinol device having four to six return coils. The device is manufactured from wire 1.6–1.9 mm. Its size is determined by the length of tumoral segment. The authors applied the device through a gastrostomy in one patient with a tumor in the cardiac portion of esophagus and in four patients with carcinoma of distal esophagus; of them, two patients were stented to prepare them for radical surgery. The authors report in all cases a positive result, including restoration of patency of esophagus. Follow-up of the patients lasting for 1 year showed maintained patency and no migration of the devices in the tumorous canal [133].

In this manner, investigations confirmed the need for a new type of endoesophageal stenting under fluoroscopy and biological compatibility of Nitinol in the gastrointestinal tract. The first clinical experience permits recommending endoesophageal stenting as a low-traumatic, anesthesia-free, bloodless method of improving patency of esophagus. Subsequent accumulation of experience and improvements introduced in the design of endoprosthesis allow determining the possibility of endoesophageal stenting for esophageal strictures of different etiology.

Genitourinary Stenting with Spiral Nitinol Stents

The gained experience in endovascular, endobiliary, endotracheal, and endoesophageal stenting based on the principle of shape memory of Nitinol endoprosthesis of various modifications was applied on the initiative of I.Kh. Rabkin in endostenting of other hollow organs, such as urethra and uterus. So, endometrial stenting under fluoroscopy was successfully performed in the patients with narrowing of uterus after surgery and radiotherapy [18].

Although in every specific case, use was made of endoprostheses of different designs, the principle thermoplastic deformation of metal with shape memory was common for all prostheses. Such a prosthesis possesses the following advantages: biological inertness, corrosion resistance, self-fixation, elasticity, possibility of passing in the narrow lumen of the vessel or hollow organ, incompressibility, functional mobility, proportioned separation of tissues, and implantability in the tissues [2, 3, 17, 18].

References

1. Rabkin IK, Zaymovsky VA, Khmelevskaya IY, et al. Experimental basis and early experience in intravascular stenting of vessels. Vestn Rentgenol Radiol. 1984;(4):57–61. Russian.
2. Rabkin IK, Germashev VG. Five-year experience in intravascular stenting of main arteries by shape-memory stents. In: Shape memory and superelasticity effects and their employment for medical purposes. Tomsk; 1989. p. 115–6. Russian.
3. Rabkin IK, Germashev VG. Five-year experience in intravascular stenting of main arteries. In: New technologies in interventional radiology. Moscow; 1989. p. 14–8. Russian.
4. Rabkin IKh, Sokolov VI, Astrozhnikov YV, et al. Interventional radiology: state of the art and perspectives. In: Review of most critical medicine problems, issue 1. Moscow: VNIIMI; 1985. p. 96. Russian.
5. Rabkin DI. Endovascular stenting of arterial vessels in experimental use. In: Endovascular revascularization. Theses of the All-Union Symposium, No. 8. Moscow–Yerevan; 1987. p. 9–13. Russian.
6. Rabkin DI. Experimental substantiation of endovascular stenting. Abstract of the candidate's dissertation. Moscow; 1987. 25 p. Russian.
7. Rabkin IK, Knyazev MD, Matevosov AL. Experience in treatment of renovascular hypertension by angioplasty of stenotic renal arteries. Khirurgiia (Mosk). 1989;(9):69–74. Russian.
8. Rabkin IK. Endovascular stenting. Khirurgiia (Mosk). 1988;(6):137–41. Russian.
9. Rabkin DI, Minkina SM, Kadnikov AA, Khasenov BP. Experimental and morphological substantiation of endovascular stenting of vessels. Med Radiol (Mosk). 1986;(10):55–63. Russian.
10. Petrovski BV, Rabkin IK. A new trend in vascular surgery—endovascular stenting. In: 31st All-Union Congress of Surgeons. Theses. Tashkent: Meditsina (Uzbek SSR); 1986. p. 369–70. Russian.
11. Petrovski BV, Rabkin IK. Endovascular stenting of vessels. Khirurgiia (Mosk). 1986;(3):3–6. Russian.
12. Petrovski BV, Rabkin IK. Today and tomorrow of endovascular surgery. In: Endovascular revascularization. Theses of the All-Union Symposium, No. 8. Moscow–Yerevan; 1987. p. 4–7. Russian.
13. Smirnova LA, Rabkin DI. Hemocoagulation system changes in intravascular stenting: experimental data. In: Endovascular revascularization. Theses of the All-Union Symposium. 8th

ed. Moscow–Yerevan: AMS USSR, National Research Center of Surgery; 1987. p. 14–5. Russian.

14. Galperin EI, Kuzovlev NF, Karugyulyan SR. Cicatricial strictures of the bile ducts. Moscow: Meditsina; 1982. Russian.
15. Petrovski BV, Milonov OB, Smirnov VA, Movchun AA. Reconstructive surgical treatment of injured extrahepatic bile ducts. Moscow: Meditsina; 1980. 304 p. Russian.
16. Shalimov AA, Shalimov SA, Domansky BV, et al. Percutaneous transhepatic dilatation and electrodissection for strictures of the bile ducts. Klin Khir (Kiev). 1985;(9):33–6. Russian.
17. Rabkin IK. Technology in roentgen endoprosthetics of the vessels, biliary ducts, bronchi, trachea and uterus with nitinol prosthesis. In: Radiological symposium. Graz; 1989. p. 63–4.
18. Konstantinov BA, Rabkin IK. New types of technology in roentgenosurgery. In: New technologies in roentgenosurgery. Moscow; 1989. p. 5–11. Russian.
19. Rabkin IK, Mednik GI, Morozova MM, et al. Endobiliary stenting with a nitinol spiral. In: Endovascular revascularization. Moscow–Yerevan: Academy of Medical Sciences; 1987. p. 231–2. Russian.
20. Rabkin IK, Timoshin AD, Mednik GI, Nelyubin SP. Early clinical application of nitinol endobiliary stent for cicatricial and tumoral bile duct strictures. In: New technologies in interventional radiology. Moscow; 1989. p. 28–9. Russian.
21. Rabkin IK, Timoshin AD, Nelyubin SP, Mednik GI. Reconditioning of bile drainage by endobiliary stenting with special nitinol structures. In: Shape memory and superelasticity effects and their employment for medical purposes. Tomsk; 1989. p. 119–20. Russian.
22. Rabkin IK, Timoshin AD, Mednik GI, et al. Biliary stent using a nitinol spiral: an experimental-clinical study. J Interv Radiol (Russ). 1989;4(3):1–5. Russian.
23. Rabkin IK, Natsvlishvili ZG, Kavteladze ZA, Babunashvili AM. Single-step laser recanalization, balloon dilatation and nitinol stent implantation in occluded abdominal artery: early clinical experience. Khirurgiia (Mosk). 1989;(6):130–1. Russian.
24. Danilov MV, Vishnevski VA, Kotovski AY, et al. Bile-removing operations for malignant strictures of the bile ducts. Khirurgiia (Mosk). 1983;(11):54–9. Russian.
25. Galperin EI, Tatishvili GG, Ivanov AY, et al. Plasty of bile ducts with a vascularized autovenous patch in experimental and clinical use. Khirurgiia (Mosk). 1980;(6):10–5. Russian.
26. Molnar W, Stockman AE. Relief of obstructive jaundice through percutaneous transhepatic catheter: a new therapeutic method. AJR Am J Roentgenol. 1974;122:356–67.
27. Molnar W, Stockman AE. Dilatation of choledochoenterostomy strictures. Radiology. 1978;129:59–64.
28. Gibson RN, Yeung E, Hadjis N, et al. Percutaneous transhepatic endoprostheses for hilar cholangiocarcinoma. Am J Surg. 1988;156:363–7.
29. Huibregtse K, Tytgat GN. Palliative treatment of obstructive jaundice by transpapillary introduction of large-bore bile duct endoprosthesis. Gut. 1982;23:371–5.
30. Huibregtse K, Katon RM, Tytgat GN. Endoscopic treatment of postoperative biliary strictures. Endosc Med. 1989;1:21–8.
31. Tytgat GN. Möglichkeiten und Grenzen der endoskopischen Therapie von Ösophagusstenosen. In: Demling L, Lux G, Domschke W, editors. Therapie postoperativer Störungen. Stuttgart: Thieme; 1983. German.
32. Tytgat GH. Upper intestinal and biliary prostheses: possibilities, results, complications. NYSGE Lecture; 1985.
33. Tytgat GH, Bartelsman JF, Den Hartog JF, et al. Upper intestinal and biliary tract endoprosthesis. Digestion Diseases and Sciences. 1986;31(Suppl9):57S–76S.
34. Vogel SB, Howard RJ, Goudi J, et al. Balloon dilatation of benign biliary strictures in high-risk patients. Am J Surg. 1985;149:73–6.
35. Kron B. Replacement of extrahepatic bile ducts in dogs with silicone elastomer prosthesis. Chirurgie. 1977;103:470–4. French.
36. Kron B. Place des prothèses de Kron le traitement des cancers des voies biliaires extrahépatiques. In: Congrès algérien de chirurgie; 1986. French.

37. Kron B, Reynier J. Prothèse cholédocienne en élastomère de silicone: technique opératoire. Nouv Presse Med. 1981;23:1933–5. French.
38. Kron B, Reynier J. Complications et limites des prothèses en silicone dans le traitement des obstructions biliaires néoplasiques: à propos de 33 cas et de 500 observations. Chir Mém Acad Chir. 1987;113(7–8):709–16. French.
39. Siegel JH. Improved biliary decompression using large caliber endoscopic prostheses. Gastrointest Endosc. 1984;30:21–3.
40. Siegel JH, Daniel SJ. Endoscopic and fluoroscopic transpapillary placement of large caliber biliary endoprosthesis. Am J Gastroenterol. 1984;79:461–5.
41. Siegel JH, Harding GT, Chateau F. Endoscopic decompression and drainage of benign and malignant biliary obstruction. Gastrointest Endosc. 1982;28:79–82.
42. Siegel JH, Pulliano W, Wright G, et al. The ultimate large caliber endoprosthesis—12F: Poiseuille was right. Gastrointest Endosc. 1985;31:158. Abstract.
43. Siegel JH, Ramsey WH, Pulliano W. Cost effectiveness of two endoscopic biliary procedures. Gastrointest Endosc. 1986;32:181–2. Abstract.
44. Siegel H, Snady H. Endoscopic biliary prostheses for carcinoma of the pancreas: nonoperative decompression in 277 patients. Am J Gastroenterol. 1986;81(8):634–41.
45. Burcharth F. Nonsurgical drainage of the biliary tract. Semin Liver Dis. 1982;2:75–86.
46. Ferrucci JT, Mueller PR, Harbin WP. Percutaneous transhepatic biliary drainage. Radiology. 1980;135:1–13.
47. Hoevels J, Lunderquist A, Ahse I. Percutaneous transhepatic intubation of the bile ducts for combined internal-external drainage in obstructive jaundice. Gastrointest Radiol. 1978;3:23–31.
48. Kautz G. Transpapillary bile duct drainage with a large-caliber endoprosthesis. Endoscopy. 1983;15:312–5.
49. McPherson GA, Benjamin IS, Habib NA, et al. Percutaneous transhepatic drainage in obstructive jaundice: advantages and problems. Br J Surg. 1982;69:261–4.
50. Nakayama T, Ikeda A, Okuda K. Percutaneous transhepatic drainage of the biliary tract. Gastroenterology. 1978;74:554–9.
51. Neff RA, Fankuchen EI, Cooperman AM, et al. Radiological management of malignant biliary obstruction. Clin Radiol. 1983;34:143–6.
52. Ring EG, Oleaga JA, Freiman DB, et al. Therapeutic applications of catheter cholangiography. Radiology. 1978;128:333–8.
53. Smale BF, Ring EJ, Freiman DB, et al. Long-term percutaneous decompression of the biliary tract. Am J Surg. 1981;141:73–6.
54. Classen M, Hagenmueller F. Biliary drainage. Endoscopy. 1983;15:221–9.
55. Haber GB, Kortan PP. Complications of endobiliary prostheses. Gastrointest Endosc. 1985;31:169. Abstract.
56. Herter FP, Cooperman AM, Ahlborn TN, et al. Surgical experience with pancreatic and periampullary cancer. Ann Surg. 1982;195:274–81.
57. Speer AG, Leung JW, Yin TP, et al. 10 French straight biliary stents vs 8 French pigtail stents. Gastrointest Endosc. 1985;31:140. Abstract.
58. Stoker J, Dees J, Van Blankenstein M, et al. Endoscopic stenting in malignant biliary strictures. Gut. 1985;26:1135. Abstract.
59. Ahlström H, Lorelius LE, Jacobson G. Inoperable biliary obstruction treated with percutaneously placed endoprosthesis. Acta Chir Scand. 1986;152:301–3.
60. Dooley JS, Dick R, Irving D, et al. Relief of bile duct obstruction by percutaneous transhepatic endoprosthesis. Clin Radiol. 1981;32:163–72.
61. Hao N, Lai P, Chung F. Percutaneous transhepatic internal drainage using polyurethane double-pigtail endoprostheses. Clin Radiol. 1986;36(1):57–9.
62. Cameron JL, Broc P, Zuidema CD. Proximal bile duct tumors: surgical management with silastic transhepatic biliary stents. Ann Surg. 1982;196:412–5.
63. Goldin E, Libson E, Rachmilewitz D. Endoscopic insertion of endoprostheses in postoperative cutaneous biliary fistula. Surgery. 1987;102(1):88–90.

64. Patelli G, Sonato R, et al. Traitement palliatif des ictères néoplasiques par prothèse biliaire en silicone. Lyon Chir. 1986;82:195–7. French.
65. Sezeur A, Kracht M, Fagniez PL, et al. Proximal stenosis of the bile ducts: results with a new surgical endoprosthesis. World J Surg. 1989;13(1):100–4.
66. Braash J. Comment to the article by A. Sezeur et al. World J Surg. 1989;13(1):104–5.
67. Bengtsson HJ, Broome AE, Rime U. Repair of bile duct defect with full-thickness vascularized jejunal patch. World J Surg. 1986;10:510.
68. Dragojevich B, Landes T, Horsen S, et al. Gallengangsplastik mit gestieltem Jejunum-Transplantat. Langenbecks Arch Chir. 1978;346:167. German.
69. Junginger T, Bottger T, Augustin N. Das gestielte Jejunumtransplantat: Möglichkeit zum partiellen Gallengangersatz. Chirurg. 1988;59(4):284–6. German.
70. Landes T, Dragojevich B, Pichlmaier H. Rekonstruktion benigner Gallengangsstenosen. MMW. 1980;112:1511. German.
71. Prokubovski VI, Koshkin VM, Farber AY. Short- and long-term results of endovascular dilatation in obliterative disease of extremity arteries. In: Endovascular surgery. Theses of the All-Union Symposium. Moscow; 1985. p. 49–51. Russian.
72. Papanicolaou N, Dawson SL, Mueller PR, et al. Biliary endoprosthesis using a balloon dilatation catheter. Gastrointest Radiol. 1985;10:394–6.
73. Rossi P. Dilatation and stenting in benign biliary strictures. In: 17th international congress of radiology. Paris; 1989. p. 444.
74. Rossi P. Metallic biliary stents: technical considerations. In: 17th international congress of radiology. Paris; 1989. p. 3028.
75. Rossi P, Salvatori F, Santoro P, et al. Self-expanding stainless steel stents in malignant biliary strictures: early experience. In: 17th international congress of radiology. Paris; 1989. p. 3030.
76. Vallon AG, Mason RR, Laurence BH, Cotton PB. ERCP in postoperative bile duct strictures. Br J Radiol. 1982;55:32.
77. Selcuk B, Arbal E, Sanin BS, et al. Percutaneous transhepatic and nasobiliary drainage and stenting in 120 cases of obstructive jaundice. In: 17th international congress of radiology. Paris; 1989. p. 138.
78. Passarello R. Palliative drainage for malignant obstruction. In: 17th international congress of radiology. Paris; 1989. p. 443.
79. Wong K, Little J, Lee A. Experience with the biliary Mueller endoprosthesis. In: 17th international congress of radiology. Paris; 1989. p. 3743.
80. Friedrich J, Link K, Schumacher K. Endoprothèse biliaire avec raccord sous-cutané permanent. In: 17th international congress of radiology. Paris; 1989. p. 791. French.
81. Rabkin IK, Zaymovsky VA, Khmelevskaya IY, et al. Superelasticity, shape-memory effect and their new applications. Tomsk; 1985. p. 185–6. Russian.
82. Rabkin IK, Zaymovsky VA, Khmelevskaya IY, et al. Intravascular stenting of vessels. In: Interventional radiology. Theses of the All-Union Symposium. 7th ed; 1985. p. 16–8. Russian.
83. Ovchinnikov AA, Vaysberg AA, Druzhinenko AV, et al. Electrosurgical endotracheal interventions in treatment of stenosis of various genesis. In: Diagnostics and treatment of stenoses of trachea and bronchi. Alma-Ata; 1986. p. 17–22. Russian.
84. Petrovski BV, Perelman MI, Koroleva NS. Tracheobronchial surgery. Moscow: Meditsina; 1978. 295 p. Russian.
85. Vishnevski AA, Adamyan AA, Nikishin AA. Peculiarities of techniques in operations on trachea and bronchi. Grudn Khir. 1984;1:40–4. Russian
86. Koroleva NS, Samokhin AY, Zenger VG. Selection of treatment method for cicatricial stenoses of trachea. In: 31st All-Union Congress of Surgeons. Theses of reports. Tashkent: Meditsina; 1986. p. 401–2. Russian.
87. Perelman MI. Tracheal surgery. Moscow: Meditsina; 1972. 208 p. Russian.
88. Kharchenko VP, Chkhikvadze VD, Bryusov PO, et al. Resection of trachea and its bifurcation. In: Surgery of trachea and bronchi. Moscow; 1986. p. 116–8. Russian.
89. Grillo HC, Zannini P, Michelassi F. Complications of tracheal reconstruction: incidence, treatment and prevention. J Thorac Cardiovasc Surg. 1986;91(3):322–8.

90. Meyer R. Reconstructive surgery of the trachea. Stuttgart/New York: Thieme; 1982. 148 p.
91. Samokhin AY. Reconstruction and reconditioning tracheal surgery with temporary T-tube dilatation. Abstract of candidate's dissertation. Moscow; 1984. 170 p. Russian.
92. Laccoureye H, Brasnu D, Guily JL, et al. Étiologie des sténoses laryngotrachéales de l'adulte. Ann Otolaryngol (Paris). 1984;101(1):35–7. French.
93. Robillard T, Piquet JJ. Sténoses laryngo-trachéales de l'adulte. Acta Otorhinolaryngol Belg. 1984;38(2):198–207. French.
94. Rodgers BM, Moazam F, Talbert JL. Endotracheal cryotherapy in refractory airway strictures. Ann Thorac Surg. 1983;35(1):52–7.
95. Simpson GT, Strong MS, Healy GB. Predictive factors in endoscopic management of laryngeal and tracheal stenosis. Ann Otol. 1982;91(4 Pt 1):384–8.
96. Biryukov YV, Koroleva NS, Zenger VG, Samokhin AY. Application of T-shaped silicon tube in tracheal surgery. Methodological recommendations. Moscow; 1986. 15 p. Russian.
97. Biryukov YV, Koroleva NS, Zenger VG, Samokhin AY. Reconstructive operations in treatment of cicatricial laryngotracheal stenoses. In: Surgery of trachea and bronchi. Moscow; 1986. p. 23–4. Russian.
98. Aboulker P, Sterkers JM, Demaldent JE. Modifications apportées à l'intervention de Rethi, intérêt dans les sténoses laryngotrachéales et trachéales. Ann Otolaryngol (Paris). 1966;83:98–106. French.
99. Perelman MI, Biryukov YV, Koroleva NS, et al. Surgical treatment of cicatricial laryngotracheal stenoses. In: Diagnostics and treatment of stenoses of trachea and bronchi. Alma-Ata; 1986. p. 12–7. Russian.
100. Svetysheva ZA, Ioffe LT, Rekhtman AG. Diagnostic and operative endoscopy in organic stenoses of trachea and bronchi. Grudn Khir. 1987;(6):47–52. Russian.
101. Svetysheva ZA, Kirsh VA, Gyunter VE, et al. Porous implants for tracheoplasty: experimental use. In: Shape memory and superelasticity effects and their employment for medical purposes. Tomsk; 1989. Russian.
102. Sokolov VI, Astrozhnikov YV, Gureeva KF, Starikova VB. Role of angioplasty in surgical patients: review of domestic and foreign publications. In: Interventional radiology. Theses of the All-Union Symposium. 7th ed. Moscow: AMS USSR, National Research Center of Surgery; 1985. Russian.
103. Cevese PG, D'Amigo G, et al. Reoperations in tracheal surgery. Ann Chir. 1981;35(8):627–8. French.
104. Martin LG, Casarella WJ, Alspaul JP, et al. Renal artery angioplasty: increased success and decreased complications in the second 100 patients. Radiology. 1986;159:631–4.
105. Crysdale WS, Crepeau J. Surgical correction of subglottic stenosis in children. J Otolaryngol. 1982;11:209–13.
106. Evans JN. Laryngotracheoplasty. Otolaryngol Clin N Am. 1977;10:119–23.
107. Kurmayev ShM. Endovascular stenting in the treatment of cicatricial stenoses of trachea. Candidate's dissertation. Moscow; 1988. Russian.
108. Yunina AI, Lapchenko MN, Zenger VG, et al. Stenting in reconstructive laryngology. Methodological recommendations. Moscow; 1982. 13 p. Russian.
109. Westaby S, Shepherd MP. Palliation of iatrogenic tracheal compression with Silastic stent. Thorax. 1983;38(4):314–5.
110. Grillo HG. Reconstructive techniques for extensive postintubational tracheal stenosis. Int Surg. 1982;67(3):215–20.
111. Harkins WB. An endotracheal metallic prosthesis in treatment of stenosis of the upper trachea. Ann Otol Rhinol Laryngol. 1952;61(3):663–76.
112. Carlens E. Plasties tracheobronchiques: greffes et anastomoses. Bronches. 1967;17(1):1–8. French.
113. Wallace MJ, Charnsangavej C, Ogawa K, et al. Tracheobronchial tree: expandable metallic stents in experimental and clinical use. Radiology. 1986;158(2):309–12.
114. Pagliero KM, Shepherd MF. Stainless steel wire coil prosthesis for anastomotic dehiscence after cervical tracheal resection. J Thorac Cardiovasc Surg. 1974;67(6):932–5.

115. Rabkin IK, Biryukov YV, Kurmayev SM. Early clinical use of nitinol prostheses for cicatricial tracheal stenoses with tracheomalacia. In: New technologies in radiosurgery. Moscow; 1989. p. 43–4. Russian.
116. Rabkin IK. Transluminal angioplasty in the USSR. In: International symposium on transluminal angioplasty. Chicago; 1983. p. 9–11. Russian.
117. Rabkin IK. Endovascular surgery. Vestn Akad Med Nauk SSSR. 1983;1:70–3. Russian.
118. Earlam R, Cunha-Melo JR. Esophageal squamous cell carcinoma. Br J Surg. 1980;67(4):381–90.
119. Collis LH. Surgical treatment of carcinoma of the esophagus and cardia. Br J Surg. 1971;58:801.
120. Prochter D. Esophageal intubation for carcinoma. World J Surg. 1980;4(4):451–61.
121. Vantsyan EN, Chernousov AF. Surgery of the esophagus. In: Reconstructive surgery. Moscow: Mir Publishers; 1989. p. 9–87.
122. Toshchakov RA, Nechiporenko IN. Esophageal bougienage and stenting in inoperable carcinoma of esophagus and cardia. Khirurgiia (Mosk). 1989;(5):115–7. Russian.
123. Jones DB, Davis CS, Smith PM. Endoscopic insertion of palliative esophageal tubes in esophagogastric neoplasms. Br J Surg. 1981;68(3):197–8.
124. Lishman AH, Delliphiani AW, Devlin HB. Insertion of esophagogastric tube in malignant strictures: endoscopy or surgery? Br J Surg. 1980;67(4):257–9.
125. Lux G, Groith H, Reimann JF, Demling L. Tumor stenosis of the upper gastrointestinal tract: nonsurgical therapy by bridging tube. Endoscopy. 1983;15(Suppl 1):207–12.
126. Toshchakov RA, Volokitin AS, Nechiporenko IN. Bougienage and stenting of esophagus in inoperable cancer. In: Operative endoscopy of the digestive tract. Moscow; 1989. p. 27–8. Russian.
127. Oskretkov VI, Shel AI, Prokhorov VI, Trop VF. Esophagoscopy in endovascular stenting of cicatricial strictures of the esophagus. In: Operative endoscopy of the digestive tract. Moscow; 1989. p. 19–20. Russian.
128. Frimberger E. Expanding spiral—a new type of prosthesis for palliation of malignant esophageal stenoses. Endoscopy. 1983;15(Suppl 1):213–4.
129. Rabkin IK, Bernshtein ML, Zaymovsky VA, et al. Use of shape-memory alloys in interventional radiology. In: Shape memory and superelasticity effects and their employment for medical purposes. Tomsk; 1989. p. 117–8. Russian.
130. Rabkin IK, Gigauri VS, Sheremetyeva GF, et al. Intravascular stenting of esophagus in experimental use. In: Endovascular revascularization. Moscow–Yerevan; 1987. p. 233–4. Russian.
131. Rabkin IK, Gigauri VS, Mamontov AS. Intravascular stenting of esophagus. Khirurgiia (Mosk). 1989;(3):118–21. Russian.
132. Rabkin IK, Mamontov AS, Prozorov SL, Mednik GI. Intraesophageal stenting by self-locking shape-memory spiral. In: Proceedings of the 1st All-Union Conference: shape memory and superelasticity effects and their employment for medical purposes. Tomsk; 1989. p. 118–9. Russian.
133. Ziganshin RV, Kecherukov AI, Monasevich LA, et al. Method of recanalization of the cardiac part of the esophagus and rectum in stenotic tumors. In: Effects of shape memory and superelasticity and their use in medicine. Tomsk; 1989. p. 114–5. Russian.

4 Second Generation

Non-spiral Nitinol Stents

Pioneering Innovative Non-spiral Nitinol Stents

Use of Nitinol wire for spiral stents was a revolution and a breakthrough in interventional radiology. Due to Nitinol characteristics, it is an ideal material for interventional devices that can be delivered into the body in a constrained form in a low-profile delivery system and expand to its intended shape and size when released from the delivery system inside the body. It has marked the birth of a completely new concept in treating different diseases and conditions without a need for major open surgery. This is the best example of the "disruptive technology," the term that has been originally introduced by the Harvard Business Professor Clayton Christensen in 1995 in the *Harvard Business Review* article [1]. Christensen later expanded on the topic in the "Innovator's Dilemma", published in 1997 by Harvard Business School Press [2]. It has since become a buzzword in start-up businesses that seek to create a product with mass appeal. Disruptive technology is an innovation that significantly alters the way that consumers, industries, or businesses operate. A disruptive technology sweeps away the systems or habits it replaces, because it has features that are recognizably superior. The wheel, the light bulb, and the cellphones are three examples of disruptive technologies. At the time, these innovations caused a profound break with previous patterns, bringing about major changes in people's lives. Medical stents can be fairly justified to be in the line of these breakthrough developments and technologies.

Stents shook up the medical industry in a big way. The standard of care completely changed and a whole new field of medicine was generated, namely Interventional Radiology, Interventional Cardiology, and Endovascular Surgery. The rate of open surgeries for many conditions that could be now treated with stents, decreased dramatically, while the rates of stenting soared. This is a disruptive technology that really reinvented cardiovascular care.

I. Rabkin, D. J. Rabkin, *Bloodline of Nitinol Stents*,
https://doi.org/10.1007/978-3-032-25697-3_4

Spiral Nitinol stents have made history and marked the inception of a new dynasty of interventional devices. With all the advantages and the historical value of the spiral stents, that have been described above, they certainly had some limitations. In order to be introduced into the body through a percutaneous access, the spiral stents had to be stretched into a straight wire and pushed or pulled through the catheter. Once released from the delivery system, the straight wire starts forming the coil shape inside the targeted vessel or a tubular structure, therefore, shortening significantly and making precise deployment sometimes challenging. The other way of delivering a spiral stent is to make it into a tight coil of much smaller diameter and restrain it mechanically for the introduction through a catheter. When it is released inside a tubular structure within a body and unlocked, it expands into its final pre-set diameter. With this technique the turns of the coil can sometimes entangle during the removal of restraint and expansion. If the coil diameter exceeds too much the diameter of a vessel where it is released, the turns of the spring can lodge under an angle to the axis of a vessel, rather than being perpendicular to it, creating suboptimal scaffolding affect and less radial force.

The limitations of the spiral Nitinol stents triggered the development of a new generation of devices. Some of the advantages of non-spiral stents are summarized in Table 4.1.

Having substantial prior experimental experience with spiral Nitinol stents and realizing the advantages and the need for non-spiral design of these devices, we (Dmitry Rabkin) have started working on the development of the new generation of Nitinol scaffolds in 1990. We teamed up with Dr. Morris Simon and Mr. Stephen Kleshinski at Beth Israel Hospital in Boston, Harvard Medical School. They have previously invented and developed Simon Nitinol Inferior Vena Cava (IVC) Filter. This unique device was designed by Dr. Morris Simon, who was a radiologist in Boston, Massachusetts, in the early 1980s and introduced as the first self-expanding IVC Filter made from Nitinol [3]. It was approved by FDA in 1985 and was revolutionary for its use on Nitinol's shape memory and superelasticity, allowing minimally invasive deployment. It was the first interventional device from Nitinol that was used in the clinical practice. It has marked a shift away from rigid stainless steel filters like the Mobin-Udin and Greenfield filters, offering much lower profile of the delivery system, greater flexibility, and adaptability to different vein diameters.

The Simon Nitinol Filter (SNF) is composed of multiple legs with a conical shape, designed to trap emboli while allowing normal blood flow (Fig. 4.1).

Table 4.1 Comparison of spiral and non-spiral stent characteristics

Feature	Spiral stents	Non-spiral stents
Radial strength	Lower	Higher
Precision	Lower	Higher (customizable)
Flexibility	Higher	Variable (design)
Vessel coverage	Lower	Higher
Deployment control	Less predictable	More controlled

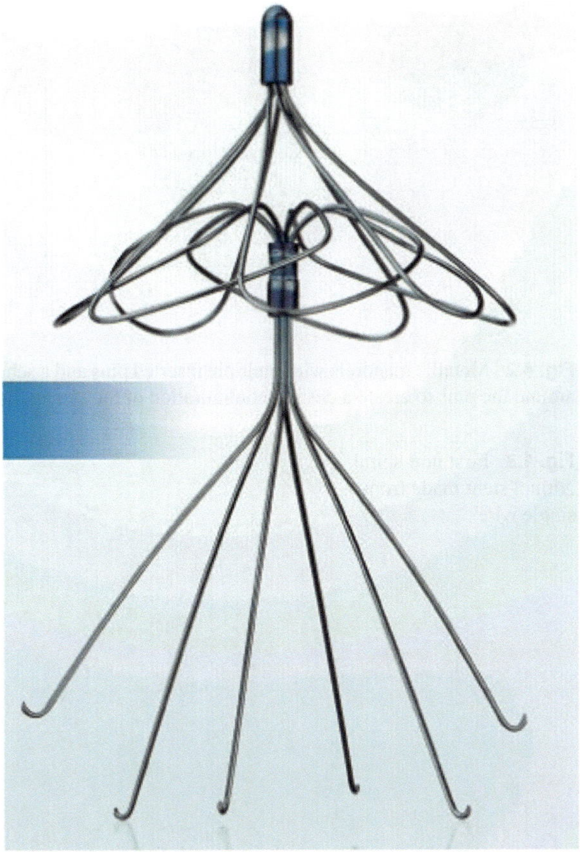

Fig. 4.1 Simon Nitinol Filter, manufactured by Bard. (Courtesy of Dr. Morris Simon)

The Simon Nitinol Filter and the Spiral Nitinol Stents played a foundational role in the development of modern endovascular devices and paved the way for the widespread use of Nitinol in Interventional Radiology and Vascular Surgery. Although not currently used in the clinical practice, they remain milestones in the evolution of minimally invasive approaches to the treatment of many diseases and conditions.

Together with Dr. Morris Simon and Mr. Stephen Kleshinski, we (Dmitry Rabkin) have designed the first non-spiral stent, made from a single Nitinol wire.

This new Nitinol stent constitutes a tubular prosthesis constructed from a single strand of thermal memory nickel titanium alloy filament (0.23 mm in diameter). The wire is formed into several axially arranged hexagonal cells welded together at specified locations to form an integral structure. In order to build the prototypes, we have made cylindrical mandrels of different diameter and length and inserted multiple pins circumferentially (Fig. 4.2).

A single continuous Nitinol wire was wound around the pins of the mandrel to the desired shape and size of the cells and secured on the mandrel. The mandrel was then placed into the furnace for the heat treatment annealing at around 700 °C for

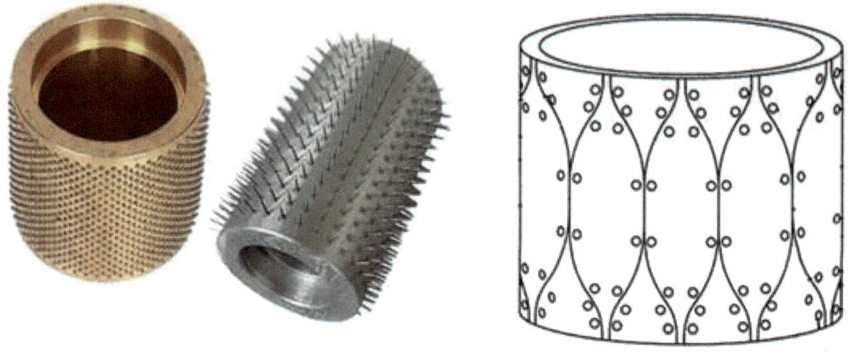

Fig. 4.2 Metallic mandrels with multiple inserted pins and a schematic drawing of winding a wire around the pins to create a desired configuration of the stent cells

Fig. 4.3 First non-spiral Nitinol stent made from a single wire

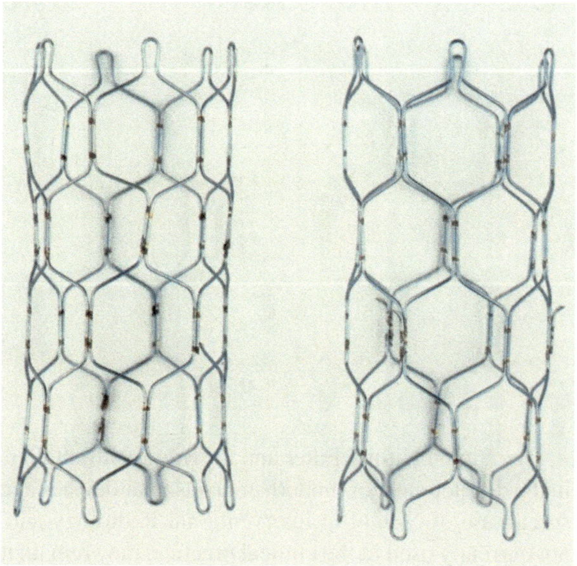

1 h. The mandrel was then taken out of the furnace and cooled down. The wire carefully removed from the mandrel and the parallel touching elements of the stent were welded manually with an electrical spot welder. The final configuration of the stents is demonstrated in Fig. 4.3.

The stents have wide hexagonal-shaped cells. A hexagon is a plane figure with six sides, six vertices, and six angles. The design resembles honeycomb sheets of the honeybee nest (Fig. 4.4). The reasons we choose a hexagon pattern: efficient use of space—most cells in the smallest area, strength and stability, and ease of construction.

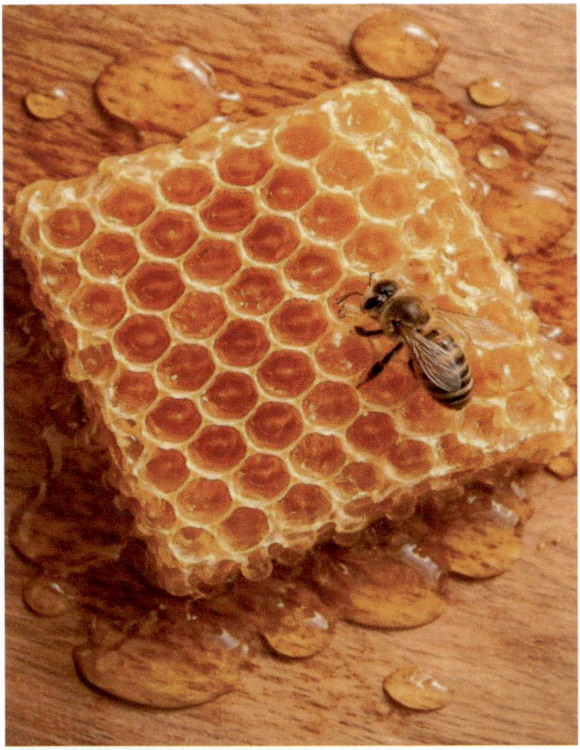

Fig. 4.4 Honeycomb pattern

The devices are cooled and collapsed into much smaller diameter in order to fit into the delivery system for percutaneous insertion. Once released inside the body from the loading chamber at the end of the catheter, they instantly expand to their original size and shape after warming to body temperature. There is minimal shortening of the stent length with expansion, making the deployment highly precise. These stents exhibit an incredibly high radial force with their expansion. The design of the stent is rather rigid with limited flexibility. For the application in the tortuous structures, several stents can be deployed in tandem. Alternatively, we have designed more flexible modular stent with interconnecting wire couplings (Fig. 4.5).

We were granted the US Patent for the unique design and characteristics of the innovative stents (Fig. 4.6) [4, 5].

We have tested in-vitro and in animals several variations of the stents with different configurations and variations of cell geometry along the length of the devices (Fig. 4.7).

Clinical Application of Symphony Nitinol Stents

Following the extensive pre-clinical studies of the above stent with an in-vitro testing and animal experiments, this stent became available on the market under the

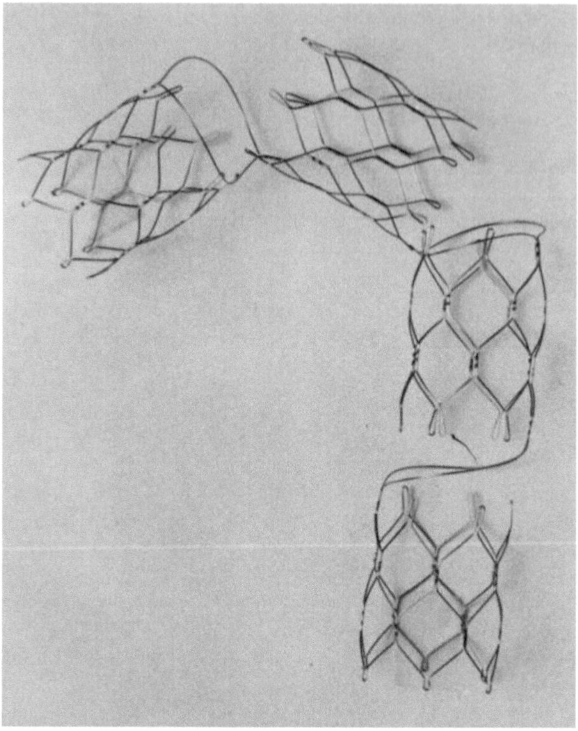

Fig. 4.5 Stent design for use in tortuous structures

name of Symphony™ Nitinol Stent with manufacturing and distribution by the Boston Scientific Corporation.

From a design classification perspective, Symphony sits within the family of wire-formed, closed-cell Nitinol stents. In Stoeckel's widely cited survey and later design monograph, Symphony is explicitly listed among "popular Nitinol self-expanding stents" as a wire-formed hexagonal cell device that is "quite rigid" compared with other wire-based stents, which are usually more flexible [6, 7]. This rigidity reflects an emphasis on radial strength and resistance to recoil at the cost of some conformability in highly mobile segments such as the distal superficial femoral artery (SFA) or popliteal artery. In practical terms, Symphony behaves more like a robust iliac scaffold.

Unlike handmade original devices, the manufactured by Boston Scientific Symphony stents had laser welded parallel struts instead of manual electric spot welding. The Symphony™ Nitinol Stent is delivered on the tip of a catheter covered with an outer sheath to protect and constrain the stent prior to deployment (Fig. 4.8a).

The outer diameter of the stent delivery system is 7 French. For exact placement of the stent, there are four radiopaque markers on the proximal and distal ends of the outer sheath and the stent, respectively.

The delivery system has a unique shape (Fig. 4.8b) with a double lumen structure: one is the guidewire lumen and the other is a flushing lumen, used for priming the stent capsule prior to use. The outer sheath is retracted by pulling a trigger on the

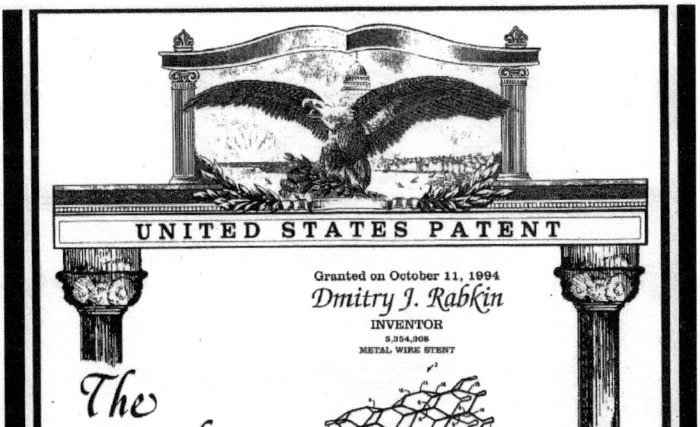

Fig. 4.6 US Patent 5,354,308 Nitinol Metal Wire Stent

proximal handle of the delivery system and as the outer sheath retracts, the stent begins to expand radially (Fig. 4.8c). After removing the outer sheath completely, the stent undergoes "shape recovery" (Fig. 4.8d) and expands within the vessel. The stent design and the delivery system ensured precise deployment of the stent within the target segment without any shortening. It provided a uniform coverage of the diseased vessel, creating a steady scaffold with equally redistributed substantial radial force to keep the vessel open.

Symphony™ stent was a big advancement in the evolution of Nitinol stents. They were successfully used in the clinical practice worldwide for different applications with excellent short- and long-term results [8, 9].

In the Kinoshita's publication [8], 74 stents were implanted in 39 lesions during this study (35 stents in 23 iliac artery lesions; 34 stents in 11 superficial femoral artery lesions, and 5 stents in 5 subclavian artery lesions). The initial procedural

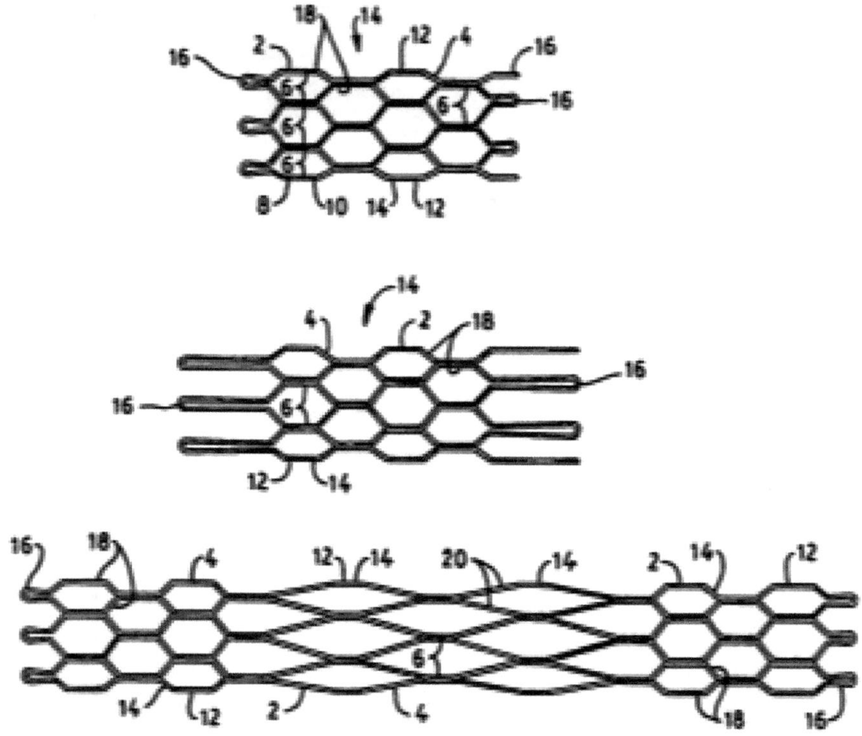

Fig. 4.7 Different stent configurations and cell geometry (US Patent 5,354,308)

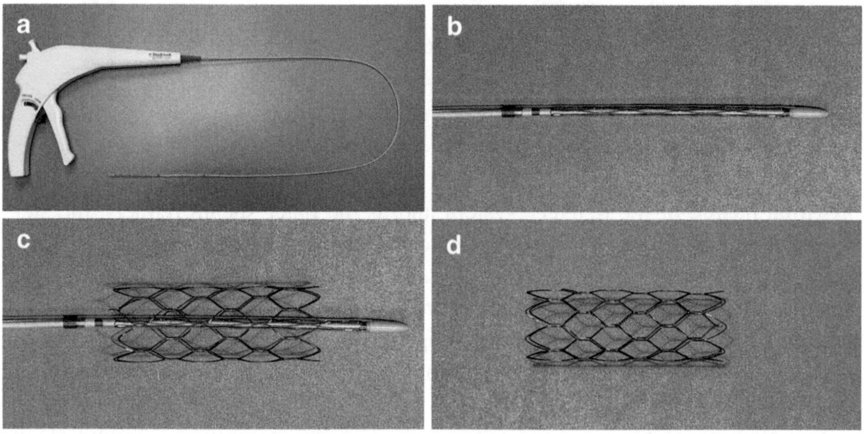

Fig. 4.8 (**a**) Delivery system of the Symphony™ Stent with proximal handle for opening the chamber with preloaded stent at the tip of the catheter. (**b**) Constrained Symphony™ Stent in the delivery catheter. (**c**) Expansion of the stent by retraction of the outer sheath, controlled from the handle. (**d**) The stent released from the outer sheath recovers its original shape [8]

success rate was 95%, and the mean percentage diameter stenosis improved to a significant degree before and after the procedure. The mean pressure gradient across the lesion also improved from 52 ± 39 mmHg to 2 ± 4 mmHg.

The initial clinical success rate was 89%. In all patients with subclavian artery disease, the symptoms caused by limb ischemia disappeared.

The initial hemodynamic success rate was 92%.

The mean follow-up period was 6.3 ± 1.4 months: follow-up angiography was performed in 33 lesions (85%; 20 iliac artery lesions, 8 superficial femoral artery lesions, and 5 subclavian artery lesions) of 27 patients. Angiographical findings showed that the lumen of the stent was maintained; patency was 97.0% and restenosis occurred in five lesions (15.2%). All restenosis lesions were localized in the superficial femoral artery. There was no significant increase in the mean pressure gradient (16 ± 3 mmHg).

Carreira et al. have evaluated the long-term results of iliac artery stent placement with use of the Symphony™ stent for the treatment of patients with intermittent claudication [9]. In a prospective study, 31 cases of iliac occlusive arterial disease were treated in 26 patients. Stenoses ($n = 27$) were treated after failed angioplasty, and occlusions ($n = 4$) were treated with primary stent placement. The follow-up period ranged between 9.5 months and 7.5 years (median = 5.9 years). Data were analyzed using the univariate analysis (Kaplan-Meier method). The mean + SD ABI pre-, post-procedure and in the last control was 0.70 + 0.17, 0.97 + 0.15, and 0.96 + 0.20, respectively. Primary patency rates (%) + SE were 83 + 7 after three years, 75 + 8 after five years, and 67 + 9 after seven years, and secondary patency rates were 93 + 5 after three years, 86 + 7 after five years, and 86 + 7 after seven years. In this study, the authors have concluded that Symphony™ stent has been proven to be a good device to treat lesions in the iliac region with acceptable patency rates and low morbidity and mortality.

The design of Symphony™ stent provides substantial radial force, which is beneficial for treating fibrotic and calcified lesions. However, due to its rigidity, the Symphony stent is not recommended for lesions located at joint flexions or in very tortuous segments of the vessels, where more flexible stents are preferable to accommodate the dynamic movements, conform to the vessel geometry, and reduce the risk of stent fracture or migration.

The design of the Symphony™ stent and material properties provide effective arterial support and have demonstrated positive clinical outcomes. However, careful consideration of lesion location and characteristics is essential to optimize stent selection and ensure the best patient outcomes.

In addition to its vascular applications, Symphony has a biliary variant that was cleared by the US Food and Drug Administration as a self-expanding metal stent for malignant biliary obstruction. The Symphony biliary stent system (Boston Scientific) received 510(k) clearance in the late 1990s as a Nitinol wire-formed device intended for endoscopic or percutaneous placement across malignant strictures of the common bile duct [10].

Symphony™ stents are no longer widely used primarily due to technological advancements of the next-generation stents and market development. Nevertheless, from a historical and didactic standpoint, Symphony stent remains an important example of a wire-formed, hexagonal-cell Nitinol stent that illustrates how specific choices in geometry and manufacturing translate directly into clinical behavior and into the selection of vascular and non-vascular indications. The development of the Symphony stent was a substantial step forward toward the development of next-generation devices based on newer technologies.

References

1. Bower JL, Christensen CM. Disruptive technologies: catching the wave. Harv Bus Rev. 1995.
2. Christensen CM. The innovator's dilemma: when new technologies cause great companies to fail. Boston: Harvard Business School Press; 1997.
3. Simon M, Athanasoulis C, Kim D, et al. Simon nitinol inferior vena cava filter: initial clinical experience. Radiology 1989;172(1).
4. Simon M, Rabkin DJ, Kleshinski S. Metal wire stent. US Patent 5,354,308. 1994.
5. Kleshinski S, Simon M, Rabkin DJ. Stent and method and apparatus for forming and delivering the same. US Patent 5,540,712. 1996.
6. Stoeckel D, Pelton A, Duerig T. Self-expanding nitinol stents: material and design considerations. Eur Radiol 2003;13.
7. Stoeckel D, Bonsignore C, Duda S. A survey of stent designs. Minim Invasive Ther Allied Technol. 2002;11(4):137–47.
8. Kinoshita Y, et al. Usefulness of the symphony nitinol stent for atherosclerosis obliterans. Circ J. 2002;66:100–2.
9. Carreira JM, Reyes R, Gude F, et al. Long-term follow-up of symphony nitinol stents in iliac arteriosclerosis obliterans. Minim Invasive Ther Allied Technol. 2008;17(1):34–42.
10. US Food and Drug Administration. 510(k) summary K963254: symphony biliary stent system. Silver Spring: FDA; 1997.

5 Third Generation

Current Manufacturing Process of Nitinol Stents

The evolution of Nitinol stent designs is clearly linked to the development of the material itself [1–4]. Early on, Nitinol was only available in wire form. Consequently, initial Nitinol stents were wire coils, like Rabkin Spiral Nitinol stent or wire-based non-spiral Symphony stent.

When Nitinol sheet became available, Angiomed (Bard) developed the first laser-cut Nitinol stent in 1997 by cutting a pattern from sheet, rolling it up and welding at specific strut locations.

The next breakthrough technology in the evolution of self-expanding stents was the development of the Nitinol superelastic seamless tubing in mid-1990s and it has since been the material of choice for endoluminal implants such as self-expanding stents [2, 7]. With it came laser cutting of tubular Nitinol components [3, 4, 7]. In 1998 Cordis has introduced its S.M.A.R.T. Nitinol stent, which was laser cut from the tubing and had an innovative flexible design. SMART Stent is a one-piece laser cut, self-expanding Nitinol stent combining a micromesh design with a multi-segmental construction.

The construction of the SMART stent provides an optimal wall apposition. Stent design offers crush recoverable endovascular stent that facilitates high radial resistive support while maintaining flexibility. It was available in a broad portfolio of sizes for the treatment of iliofemoral lesions. The stent had built-in tantalum radiopaque markers (six at each end) to enhance fluoroscopic visibility during deployment (Fig. 5.1).

Today, by far most self-expanding Nitinol stents are produced by laser cutting of Nitinol tubing.

The current manufacturing process of Nitinol stents involves several precise and controlled steps to ensure the final product meets stringent medical standards. Below is a detailed step-by-step guide to the production of Nitinol stents.

I. Rabkin, D. J. Rabkin, *Bloodline of Nitinol Stents*,
https://doi.org/10.1007/978-3-032-25697-3_5

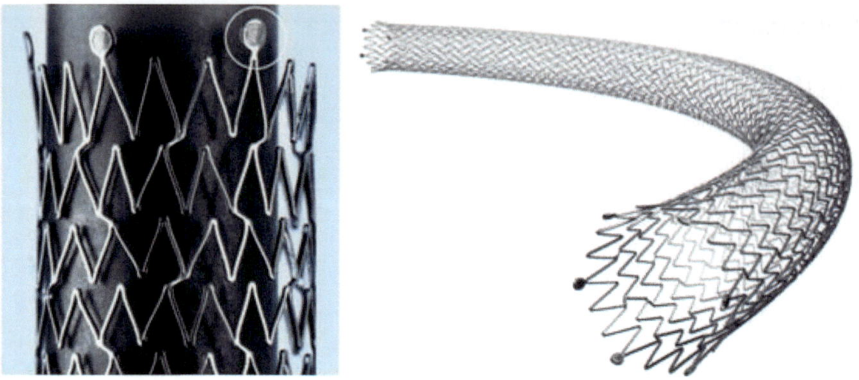

Fig. 5.1 Cordis S.M.A.R.T. Nitinol stent with built-in tantalum radiopaque markers

1. Raw Material Preparation
   1.1. Alloy Selection and Composition Control
      - Nitinol is composed of approximately 55–56% nickel and 44–45% titanium.
      - The exact ratio is carefully controlled to achieve the desired transformation temperature (typically body temperature for self-expanding stents).
      - High-purity raw materials are used to avoid contamination.

   1.2. Ingot Production
      - The nickel and titanium metals are melted together using vacuum induction melting (VIM) or vacuum arc remelting (VAR).
      - The resulting ingot is remelted multiple times to ensure homogeneous composition and minimize impurities.
      - The ingot is then forged into billets or rods for further processing.
2. Tube Formation
   2.1. Extrusion and Drawing
      - The Nitinol billet is hot-extruded to form cylindrical rods.
      - These rods are then drawn through precision dies to reduce the diameter to the required size for stent tubing.
      - Multiple passes with intermediate annealing at 500–600 °C are used to avoid work hardening.

   2.2. Tube Annealing
      - The drawn Nitinol tubes are annealed in a controlled atmosphere furnace (typically argon) at 500–600 °C.
      - This process relieves stresses and restores the material's shape memory properties.
3. Stent Fabrication
   3.1. Laser Cutting
      - The Nitinol tube is loaded into a CNC-controlled femtosecond or nanosecond fiber laser system.

- The laser precisely cuts the stent pattern (typically a mesh or lattice design) based on a CAD model.
- A special coolant or inert gas environment (argon or nitrogen) prevents oxidation and thermal damage.

3.2. Surface Cleaning and Deburring
- After cutting, the stents have sharp edges and burrs, which are removed using:
  - Ultrasonic cleaning with solvents to remove debris.
  - Electropolishing (anodic treatment in an electrolyte bath) to smoothen and passivate the surface.
  - Mechanical polishing (if necessary) to further refine the finish.

4. Shape-Setting and Heat Treatment

4.1. Crimping onto a Mandrel
- The stent is placed onto a mandrel with the desired final expanded shape (Fig. 5.2).
- The mandrel is designed based on the patient's vascular geometry.

4.2. Heat Treatment for Shape Memory
- The stent and mandrel assembly is placed in a vacuum furnace and heated to 450–550 °C for a specific time.
- Rapid quenching (cooling in a controlled environment) helps "lock in" the desired shape memory characteristics.
- Post-heat treatment, the stent automatically expands when exposed to body temperature.

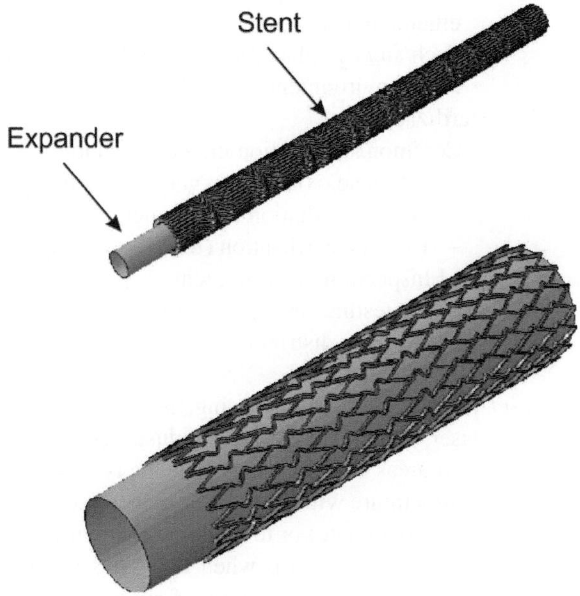

Fig. 5.2 Nitinol microtube with laser-cut slots along its length placed on an expander. The stent is then expanded to its desired diameter for heat treatment to achieve the final cell configuration and pattern

5. Surface Finishing and Passivation
   5.1. Final Electropolishing
      - The stent is further electropolished to remove microscopic imperfections and improve corrosion resistance.
   5.2. Passivation
      - The stent is soaked in nitric acid or citric acid baths to remove free nickel from the surface and create a titanium-rich oxide layer.
      - This step enhances biocompatibility and minimizes nickel leaching into the bloodstream.
6. Mechanical and Functional Testing
   6.1. Dimensional Inspection
      - The stents are measured with laser micrometers and optical inspection systems to verify wall thickness, length, and strut dimensions.
   6.2. Mechanical Testing
      - Radial force testing ensures the stent has adequate outward force for arterial support.
      - Fatigue testing simulates millions of expansion-contraction cycles to confirm long-term durability.
   6.3. Corrosion and Biocompatibility Testing
      - Electrochemical tests ensure the stent resists corrosion.
      - Cytotoxicity and hemocompatibility tests confirm that the stent does not provoke an immune response.
7. Sterilization and Packaging
   7.1. Cleaning and Packaging
      - The stents undergo final ultrasonic cleaning in high-purity water and ethanol baths.
      - Each stent is placed into a sterile packaging unit, often under a clean-room environment (ISO Class 5).
   7.2. Sterilization
      - Common sterilization methods include:
         – Ethylene oxide (EtO) gas sterilization (most common).
         – Gamma radiation (if polymer coatings allow).
         – E-beam sterilization (for drug-eluting stents).
   7.3. Final Inspection and Shipment
      - Batch testing and visual inspection are conducted before shipping to hospitals or distributors.

Laser machining works by using the neodymium:yttrium-aluminum-garnet or Nd:YAG laser, which is the current industry standard to precisely remove material from selected areas of a tubing [3, 4]. This is done by heating the tube locally to a very high temperature with the laser, which causes the material in that area to either evaporate quickly (ablate) or to melt, or react with oxygen if it is present.

The main quality concerns when using this method are the redeposition of the removed material, the accumulation of contamination products (dross) or burrs on the part, and the formation of heat-affected zones (HAZ), which are areas where material was not removed, but the part was affected by the high temperature from the laser [1, 4, 6].

Due to its shape memory and superelasticity, Nitinol is particularly sensitive to forming HAZ. For this reason, Nitinol is usually laser machined using a pulsed laser. In this type of laser machining, the laser is pulsed on for just a small fraction of a second, causing ablation, then is switched back off, which allows the part time to dissipate heat and cool, then the pulse is repeated.

Picosecond and femtosecond laser technology is best for cutting stents. Medical laser cutting is an integral part in many medical devices and advancements in this industry. While there are different laser systems that can cut stents like nanosecond, picosecond, femtosecond, and fiber laser technology, it is the picosecond and femtosecond laser systems that have proved to be the best choice in laser technology. A high-energy density laser beam is focused on the surface of the workpiece and the material vaporizes leaving the desired stent mesh. The remaining material is then blown away by a pressurized air flow [3–5].

Another topic of active research and development in this area is the intentional use of laser heating during the cutting process to locally control the mechanical properties of the Nitinol device. The mechanical properties of Nitinol are highly sensitive to the Ni:Ti ratio, and thermal history. Ni is preferentially removed by laser heating, so for this reason, controlled laser exposure can be used to change the local Ni:Ti ratio and affect mechanical properties [3, 7].

Once shape-setting is complete, extensive post-processing is needed to remove oxides, recast layers, and microburrs created during laser cutting or braiding, and to create a smooth, corrosion-resistant, fatigue-friendly surface [3, 4, 7, 8]. The first step is cleaning and pickling: the stents are degreased and then exposed to acid baths (often mixtures containing hydrofluoric and nitric acids in tightly controlled conditions) to dissolve recast Nitinol, remove sharp edges, and strip the thick, non-uniform oxide formed during cutting or heat-setting [2–4]. This is followed by electropolishing, in which the stent functions as the anode in an electrolytic cell and the surface is uniformly dissolved at the microscopic level [3, 4, 8, 9]. Electropolishing smooths strut edges, rounds laser kerfs, and thins the oxide to a controlled, adherent titanium-rich layer that improves corrosion resistance and reduces nickel ion release [2–4, 8]. The combination of pickling and electropolishing dramatically reduces surface defects that otherwise concentrate stress and serve as fatigue crack initiation sites [3, 8]. A valuable illustration here would be a before-and-after micrograph comparison: one panel showing a rough laser-cut edge with recast droplets and microcracks, the other showing a smooth, rounded, and electropolished strut with uniform oxide [3, 8, 9].

Less common method for fabricating Nitinol medical devices is *photochemical etching*. In this method, a piece of Nitinol tube, wire, or other shape is selectively masked, then exposed to a chemical etchant [3].

The main advantages of this technique are that it avoids the formation of burrs and redeposited material that can be an issue with laser machining, and does not involve the exposure of any area of the stent to high temperature. However, the processing speed is generally slower than laser machining, and is best suited for making 2D shapes, unless the desired 3D shape can be made by folding or rolling.

One trend in this area involves the use of alternate and less hazardous chemicals in the etching procedure. A second is the incorporation of microfabrication techniques, including photolithography and thin film deposition, to fabricate more intricate, precise, and three-dimensional shapes.

Braided or woven Nitinol stents are less commonly used and are made from a Nitinol wire, rather than a tubing [3–5]. Braiding or weaving for wire-based stents is done by interlacing wires into a mesh structure (Fig. 5.3), but the shape setting and heat treatments are similar as described above. Braided stents have a simple shape, very high torsional stiffness, and do not buckle even under high-axial compression. However, their main drawback is a low-radial force and substantial shortening during deployment (Fig. 5.4).

Fig. 5.3 Braiding technique of stent manufacturing

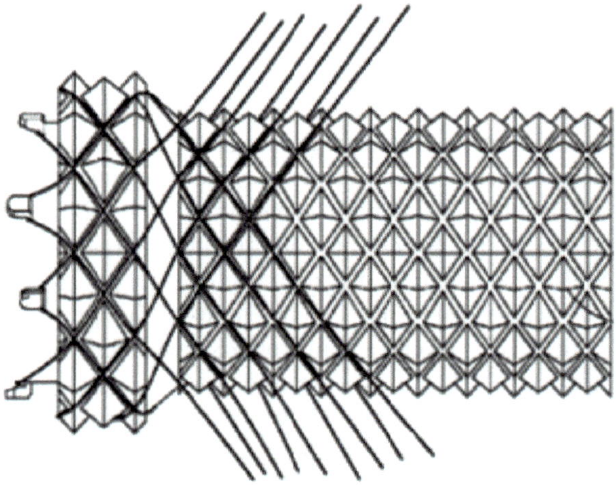

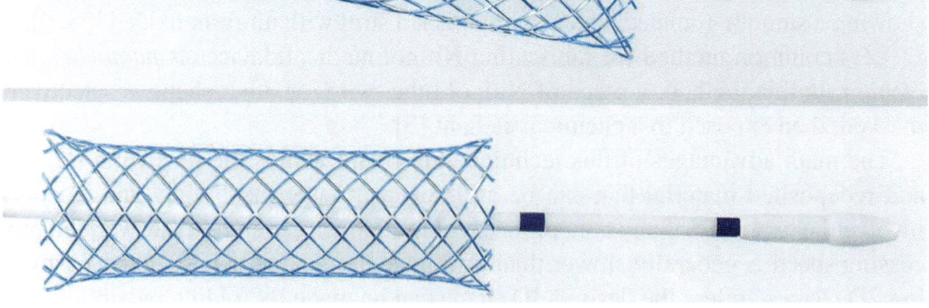

Fig. 5.4 Illustration of braided stent shortening during delivery [10]

Additive manufacturing (AM) of stents is an area of growing research that has the potential to lead to substantial improvements in patient outcomes due to its ability to rapidly develop custom stents [6]. Laser beam technology has developed to the point that today laser beams are very small (typically 20–80 μm); therefore, they can provide not only the means for developing stents through subtractive manufacturing, but also AM through laser powder bed fusion [6]. Nowadays, only laser-based powder bed fusion (LB-PBF), sometimes also called selective laser melting, is a viable manufacturing technique for NiTi stents.

The most important advantage of applying AM to stent manufacture is the ability to produce fully customizable stents and, in general, medical devices based on patient-specific 3D models. These stents would have a variable geometry that is consistent with the anatomy of the patient. Another advantage of AM of stents is that the production is not dependent or limited by the availability of suitable commercially available tubes for laser cutting. Furthermore, one last advantage not to be overlooked in utilizing the LB-PBF techniques is waste minimization during production, compared to laser cutting.

However, there are also some significant limitations in the manufacture of AM stents. A main issue regards the low-surface quality of the as-built surfaces, especially since the required strut thicknesses of NiTi stents are very small, in the order of 100–500 μm, which is comparable to the size of the powder particles (10–60 μm) and the laser beam. This requires careful control of the energy release but also the scan vector accuracy [6]. In addition, shape memory and superelasticity properties are highly dependent on the powder composition and process settings. Any slight changes in the nickel content due to the laser melting during the process in the composition can change the transformation temperatures and, subsequently, the superelastic behavior of the AM stents.

Manufacturing process of the stents is not simple. Their strut thickness is in the order of magnitude of hundreds of microns; therefore, they need careful and precise tolerances. Moreover, being medical devices, they need to be compliant with strict guidelines and rules, for example, in Europe they need to have the CE (Conformite Europeenne) mark and in the Unites States the FDA (Food and Drug Administration) approval is required. The production of Nitinol stents is a highly controlled process requiring precision engineering, material science, and medical expertise. The combination of laser machining, heat treatment, electropolishing, and rigorous testing ensures a reliable and biocompatible medical device ready for life-saving applications.

Fabrication of intravascular Nitinol stents is a highly demanding process. It is typically done using laser machining, using fast pulses to reduce the heat load on the part, or less commonly by selective chemical etching, braiding or additive manufacturing. Recent trends in this area include the use of more advanced laser pulsing technology, laser processing to control material properties while cutting, and the incorporation of microfabrication techniques.

Medical stents are a great example of how technology and the medical industry have cooperated to fulfill a need that so many people have benefited from using these life-saving devices.

Stent Design: Open and Closed Cells

The structural design of the stents plays a crucial role in their performance, flexibility, and effectiveness. Stents can be broadly categorized based on their cell structure into open-cell and closed-cell designs. Closed-cell designs are characterized by interconnected stent strut with smaller free area, while the open-cell designs have larger free cell area with fewer interconnections (Fig. 5.5). These two designs offer different mechanical and biological properties, making them suitable for specific clinical applications [12, 13, 17].

Open-Cell Stent Design

Definition

Open-cell stents have an interconnected structure with larger gaps between the struts. The design allows for more flexibility and vessel conformability, making them ideal for tortuous or curved vascular structures [15, 17].

Characteristics

1. Larger Openings between Struts—The strut connections do not fully enclose each segment, resulting in larger open spaces [11, 20].
2. Higher Flexibility—Due to the larger gaps, these stents can bend more easily, adapting better to curved arteries [15].
3. Better Vessel Wall Conformability—The design allows the stent to adjust more effectively to the shape of the vessel [11, 13].
4. Less Radial Strength—The open design reduces the overall structural strength, making the stent less resistant to external forces [17].
5. Higher Metal Fatigue Resistance—The flexibility helps in reducing stress concentrations that could lead to fractures [18].
6. Better Side-Branch Access—The larger open areas allow easier access to side branches, which is especially useful in bifurcated lesions [1].
7. Increased Risk of Plaque Prolapse—Due to the larger openings, arterial plaque may protrude through the gaps, potentially leading to restenosis [13, 14, 20].

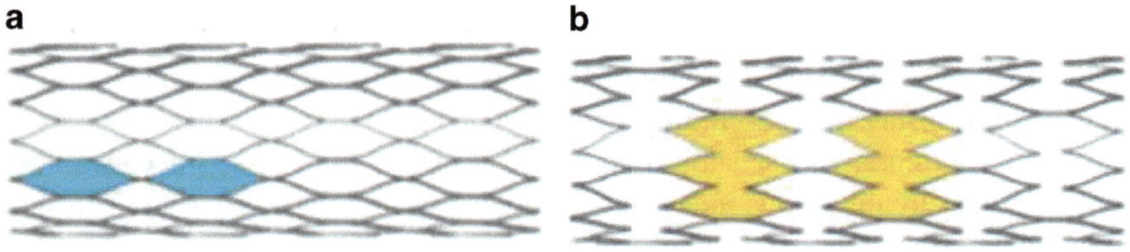

Fig. 5.5 Schematic drawing of the closed-cell (**a**) and open-cell (**b**) design of the stents

Clinical Applications

- Used in tortuous or curved vessels.
- Preferred when access to side branches is critical.
- Suitable for vessels requiring high flexibility.

Closed-Cell Stent Design

Definition

Closed-cell stents have a more continuous, uniform structure with smaller gaps between the struts. This design provides better radial strength and coverage, making them suitable for high-pressure areas and reducing the risk of plaque prolapse [12, 14].

Characteristics

1. Smaller Openings between Struts—The strut connections are more tightly linked, resulting in smaller gaps [12].
2. Higher-Radial Strength—Due to the tighter structure, these stents provide greater resistance against vessel recoil and external forces [17].
3. Less Flexibility—The design sacrifices flexibility, making it less adaptable to highly curved vessels [15, 17].
4. Better Plaque Coverage—The smaller gaps reduce the likelihood of plaque protruding through the stent struts, lowering the risk of restenosis [13, 14].
5. More Rigid Structure—The design makes it less adaptable to dynamic vessel motion [12].
6. Limited Side-Branch Access—The tighter structure can hinder access to side branches, potentially complicating interventions in bifurcated lesions [11].

Clinical Applications

- Used in straight or less curved vascular segments.
- Preferred for areas requiring high-radial force.
- Suitable for lesions with a high risk of plaque prolapse.

Comparison of Open-Cell and Closed-Cell Stents

Feature	Open-cell design	Closed-cell design
Strut arrangement	Larger open spaces between struts	More closely connected struts
Flexibility	High (adapts to curved vessels)	Low (more rigid structure)
Radial strength	Lower	Higher
Side-branch access	Easy	Limited
Plaque prolapse risk	Higher	Lower
Conformability	Better for tortuous vessels	Less adaptable to vessel curvature
Clinical use	Curved, or bifurcated arteries	Carotid, iliac, and straight vessels

Both open-cell and closed-cell stents have advantages and disadvantages, and the choice between them depends on the patient's specific needs [19]. Open-cell stents offer greater flexibility and better access to side branches but may have lower-radial strength and a higher risk of plaque prolapse. On the other hand, closed-cell stents provide better radial strength and plaque coverage, but are less flexible and may obstruct side-branch access [17, 20]. When a stent with open-cell design is bend or placed into a curved segment of a vessel, the cells on the lesser curvature change geometrical configuration with decrease in the overall area of the cell, while the area of the cells on a greater curvature increases, allowing for more flexibility of the stent and better conformability to the vessel's shape (Fig. 5.6a). When a stent with closed-cell design is bend, the cells on the lesser and greater curvature change their configuration, but the overall area of each cell remains the same, making the stent more rigid (Fig. 5.6b) [15]. The selection of the stent type should be based on vessel anatomy, lesion characteristics, and the intended clinical outcome.

Practically most current Nitinol self-expanding laser-cut stents have open-cell design. Understanding and taking into consideration that there are beneficial features of both designs for certain applications, in 2002 we (Dmitry Rabkin) together with Dr. Eyal Morag and Mr. Ophir Perelson have developed a new modular multi-segment stent, combining and alternating closed and open cells along the length of the same device (Fig. 5.7) [11, 18].

We have investigated different modifications with alternating open- and closed cells in various combinations (Fig. 5.8).

Depending on the clinical needs and applications, these stents can provide optimal radial force of the closed cells in the mostly needed areas of the covered lesions with high flexibility of the open cells to adapt to the tortuous anatomy of the stented segments (Fig. 5.9) [16].

We have built and tested different embodiments of the modular multi-segment stents, depending on their anatomical applications and intended use (Fig. 5.10).

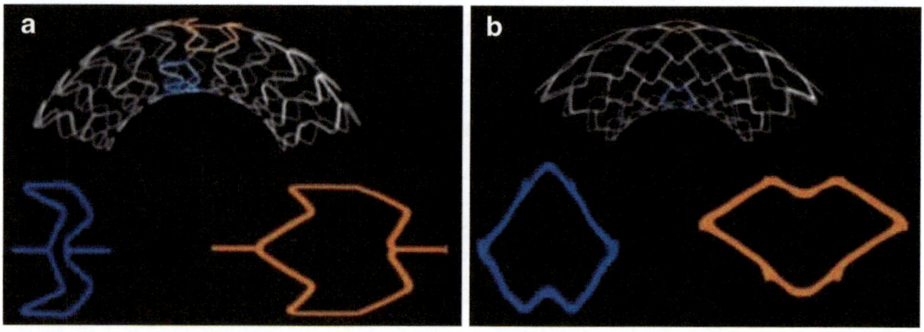

Fig. 5.6 Open (**a**) and Closed (**b**) Cells: The area and configuration of the open cell change, depending if it is located on a lesser or greater curvature of the bended stent. The configuration of the closed cell changes, depending on its location on the lesser or greater curvature, but the area of the cell remains the same

(12) INTERNATIONAL APPLICATION PUBLISHED UNDER THE PATENT COOPERATION TREATY (PCT)

CORRECTED VERSION

(19) World Intellectual Property Organization
International Bureau

(43) International Publication Date
12 June 2003 (12.06.2003)

PCT

(10) International Publication Number
WO 03/047464 A3

(51) International Patent Classification[7]: A61F 2/06

(21) International Application Number: PCT/US02/38456

(22) International Filing Date: 3 December 2002 (03.12.2002)

(25) Filing Language: English

(26) Publication Language: English

(30) Priority Data:
60/337,060 3 December 2001 (03.12.2001) US

(71) Applicant (*for all designated States except US*): **INTEK TECHNOLOGY L.L.C.** [US/US]; 2711 Centerville Road #400, Wilmington, DE 19808 (US).

(72) Inventors; and
(75) Inventors/Applicants (*for US only*): **RABKIN, Dimitry, J.** [US/US]; 79 Wallis Road, Chestnut Hill, MA 02467 (US). **MORAG, Eyal** [US/US]; 19 Park Street, East Hampton, MA 01027 (US). **PERELSON, Ophir** [US/US]; 8730 Wilshire Blvd., Suite 520, Beverly Hills, CA 90211 (US).

(74) Agent: **RASKIN, Martin, G.**; STEINBERG & RASKIN, P.C., 1140 Avenue of the Americas, 15th Floor, New York, NY 10036-5803 (US).

(81) Designated States (*national*): AE, AG, AL, AM, AT, AU, AZ, BA, BB, BG, BR, BY, BZ, CA, CH, CN, CO, CR, CU, CZ, DE, DK, DM, DZ, EC, EE, ES, FI, GB, GD, GE, GH, GM, HR, HU, ID, IL, IN, IS, JP, KE, KG, KP, KR, KZ, LC, LK, LR, LS, LT, LU, LV, MA, MD, MG, MK, MN, MW, MX, MZ, NO, NZ, OM, PH, PL, PT, RO, RU, SD, SE, SG, SK, SL, TJ, TM, TN, TR, TT, TZ, UA, UG, US, UZ, VN, YU, ZA, ZM, ZW.

(84) Designated States (*regional*): ARIPO patent (GH, GM, KE, LS, MW, MZ, SD, SL, SZ, TZ, UG, ZM, ZW),

[Continued on next page]

WO 03/047464 A3

(54) Title: MULTI-SEGMENT MODULAR STENT AND METHODS FOR MANUFACTURING STENTS

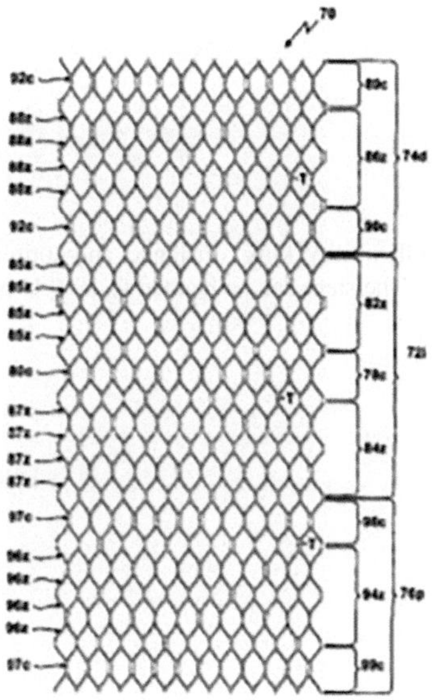

(57) **Abstract:** A modular stent (70) having at least one stent module including an intermediate segment consisting of one of either a closed-cell segment (78c) or a Z-segment (82z) and a pair of end segments connected to respective longitudinal ends of said intermediate segment, each end segment consisting of the other of said closed-cell segment (78c) or Z-segment (82z), each said closed cell segment (78c) consisting solely of at least one annular closed cell ring (80c) and each Z-segment consisting solely of at least one annular ring. A method of manufacturing a stent from a small diameter tube to includes laser-cutting the small diameter tube to define a plurality of longitudinally adjacent Z-rings, expanding the small diameter tube, and removing predetermined interconnector portions from the expanded tube to provide the predetermined desired arrangement of interconnected closed-cell rings and Z-rings.

Fig. 5.7 European patent for multi-segment modular stent

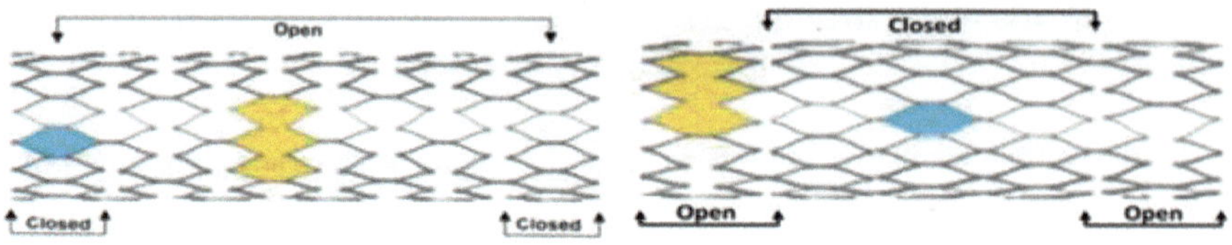

Fig. 5.8 Modular stent designs with combinations of open- and closed cells

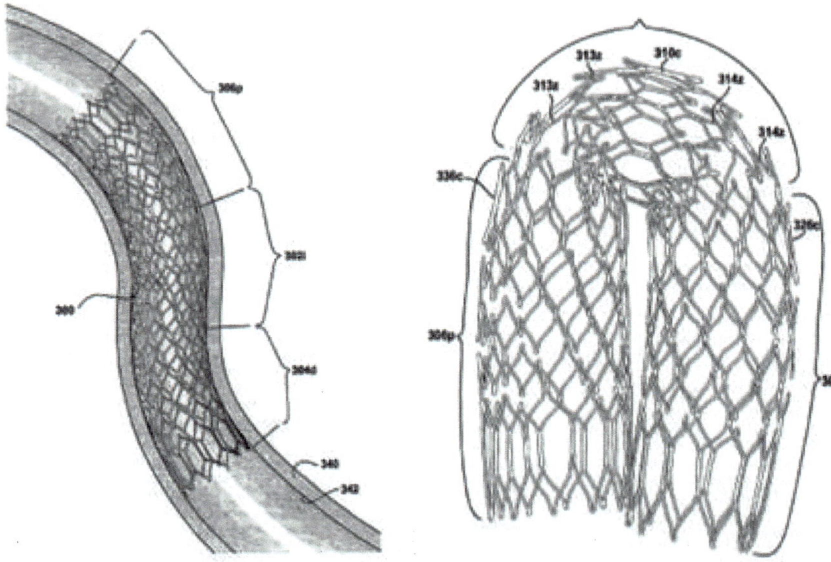

Fig. 5.9 Multi-segment stents provide exceptional flexibility, kink resistance, and optimal radial force in the strategic areas (EP WO 03/047464 A3). The stent can be bended to 180° U-turn configuration without any kinking

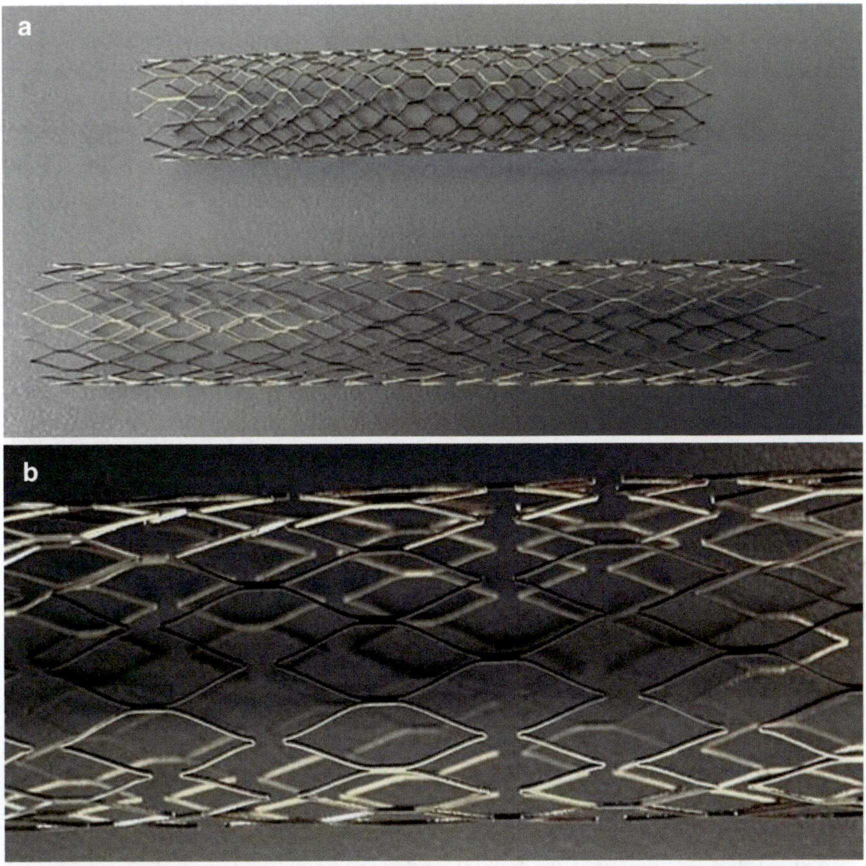

Fig. 5.10 Actual representative stents of our design with incorporated rows of closed cells along the length of the devices

Family of Modern Nitinol Stents

Arterial Nitinol Self-Expanding Stents

Bare-metal Nitinol self-expanding stents occupy a central and historically important position in endovascular treatment of arterial disease. They represent the earliest successful marriage of shape memory metallurgy with catheter-based vascular reconstruction, and—despite the rapid rise of drug-eluting and covered alternatives—bare-metal Nitinol stents remain widely used because of their mechanical reliability, flexibility, fatigue resistance, and predictable long-term behavior.

The dominance of Nitinol as a stent material emerged from its unique combination of superelasticity, shape memory, and high-fatigue endurance. Nitinol can be crimped into a small sheath and yet regain a prescribed expanded geometry owing to a stress-induced transformation between martensite and austenite phases. This characteristic permits self-expansion at body temperature with relatively constant radial force over a range of diameters. In arteries that bend, twist, elongate, or compress—such as the femoropopliteal segment, popliteal artery, external iliac artery, and carotid artery—these properties make Nitinol far superior to rigid stainless steel or cobalt-chrome alloys [22]. As a result, bare-metal Nitinol stents became the default devices for many peripheral vascular territories [21].

The design landscape of bare-metal Nitinol self-expanding stents can be thought of in several families. The most traditional devices are laser-cut Nitinol tubes with a repeating pattern of rings and connectors. Over the last 20 years, these designs have evolved substantially. Early generations had relatively thick struts and stiff connectors, and stent fracture was a major challenge, particularly in the high-motion environment of the femoropopliteal artery. Contemporary laser-cut Nitinol stents, however, use optimized geometries with thinner struts, more flexible bridges, and tailored heat treatment. These advancements greatly improved fatigue resistance, flexibility, and conformability, while preserving adequate radial support [21].

A second major family consists of interwoven or braided Nitinol stents. These devices are constructed from multiple Nitinol wires braided into a tubular scaffold rather than being laser cut from a single tube. The result is a structure with exceptional flexibility and ability to deform, compress, and recover without fracture. Because the wires can slide minutely relative to one another, strain is distributed along the construct rather than concentrated at specific hinge points. These stents are particularly attractive for the distal superficial femoral artery and popliteal artery—regions exposed to extreme bending, torsion, and muscular compression [23]. Their mechanical resilience has contributed to a significant shift in practice, with many operators preferring interwoven bare-metal stents whenever the treatment zone includes the knee joint [24].

A third design concept is the helical or three-dimensional centerline bare-metal Nitinol stent. These stents deliberately impose a gentle helical geometry on the arterial lumen after implantation. The purpose is to restore physiologic swirling flow patterns and increase uniform wall shear stress, conditions believed to suppress neointimal hyperplasia. Although still bare metal, they represent a biologically inspired strategy aimed at modifying blood flow rather than relying on drugs or graft coverings. Registry data suggest promising long-term performance in the femoropopliteal segment, especially in complex or long lesions [25].

In the carotid circulation, bare-metal Nitinol stents are also standard. The vast majority of carotid stents are self-expanding Nitinol devices, many with either open-cell or closed-cell patterns. A more recent evolution introduces dual-layer or micromesh Nitinol constructs. These remain completely bare metal but incorporate an ultra-thin inner mesh designed to reduce plaque prolapse and microembolization. Because carotid stenting demands embolic protection and meticulous technique, the highly flexible and self-expanding behavior of Nitinol is especially advantageous [26]. Unlike in the femoropopliteal territory, drug-eluting or covered stents have not displaced bare-metal Nitinol in carotid procedures; instead, refinements have remained entirely within the bare-metal domain [27].

The role of bare-metal Nitinol stents varies by arterial territory. In the femoropopliteal artery, they were once the universal solution to restenosis that followed balloon angioplasty. Modern practice, however, recognizes the limits of bare-metal scaffolding in very long, heavily calcified, or high-risk lesions. In these situations, drug-coated balloons, paclitaxel-eluting Nitinol stents, and covered stent-grafts have demonstrated superior patency. Nevertheless, bare-metal Nitinol stents remain widely used for de novo lesions of moderate length, particularly when cost, simplicity, or avoidance of paclitaxel is desirable. Interwoven stents and helical stents broaden the bare-metal family and serve important roles in the popliteal artery and tortuous segments where fatigue resistance is critical. For short dissections after balloon angioplasty, bare-metal Nitinol stents are also used as "spot scaffolds" in combination with drug-coated balloons, an increasingly popular hybrid strategy.

In the iliac arteries, the position of bare-metal Nitinol stents is even stronger. In the external iliac artery—a long, mobile, and often tortuous vessel—self-expanding Nitinol stents routinely demonstrate excellent long-term patency. They tolerate hip flexion and external compression far better than balloon-expandable stainless steel devices. In the common iliac artery, both balloon-expandable and Nitinol stents are used, with the choice depending on the need for precise ostial placement. Yet, for many iliac lesions, bare-metal Nitinol remains a primary and durable option. Covered stents are used for complex occlusions or aneurysmal disease, but most routine iliac revascularization still relies on bare-metal Nitinol devices.

Beyond the major territories, Nitinol bare-metal stents are used in renal, mesenteric, subclavian, and vertebral arteries when the vessel segment is mobile, tortuous, or subject to compression. Balloon-expandable stents remain favored for ostial, rigid, or heavily calcified lesions where high-deployment precision is essential, but Nitinol stents are preferred whenever flexibility and fatigue resistance are priorities. Their use in intracranial and coronary arteries is limited because those environments demand extremely thin struts, precise balloon-expandable deployment, and different mechanical characteristics.

In evaluating the performance of bare-metal Nitinol stents, restenosis, patency, and stent fracture are key considerations. Bare-metal Nitinol stents perform very well in territories with low-mechanical stress such as the iliac arteries [21]. In the femoropopliteal segment, their patency is acceptable in shorter lesions but declines as lesion length increases [28, 29]. Neointimal hyperplasia remains the primary cause of restenosis, and while improved geometry, helical flow, and optimized radial force have made progress, no bare-metal design fully prevents proliferative responses in long, calcified, or high-risk segments. Stent fracture, once a major limitation, is now far less common due to improved engineering, though it has not been eliminated entirely. Interwoven designs have greatly mitigated this problem in the popliteal artery. Overall, stent fracture correlates strongly with restenosis and occasionally with pseudoaneurysm formation, so minimizing construct length and avoiding excessive overlap remain important principles.

From a safety perspective, thrombosis of bare-metal Nitinol stents is relatively infrequent when proper antiplatelet therapy is used. Distal embolization can occur during deployment or post-dilation in friable plaque, especially in the femoropopliteal artery, and is routinely mitigated with embolic protection in carotid interventions. Nickel hypersensitivity is a theoretical concern but clinically significant reactions to intravascular Nitinol stents are rare; most patients tolerate Nitinol implants without issue.

Considering all territories together, the current status of bare-metal Nitinol stents can be summarized as follows. They remain foundational devices in peripheral arterial intervention because of their mechanical reliability, flexibility, and long track record. In the femoropopliteal artery, they are still widely used but increasingly complemented by drug-eluting stents, drug-coated balloons, and covered stent-grafts for long or complex lesions. In the popliteal artery, interwoven bare-metal designs have effectively solved earlier fracture problems and are now preferred by many operators. In the iliac circulation, bare-metal Nitinol stents continue to represent one of the most stable and durable solutions. In the carotid artery, nearly the entire field of stenting is built on Nitinol bare-metal platforms, with micromesh and dual-layer refinements rather than drug or graft adjuncts. In renal, mesenteric, and subclavian arteries, Nitinol stents remain important whenever conformability and fatigue resistance are needed.

Future development of bare-metal Nitinol stents focuses on further refining geometry and strut thickness, improving fatigue performance in long-term physiologic simulations, and developing surface modifications that improve endothelialization without adding drug coatings. Research also continues in computational planning, using imaging-based modeling to select the optimal stent type, length, and landing zones for individual patients. Although bare-metal Nitinol stents now coexist with a wider array of drug-eluting and covered technologies, they remain integral to endovascular practice and continue to evolve through improved design and biomechanical understanding.

Currently, there are multiple self-expanding Nitinol stents from different manufacturers available for use in the arterial applications. The list of the commercially available Nitinol self-expanding stents and their comparison chart were published by the Endovascular Today Device Guide and summarized in this chart.

US Device Guide: Nitinol Self-Expanding Arterial Stents

Company name	Product name	Stent diameter (mm)	Stent length (mm)
Abbott	Absolute Pro Vascular Stent	6, 7, 8, 9, 10	20, 30, 40, 60, 80, 100
Abbott	Supera Peripheral Stent System	4.5, 5, 5.5, 6, 6.5, 7.0, 7.5	20, 30, 40, 60, 80, 100, 120, 150
BD Interventional	E-Luminexx Vascular Stent	7, 8, 9, 10	20, 30, 40, 60, 80, 100
BD Interventional	LifeStar Vascular Stent System	7, 8, 9, 10	20, 30, 40, 60, 80, 100
BD Interventional	LifeStent 5F Vascular Stent System	5, 6, 7	20, 30, 40, 60, 80, 100, 120, 150*, 170* (*only available in 5–7 mm diameters; only available in 5 mm diameter)

Company name	Product name	Stent diameter (mm)	Stent length (mm)
BD Interventional	LifeStent and LifeStent XL Vascular Stent System	5, 6, 7	20, 30, 40, 60, 80, 100, 120, 150, 170
BD Interventional	LifeStent Solo Vascular Stent System	7	200
Biotronik, Inc.	Astron	7, 8, 9, 10	30, 40, 60, 80
Biotronik, Inc.	Pulsar-18	4–7	20–150
Biotronik, Inc.	Pulsar-18 T3	4, 5, 6, 7	20, 30, 40, 60, 80, 100, 120, 150, 170, 200
Boston Scientific	Epic Vascular Self-Expanding Stent System	6, 7, 8, 9, 10, 12	20, 30, 40, 60, 80, 100, 120
Boston Scientific	Innova Vascular Self-Expanding Stent System	5, 6, 7, 8	20, 40, 60, 80, 100, 120, 150, 200
Cook Medical	Zilver 518 Vascular Stent	6, 7, 8, 9, 10	20, 30, 40, 60, 80
Cook Medical	Zilver 635 Vascular Stent	6, 7, 8, 9, 10	20, 30, 40, 60, 80
Cordis	Smart Control Iliac Stent System	9, 10	20, 30, 40, 60, 80
Cordis	Smart Control Vascular Stent System	6, 7, 8	20, 30, 40, 60, 80, 100
Cordis	Smart Vascular Stent System	6, 7, 8	120, 150
Medtronic	EverFlex Self-Expanding Peripheral Stent System	7, 8	20, 30, 40, 60, 80, 100, 120
Medtronic	EverFlex Self-Expanding Peripheral Stent System	6, 7, 8	20, 30, 40, 60, 80, 100, 120, 150, 200
Medtronic	EverFlex Self-Expanding Peripheral Stent with Entrust Delivery System	6, 7, 8	20, 30, 40, 60, 80, 100, 120
Medtronic	Protégé EverFlex Self-Expanding Stent System	5	20, 30, 40, 60, 80, 100, 120
Medtronic	Protégé GPS Self-Expanding Stent System	9, 10, 12	20, 30, 40, 60, 80
Medtronic	Protégé GPS Self-Expanding Stent System	9, 10, 12, 14	20, 30, 40, 60, 80
Terumo Interventional Systems	R2P Misago RX Self-Expanding Peripheral Stent	6, 7, 8	40, 60, 80, 100, 120, 150
Veryan Medical	BioMimics 3D Vascular Stent System	5, 6, 7	60, 80, 100, 125, 150
Vesalio	NeVa VS	4	Full length: 35 mm; working length: 30 mm (excluding the 5-mm tip)

Table 5.1 Comparison of commercial arterial Nitinol Stents: a geometric analysis [21]

Stent name/ manufacturer	Indications for use	Cell design
Zilver (Cook Medical)	Symptomatic iliac artery disease	Open cell
SMART Control (Cordis)	Iliac and femoro-popliteal disease	Open cell (micromesh multisegmental design)
Pulsar (Biotronic)	Femoral and infrapopliteal atherosclerotic disease	Open-cell (peak-to-valley design with S-connectors)
TIGRIS (Gore)	Superficial femoral and femoro-popliteal disease	Open-cell with external fluoropolymer lattice
Innova (Boston Scientific)	Superficial femoral artery lesions	Hybrid-cell (closed-cell ends, open-cell center)
Supera (Abbott)	Superficial femoral and femoro-popliteal disease	Interwoven wire technology
Absolute Pro (Abbott)	Iliac artery disease	Hybrid-cell design (closed-cell end segments)
EverFlex (Medtronic)	Superficial femoral and femoro-popliteal disease	Open cell, spiral cell connection pattern
LifeStent (BD)	Superficial femoral and femoro-popliteal disease	Open cell, helical design

The available Nitinol stents slightly differ from each other by cell geometry (Table 5.1), radial force, and flexibility (Fig. 5.11). They are offered in different ranges of diameters and lengths, but overall they are very similar in their performances and the operators make their preferences which devices are used for any specific indications and clinical scenarios.

The choice of a specific Nitinol stent depends on the clinical context, anatomical location, lesion characteristics, and mechanical demands.

Common Preferences for Nitinol Stents

1. Self-expanding behavior: Useful in areas where vessels may be compressed or bend, like the superficial femoral artery (SFA).
2. Radial force: Maintains vessel patency against external compression and recoil.
3. Flexibility and conformability: Ideal for tortuous vessels.
4. Fatigue resistance: Important in mobile or high-strain areas (e.g., femoropopliteal segment).
5. Shape memory: Enables delivery through low-profile sheaths with expansion at body temperature.

Specific Indications by Stent Type/Region

1. Superficial Femoral Artery (SFA)/Femoropopliteal Stents
   - Stents used: for example, *Zilver, Supera, Lifestent, SmartControl*
   - Indications:
     - Long, calcified, or occluded lesions

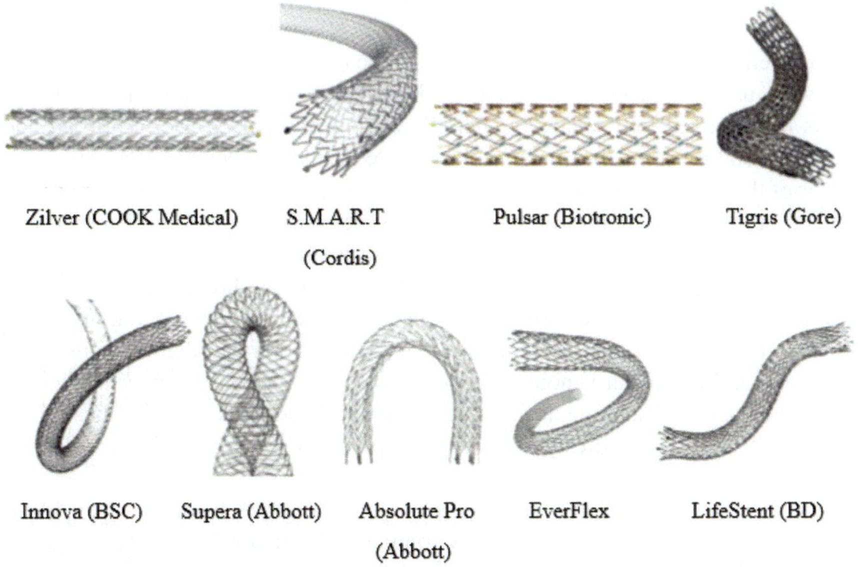

Fig. 5.11 Nitinol stents available on the market for peripheral arterial applications

  - Claudication or critical limb ischemia
  - Lesions not suitable for angioplasty alone due to elastic recoil or dissection
- Preferences:
  - High flexibility (Supera: interwoven design)
  - Resistance to fracture
  - Long lesion coverage

2. Iliac Arteries
   - Stents used: for example, *SMART Control, EPIC, Absolute Pro*
   - Indications:
     - Aortoiliac occlusive disease
     - Post-angioplasty dissection
   - Preferences:
     - High-radial strength
     - Good deployment accuracy
3. Carotid Arteries
   - Stents used: for example, *Precise Pro Rx, Protégé Rx, Rx Acculink, Xact*
   - Indications:
     - High-risk surgical patients with carotid stenosis
   - Preferences:
     - Closed-cell design for embolic protection
     - Tapered diameter for ICA-CCA transition
     - Use with embolic protection devices

Venous Nitinol Self-Expanding Stents

Until recently the arterial Nitinol stents were the only ones commercially available and were used off-label for different applications. Venous Nitinol self-expanding stents have moved in a relatively short time from improvised use of arterial and braided metallic stents to a mature class of dedicated devices that now sit at the center of therapy for symptomatic iliofemoral venous outflow obstruction. The core clinical problems are non-thrombotic iliac vein lesions such as May–Thurner syndrome, post-thrombotic chronic iliofemoral obstruction, and complex iliocaval stenosis or occlusion. These conditions are major drivers of chronic venous disease, with pain, edema, venous claudication, skin changes, and ulceration that often persist despite anticoagulation and compression. Contemporary guidelines from North American and European venous societies now regard endovascular recanalization with venoplasty and stenting as first-line treatment for patients with significant iliofemoral obstruction and lifestyle-limiting symptoms or severe post-thrombotic syndrome [30].

The rationale for dedicated venous Nitinol stents comes from the clear differences between venous and arterial environments. Iliofemoral veins are larger in diameter, often in the 12–18 mm range, and experience relatively low-shear stress but substantial external compression by the overlying right common iliac artery, spine, and pelvic structures. They must accommodate respiratory, postural, and abdominal pressure changes without losing lumen. Early venous interventions used devices such as the braided elgiloy Wallstent, which provided flexibility and fracture resistance but had pronounced foreshortening and was never engineered around venous anatomy [31]. Over the past decade, engineers and clinicians have developed stents specifically for the venous system, focusing on high-radial force over large diameters, long single-segment lengths, controlled foreshortening, flexibility across the inguinal ligament, and designs that avoid jailing the contralateral common iliac vein at the confluence [32].

Modern venous Nitinol stents are almost uniformly self-expanding and laser cut from Nitinol tubes, but their architecture varies widely. Some devices favor a closed-cell or near-closed-cell design with linked ring segments to maximize wall coverage and radial strength, while others adopt more open geometries or hybrid “flash-link” connectors to balance support with flexibility [33]. All aim to provide robust scaffolding against compressive forces, maintain diameter over the long term, and yet conform to the curvature of the iliac veins and the angulation at the iliocaval confluence. The typical size range extends to 18–24 mm in diameter and 80–160 mm in length, allowing treatment of long iliac segments with a single stent in many cases. Most systems are entirely bare metal; there are no clinically established drug-eluting venous stents, so pharmacologic modulation of neointimal hyperplasia has not yet paralleled the arterial field.

The dedicated Nitinol venous stent landscape is dominated by a handful of first-generation devices that have now accrued 3–5 years of prospective trial data. Zilver Vena (Cook Medical), Venovo (BD/Bard), Abre (Medtronic), and Vici (originally Veniti, now Boston Scientific) are the best studied. A systematic review of dedicated venous stents for iliocaval and femoral deep venous disease, along with later meta-analyses, shows that across devices, 12-month primary patency is typically in the 80–90% range, with high rates of symptom improvement and ulcer healing [34]. Prospective single-arm trials such as VIRTUS for Vici, VERNACULAR for Venovo, ABRE for the Abre stent, and VIVO for Zilver Vena consistently meet primary performance endpoints and demonstrate sustained patency and quality-of-life gains into the mid-term [35].

Abre is a self-expanding Nitinol stent with an open-cell architecture and large diameters tailored to iliofemoral anatomy. In the pivotal ABRE study, which enrolled 200 patients with symptomatic iliofemoral obstruction, 12-month primary patency was high and major adverse events within 30 days were rare; extended follow-up out to 3 years confirms durable patency, sustained reductions in Venous Clinical Severity Scores, and an absence of device-related fractures on serial radiographs [36].

The Zilver Vena stent, studied in the VIVO trial, has similarly strong data, with 12-month results showing high patency and clinically meaningful relief of pain, edema, and ulceration, and 3-year results confirming durability across post-thrombotic and non-thrombotic subgroups without an emerging fracture or migration signal [37].

The Venovo stent has now reported 3-year outcomes in patients with iliac and common femoral venous obstruction; the device was successfully deployed in the vast majority of lesions, primary patency remained favorable through mid-term follow-up, and venous clinical scores and quality of life improved significantly from baseline [38].

Vici, which has a more rigid, high-radial force closed-cell design intended for severe compression, also shows good long-term patency and clinical benefit, although mid-term imaging in the VIRTUS trial revealed some stent fractures, highlighting the trade-off between rigidity and fatigue in high-motion zones [35].

European devices from Optimed and others broaden the design spectrum. The Sinus-Venous stent uses independent ring segments linked by flexible connectors, aiming for high-radial strength with controlled foreshortening, and early and intermediate studies show excellent technical success, significant symptom relief, and relatively low loss of patency compared with historical arterial experience [39]. Sinus-XL Flex and Sinus-Obliquus extend this concept to larger diameters and oblique or tapered anatomies; the Sinus-Obliquus in particular has been used as a hybrid oblique stent at the iliocaval confluence, with good patency and safety in post-thrombotic and compression-related disease [40].

Newer platforms reflect additional refinements: the Duo Venous Stent System, for example, combines two stent components to optimize coverage of the iliac vein and common femoral vein and has shown promising 12-month safety and efficacy in the VIVID trial; the V-Mixtent and VENA-BT tapered iliac venous stent represent efforts to better match the conical geometry of the iliac vein and the iliocaval junction, supported so far by early clinical data and preclinical ovine models [41].

The core clinical indications for venous Nitinol stenting are now well defined. Patients with chronic iliofemoral obstruction due to May–Thurner anatomy or post-thrombotic scarring and who have disabling symptoms despite optimal conservative therapy are the largest group. Systematic reviews and contemporary practice guidelines emphasize that iliofemoral stenting in such patients reliably improves pain, swelling, walking capacity, and ulcer healing, with a substantial proportion of patients moving to lower-CEAP classes and reporting better quality of life [34]. Venous stents are also increasingly used after early thrombus removal procedures for acute iliofemoral deep venous thrombosis, where they serve to scaffold the compressed or damaged segment and prevent recurrent obstruction; both the Society for Vascular Surgery and American Venous Forum guidelines on acute DVT support early thrombus removal and correction of underlying iliac obstruction in selected patients [30]. In addition, iliocaval and inferior vena cava stenting with Nitinol devices is gaining traction for both benign and malignant extrinsic compression, with systematic reviews suggesting acceptable safety, good technical success, and clinically meaningful relief of lower-limb congestion [42].

Despite these successes, venous Nitinol stenting is not without complications or unanswered questions. In-stent restenosis and loss of patency, often driven by neointimal hyperplasia on a background of sluggish venous flow and continuing thrombophilic risk, remain important challenges. A recent meta-analysis of medium- to long-term outcomes with dedicated venous stents across 11 devices reported 12-month primary patency of around 83%, with secondary patency higher after reintervention, but with significant heterogeneity between post-thrombotic and non-thrombotic indications and between studies [43]. Long-term data demonstrate that patients with extensive post-thrombotic scarring, poor outflow, or ongoing thrombophilia have higher rates of restenosis and stent thrombosis, even when modern devices are used and anticoagulation is carefully managed [44]. Migration and malposition are relatively infrequent, but systematic reviews show that they do occur, particularly when undersized stents are deployed in large, dynamic venous segments or when technical errors lead to poor anchoring at the confluence or common femoral vein [45].

The safety profile of Nitinol itself in the venous system has been reassuring. Major bleeding is driven far more by the antithrombotic regimen than by the device; there are no venous analogues of paclitaxel-associated mortality debates seen in the arterial sphere because venous stents are bare metal. Stent fractures, a dominant theme in early arterial Nitinol experience, appear uncommon among modern venous devices, with pivotal trials such as ABRE, VIVO, and VERNACULAR reporting no fractures at 3 years, while VIRTUS reported a modest number of fractures mainly in heavily stressed segments without a clear adverse effect on overall safety signals [31]. Nickel hypersensitivity reactions to venous Nitinol stents are rarely reported and do not presently drive device selection in routine practice.

From an engineering standpoint, current development is focused on capturing the complex three-dimensional behavior of the iliofemoral venous system and tailoring stent geometry accordingly. Bench testing and finite-element modeling are used to optimize strut patterns and connectors for high-radial force with low-local strain, minimizing fatigue while accommodating repeated compression between the spine and artery and flexion at the hip [32]. Device designers are also refining radiopacity, delivery system trackability, and deployment precision to allow accurate landing at the iliocaval confluence and common femoral vein while maintaining the ability to re-line or extend constructs in staged procedures. Longer term, there is interest in whether surface modifications or bioactive coatings—still without drug elution—could further improve endothelialization and lower thrombosis risk, and in integrating advanced imaging such as intravascular ultrasound with machine-learning-assisted CT analysis to better define true stenosis and plan stent sizing and landing zones [21].

Clinically, the "current status" of venous Nitinol self-expanding stents can be summarized as one of consolidation and refinement rather than basic proof-of-concept. The foundational questions of whether stenting works for symptomatic iliofemoral obstruction and whether dedicated venous Nitinol stents outperform repurposed arterial devices have effectively been answered in the affirmative by multiple prospective trials, systematic reviews, and guideline statements [34]. The field is now focused on finer points: choosing among several well-performing Nitinol platforms for specific anatomies and etiologies, understanding which patients derive the largest long-term benefit, optimizing antithrombotic regimens, and managing restenosis and thrombosis when they occur. At the same time, new devices and geometries continue to appear, and medium-term data are accumulating for tapered, oblique, and modular Nitinol venous stents that attempt to better match individual venous anatomy. In this evolving landscape, self-expanding Nitinol remains the material of choice for deep venous stenting and is likely to retain that role even as techniques and device designs continue to be refined.

The average size of the venous blood vessels is larger than those of the corresponding arterial system. Accordingly, venous stents have larger diameters, compared to arterial stents. In general, the strut thickness of the venous stents is larger, providing stronger radial force, which is needed particularly in the cases of extrinsic compression of the veins. This comes at some expense of flexibility of the venous stents, but vein wall is more elastic and pliable, reducing the need for flexibility of the stents for venous applications.

The main differences between Nitinol arterial and venous stents come down to the design requirements for the different environments they're used in (Table 5.2).

The list of the commercially available dedicated venous Nitinol self-expanding stents and their comparison chart were published by the Endovascular Today Device Guide and summarized in this chart.

Table 5.2 Comparison of arterial and venous stents

Design feature	Arterial stents	Venous stents
Use	To treat arterial blockages (e.g., PAD)	To treat venous obstructions (e.g., iliofemoral DVT, May–Thurner)
Blood flow	High pressure, pulsatile	Lower pressure, steady flow
Vessel Wall	Thicker, muscular arteries	Thinner-walled, more flexible veins
Radial force	Moderate-to-high, but balanced	High-radial force to keep larger veins open
Flexibility	Prioritized for tortuous arteries	Also flexible, but often more robust
Strut thickness	Less than 200 microns	Over 300 microns
Diameter	Smaller (typically 4–8 mm)	Larger (10–20 mm)
Length	Various (usually shorter than venous)	Often longer (to cover long obstructions)
Crush resistance	Important	Very important (especially for extrinsic compression)
Cell structure	Open cell or hybrid	Usually, open cell for added flexibility to balance rigidity of thicker struts

US and EURO Device Guide: Nitinol Venous Stents

Company name	Product name	Cell design	Stent diameter (mm)	Stent length (mm)
BD Interventional	Venovo Venous Stent System	Open-cell	10, 12, 14, 16, 18, 20	40, 60, 80, 100, 120, 140, 160
Bentley InnoMed GmbH	BeYond	Open-cell design; closed-cell stent ends	10–18	60–150
Boston Scientific Corporation	Vici	Closed cell	12, 14, 16	60, 90, 120
Cook Medical	Zilver Vena	Open cell	14, 16	60, 100, 140
Medtronic	Abre Venous Self-Expanding Stent System	Open cell	10, 12, 14, 16, 18, 20	40, 60, 80, 100, 120, 150
Optimed Medizinische Instrumente GmbH	Sinus-Obliquus	Hybrid	14, 16, 18	80, 100, 150
Optimed Medizinische Instrumente GmbH	Sinus-Venous	Hybrid	10, 12, 14, 16, 18	60, 80, 100, 120, 150
Optimed Medizinische Instrumente GmbH	Sinus-XL	Closed cell	16, 18, 20, 22, 24, 26, 28, 30, 32, 34, 36	30, 40, 60, 80, 100

Company name	Product name	Cell design	Stent diameter (mm)	Stent length (mm)
Optimed Medizinische Instrumente GmbH	Sinus-XL 6F	Closed cell	14, 16	30, 40, 60, 80, 100
Optimed Medizinische Instrumente GmbH	Sinus-XL Flex	Open cell	14, 16, 18, 20, 22, 24	40, 60, 80, 100, 120, 150, 160

Dedicated venous Nitinol stents available on the market have different cell configurations and their pattern along the length of the devices, but all share similar features of improved high-radial force to resist external compression (e.g., from crossing arteries like in May–Thurner syndrome, fibrotic tissues post-radiation therapy or from the pressure of adjacent tumors) (Fig. 5.12).

They are offered in larger diameters and longer lengths than arterial stents, matching the size and the structure of the veins (Table 5.3).

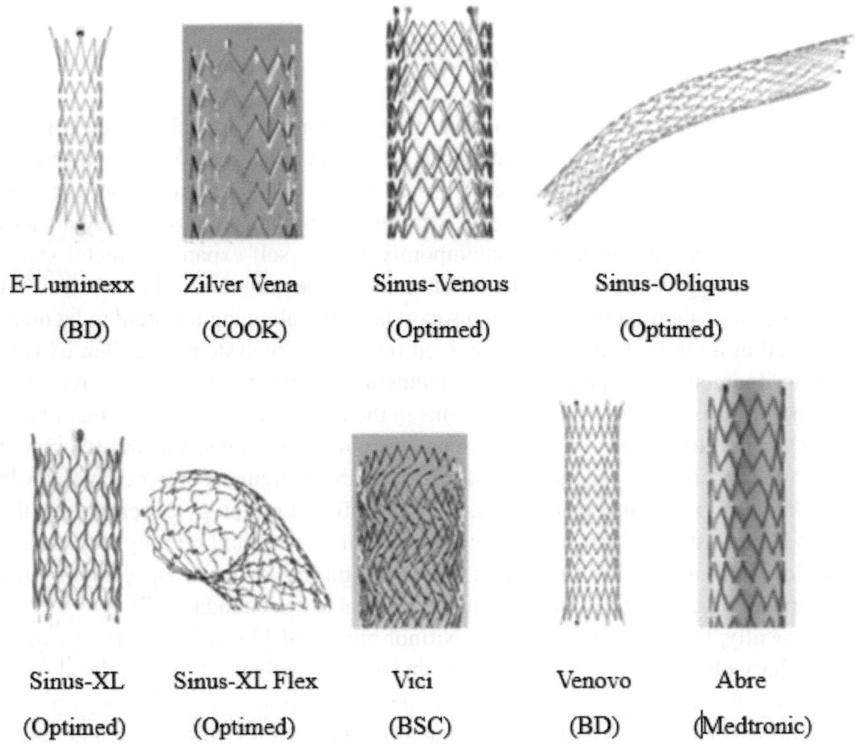

Fig. 5.12 Dedicated venous Nitinol stents available on the market

Table 5.3 Comparison of commercial venous Nitinol Stents: a geometric analysis [21]

Stent name/ manufacturer	Indications for use	Cell design
E-Luminexx (Bard)	Iliac occlusive disease	Diamond cell, open-cell design with flared ends
Zilver Vena (Cook Medical)	Obstructed iliofemoral veins	Chevron, open-cell design
Sinus Venous (Optimed)	Ileofemoral veins, post-thrombotic syndrome, DVT	Open-cell design
Sinus Obliquus (Optimed)	Iliac veins obstruction, IVC confluence obstruction	Hybrid-cell: closed-cell design at ends, open-cell middle
Sinus XL Flex (Optimed)	Obstruction of IVC, SVC, iliac and femoral veins	Open-cell design
Vici (Boston Scientific)	Ileofemoral venous obstructive disease	Close-cell design
Venovo (BD	Ileofemoral venous obstructive disease	Open-cell design with flared ends
Abre (Medtronic)	Ileofemoral venous obstructive disease	Open-cell design with 3-points connections

Biliary Nitinol Self-Expanding Stents

Nitinol self-expanding biliary stents are now the dominant metallic platforms for endoscopic and percutaneous palliation of biliary obstruction, particularly in patients with unresectable malignant disease of the distal common bile duct and hilar region. Early biliary metal stents were often stainless steel or elgiloy devices designed for vascular use, but contemporary biliary self-expanding metal stents (SEMS) are largely made of nickel–titanium alloy because Nitinol combines biocompatibility, "thermal memory," and superelasticity, allowing the stent to be manufactured at a target diameter, compressed on a delivery system, and then expand back to its intended shape under body temperature with durable radial force [46]. This behavior is particularly advantageous in the bile duct, where deployment must occur through long, tortuous endoscopic or percutaneous paths, and where gradual self-expansion reduces the risk of perforation or abrupt trauma compared with more rigid balloon-expandable designs. Early interventional radiology experience in the 1990s already showed that self-expanding Nitinol stents could reliably re-establish bile flow with acceptable patency in malignant biliary obstruction, validating the concept and opening the door to the broad clinical use seen today [47].

Clinically, the main indication for Nitinol biliary SEMS is palliation of malignant biliary obstruction, most commonly due to pancreatic head cancer, distal cholangiocarcinoma, ampullary carcinoma, or metastatic disease, although they are also used in selected benign strictures. Contemporary reviews emphasize that metal stents are preferred over plastic stents when life expectancy exceeds 3–4 months, because their larger effective lumen and longer patency translate into fewer episodes of cholangitis and reintervention [48]. A large comparative study in 2022 confirmed the superiority of SEMS over plastic stents in malignant obstruction, with metal stents achieving longer time to recurrent biliary obstruction and requiring fewer reinterventions without a significant increase in serious adverse events [49]. As a result, both endoscopic and radiologic societies now treat Nitinol SEMS as standard-of-care devices for distal malignant obstruction in patients with unresectable or borderline-resectable disease, while plastic stents are reserved for very short-term decompression, preoperative drainage, or situations where cost or anatomy preclude metal stent placement [48].

Current Nitinol biliary stents are manufactured as braided or laser-cut tubular meshes with different patterns that balance radial force, axial flexibility, foreshortening, and resistance to kinking. Their diameters typically range from 8 to 10 mm with lengths from 40 to 100 mm, which can be combined to span long strictures [48]. Design parameters such as radial force and axial force are critical: higher-radial force helps oppose tumor compression and maintain lumen, but excessive axial rigidity can increase the risk of pain, migration, or injury at the hepatic hilum or papilla. Experimental work comparing different Nitinol biliary stents has highlighted that each device family occupies a different position on this mechanical spectrum, and understanding these differences helps operators select a stent appropriate to the location and morphology of the obstruction [50].

One of the central questions in the evolution of Nitinol biliary SEMS has been whether stents should be uncovered, partially covered, or fully covered. Uncovered SEMS allow tissue ingrowth through the lattice, which helps anchor the stent and reduces migration, but this also permits tumor ingrowth and epithelial hyperplasia that eventually occlude the lumen. Covered stents add a polymer membrane—most commonly silicone, PTFE, or polyurethane—over the Nitinol scaffold to provide a smooth inner surface resistant to tumor ingrowth and bacterial biofilm formation, at the cost of higher-migration risk and potential occlusion of side branches, such as the cystic duct or pancreatic duct [51]. Early randomized trials, such as the Isayama "diamond stent" study, showed that covered stents could significantly reduce tumor ingrowth compared with uncovered designs, establishing the conceptual advantage of coverage in malignant obstruction [51]. However, when Nitinol biliary stents were specifically compared, the picture became more nuanced. A landmark randomized trial of covered versus uncovered Nitinol SEMS in malignant distal obstruction by Kullman and colleagues found no significant differences in patency time, patient survival, or overall complication rates between the two groups, although covered stents had more migration and uncovered stents more tumor ingrowth [52]. Several subsequent randomized studies and meta-analyses, including work by Almadi, Li and co-authors, and Sakai, broadly confirmed that covered and uncovered SEMS offer similar overall patency and dysfunction rates, but that their failure modes differ: uncovered stents tend to fail by tumor ingrowth, whereas covered stents more often fail by migration or sludge [53].

Partially covered Nitinol stents were developed as a compromise approach, with a central covered segment to prevent ingrowth at the stricture and bare ends to allow embedding into the duct wall for anchoring. Clinical studies comparing partially covered to uncovered Nitinol SEMS for distal malignant biliary obstruction have generally shown similar survival and overall adverse event profiles, but several series and a 2017 multicenter study reported that partially covered SEMS may achieve longer patency than both uncovered and fully covered designs, presumably because they better suppress ingrowth while reducing the tendency to migrate [54]. A 2020 retrospective analysis of percutaneous transhepatic stenting with Nitinol SEMS likewise found that partially covered stents had superior patency to uncovered or fully covered stents in distal malignant obstruction [55]. More recent trials of novel fully covered Nitinol SEMS with anti-migration features, including anchoring fins and flared ends, show that engineering strategies can mitigate migration while preserving the advantages of full coverage [56]. A 2023 study by Wu and colleagues demonstrated that modern fully covered SEMS provide a smooth inner surface that protects against both tumor ingrowth and biofilm formation, resulting in favorable patency in unresectable distal obstruction, while a 2023–2024 wave of designs continues to refine these concepts [57].

Beyond distal obstruction, Nitinol SEMS play a central role in palliation of hilar cholangiocarcinoma and other proximal biliary cancers, but the optimal strategy is more complex. In the hilum, drainage of both lobes may require placement of multiple metal stents using side-by-side or stent-in-stent techniques. Most centers favor uncovered or partially covered Nitinol SEMS for hilar disease to avoid occluding segmental bile ducts and to facilitate stent-in-stent deployment, although fully covered stents are sometimes used in more distal hilar lesions or as "inside stents" above the papilla [48]. The balance between achieving adequate drainage, avoiding cholangitis, and minimizing stent occlusion is delicate, and comparative data are less robust than for distal obstruction, but Nitinol SEMS have clearly replaced plastic stents as the mainstay of palliation for unresectable high-grade hilar strictures in patients with a reasonable life expectancy [48].

Nitinol biliary SEMS are also used in benign disease, especially chronic benign strictures after surgery, chronic pancreatitis, or liver transplantation. In this setting, the ability to remove or exchange the stent is crucial, so fully covered Nitinol SEMS are generally preferred because their membranes prevent tissue ingrowth and allow retrieval. Contemporary series and small randomized trials suggest that temporary placement of fully covered Nitinol SEMS can achieve stricture resolution rates comparable to or better than multi-plastic stent strategies, with fewer ERCP sessions, but at the cost of higher-migration risk and potential cholecystitis due to cystic duct occlusion [48]. There is still no universal consensus on optimal dwell time, stent diameter, or number of stent exchanges in benign strictures, and practice patterns vary between centers, but the trajectory is clearly toward greater use of removable covered Nitinol SEMS in selected benign conditions where the anatomical risk of migration and side-branch occlusion is acceptable [48].

Complications of Nitinol biliary SEMS largely reflect their mechanical and biological interactions with the bile duct environment. Tumor ingrowth, overgrowth at the ends, sludge formation, and bacterial biofilm can all lead to recurrent biliary obstruction, necessitating repeat endoscopic or percutaneous intervention. Covered stents eliminate tumor ingrowth but remain vulnerable to overgrowth and sludge, and several studies and reviews have described how biofilm development on irregular mucosal surfaces contributes to stent occlusion, an effect that smooth covered membranes may partially mitigate [57]. Migration is the dominant mechanical complication of covered Nitinol stents, particularly when placed across shorter strictures, in benign disease, or without adequate stent length extending beyond the narrowed segment. This problem has driven extensive research into anti-migration design features such as anchoring fins, flared ends, double-layer configurations, and partially covered designs, summarized in a 2025 review by Chun and colleagues, which concludes that no single strategy is universally superior, but that combining coverage with robust anchoring appears most effective [58]. Other adverse events include cholecystitis if the cystic duct is covered, pancreatitis when the pancreatic orifice is obstructed, and, more rarely, perforation or hemorrhage during placement or dilation [48]. Overall, however, large series and randomized trials suggest that Nitinol SEMS are safe, with serious device-related complications occurring in a minority of patients and being manageable in most cases.

From a materials science perspective, Nitinol remains the most widely used metal for biliary SEMS, but active research is exploring how to improve stent performance through coatings and alternative materials. Recent reviews on biliary stent materials and surface modification argue that nondegradable metal stents—including Nitinol, stainless steel, and cobalt–chromium—provide excellent radial strength but are intrinsically prone to long-term complications such as occlusion and bacterial colonization, inspiring interest in biodegradable stents and functional coatings [59]. Experimental and early clinical studies have investigated biodegradable polymer stents and biodegradable metal stents (e.g., magnesium alloys) for biliary applications, as well as drug-eluting or antibacterial coatings on Nitinol SEMS to suppress hyperplasia and biofilm formation [60]. While these technologies are not yet part of routine biliary practice, they represent an important direction for future development, particularly in benign disease where the presence of permanent metal may be undesirable. Even in surgical settings, such as biliary reconstruction after pancreaticoduodenectomy, biodegradable biliary stents are starting to show benefits in reducing fistulas and long-term strictures, suggesting that the long-term paradigm for benign biliary support may shift away from permanent Nitinol devices [61].

In summary, the current status of biliary Nitinol self-expanding stents is that of a mature, mainstream technology that has decisively replaced plastic stents and older metal designs for most patients requiring durable palliation of malignant biliary obstruction. Nitinol SEMS offer predictable deployment, strong radial support, and long patency in distal and hilar disease, with design variants—uncovered, partially covered, and fully covered—tailored to different anatomical and clinical priorities. Randomized trials and meta-analyses have shown that while covered and uncovered Nitinol stents have broadly similar overall patency and survival, covered stents prevent tumor ingrowth at the expense of higher-migration rates, and partially covered and anti-migration designs attempt to balance these trade-offs [52]. In benign disease, fully covered Nitinol SEMS are increasingly used as removable scaffolds that can shorten treatment courses compared with serial plastic stenting, though optimal protocols remain under active study. Parallel advances in functional coatings, anti-migration engineering and biodegradable stent technologies suggest that the next decade will see further refinement of biliary stent design, but for now, Nitinol self-expanding SEMS remain the backbone of endoscopic and percutaneous management of biliary obstruction worldwide.

Key Features of Biliary Nitinol Stents

1. Material: Nitinol
   - Nitinol provides:
     - Shape memory: The ability to return to a predetermined shape upon deployment.
     - Superelasticity: Adaptation to bile duct movement and angulation without deformation.
     - Corrosion resistance: Important due to the bile's biochemical environment.
     - Biocompatibility: Minimizes tissue reaction and inflammation.
2. Design
   - Uncovered, partially covered, or fully covered designs:
     - Uncovered: Allow tissue ingrowth (for benign strictures) but prone to restenosis.
     - Covered (with PTFE or silicone membrane): Prevent tumor ingrowth and sludge formation.
     - Partially covered: Balance between patency and anchoring.
   - Open-cell or closed-cell mesh:
     - Affects flexibility and coverage.
     - Open-cell designs conform better to tortuous ducts.
   - Anti-migration features:
     - Flares, anchoring barbs, or dog-bone ends.
     - Prevent stent displacement by bile flow or peristalsis.
   - Variable diameters and lengths:
     - Commonly 6–10 mm in diameter.
     - Lengths vary from 4 cm to 12 cm, depending on stricture size.
   - Delivery systems:
     - Compatible with endoscopic retrograde cholangiopancreatography (ERCP) or percutaneous transhepatic biliary drainage (PTBD).
     - Sheath systems designed for smooth passage through strictures.

Clinical Applications

- Malignant biliary obstruction (e.g., from pancreatic cancer, Hepatocellular carcinoma, or cholangiocarcinoma).
- Benign biliary strictures (less common for SEMS use due to tissue ingrowth issues).
- Post-surgical bile leaks or strictures.
- Palliative care for unresectable tumors.

Differences from Vascular Stents

Feature	Biliary Nitinol stents	Vascular stents
Primary use	Bile duct obstructions (malignant or benign)	Arterial or venous narrowing, aneurysms, dissections
Environment	Exposed to bile, enzymes, digestive juices	Blood (hemodynamic pressure, clotting factors)

Feature	Biliary Nitinol stents	Vascular stents
Design requirements	High resistance to corrosive bile Anti-migration features Adaptability to curved, compressible ducts	Hemodynamic compatibility High-radial force Resistance to blood pressure and thrombus
Covering	Often covered to prevent tumor ingrowth	Rarely covered; bare-metal most common
Radial force	Moderate to maintain duct patency without trauma	High to resist arterial recoil
Flexibility	High flexibility and conformability to tortuous biliary anatomy	Variable
Deployment	Via ERCP or PTBD	Typically via angiography and catheterization
Removal	Some are retrievable (esp. in benign cases)	Mostly permanent
Common complications	Migration Occlusion by sludge or tumor Cholangitis	In-stent restenosis Thrombosis Embolization

Biliary stents are tailored for a non-vascular system with low flow, exposure to enzymes and bile, and tumor compression. Vascular stents must handle high-pressure flow, thrombotic potential, and pulsatile motion.

Dedicated biliary Nitinol stents are engineered to meet the challenges of the biliary tree: flexibility, anti-corrosion, and resistance to tumor ingrowth. They are fundamentally different from vascular stents in terms of anatomy, physiology, deployment, and mechanical requirements.

Selecting the appropriate biliary stent depends on several factors, including the type of obstruction (malignant versus benign), location of the stricture, patient prognosis, and intended duration of treatment. Clinical guidelines are based on these variables, with a focus on maximizing patency, reducing complications, and improving quality of life.

Here's a comprehensive overview of current clinical guidelines for stent selection in biliary disease:

1. Malignant Biliary Obstruction (MBO)

   Goal: Palliation of obstruction, prolong stent patency, improve biliary drainage.

   Common Causes:

   - Pancreatic adenocarcinoma
   - Cholangiocarcinoma
   - Gallbladder carcinoma
   - Metastatic lymphadenopathy

Guideline-based stent selection

Expected survival	Recommended stent	Rationale
<4 months	Plastic stent (7–10 Fr)	Short-term patency is sufficient; cost-effective
≥4 months	Self-Expanding Metal Stent (SEMS)	Longer patency, fewer re-interventions

Covered versus Uncovered SEMS

- Covered SEMS:
  - Reduce tumor ingrowth
  - Slightly higher-migration risk
  - Better patency in distal obstructions (e.g., pancreatic cancer)
- Uncovered SEMS:
  - Lower migration risk
  - Allow bile duct side branch drainage
  - Preferred in hilar lesions to avoid blocking segmental ducts

Location Matters

- Distal MBO (e.g., pancreatic cancer at head):
  - Prefer covered SEMS
- Hilar MBO (e.g., Klatskin tumor):
  - Prefer uncovered SEMS
  - Bilateral stenting may be required for Bismuth type II–IV
  - Techniques: side-by-side or stent-in-stent

Guidelines Reference: ESGE (European Society of Gastrointestinal Endoscopy), ASGE (American Society for Gastrointestinal Endoscopy)

2. Benign Biliary Strictures (BBS)

Goal: Restore and maintain bile flow until stricture resolves.

Common Causes:

- Post-operative (e.g., cholecystectomy)
- Chronic pancreatitis
- Primary sclerosing cholangitis
- Liver transplant anastomotic stricture

Recommended stent types

Stricture type	Preferred stent	Duration
Post-surgical/anastomotic	Plastic stents (multiple side-by-side)	Every 3 months for 6–12 months
Resistant or complex strictures	Fully covered SEMS (removable)	6–12 months; then remove

- Plastic stents:
  - Multiple stents in parallel have better outcomes than a single stent.
  - Periodic exchange every 3 months to prevent clogging.
- Removable covered SEMS:
  - Effective for tight or recurrent strictures.
  - Avoid in strictures involving bile duct bifurcation (can block ducts).

Guidelines Reference: ESGE 2018, AASLD, EASL

3. Biliary Leaks
   Goal: Divert bile flow, allow leak to heal.
   Common Indications
   - Post-cholecystectomy leak
   - Post-liver transplant or hepatic trauma

   Recommended Stent
   - Plastic stent (7–10 Fr) with or without biliary sphincterotomy
   - Typically left in for 4–8 weeks
   - Covered SEMS generally not needed unless there's a concurrent stricture.
4. Cholangiolithiasis with Stricture
   Goal: Temporarily bypass stricture and enable stone clearance.
   Recommended Approach
   - Balloon dilatation + plastic stent
   - May need short-term SEMS if stones are recurrent or if strictures are tight

5. Summary Algorithm (Simplified)

Condition	Plastic stent	SEMS (covered)	SEMS (uncovered)
Short life expectancy MBO	✓	✖	✖
Long life expectancy MBO (distal)	✖	✓	✖
MBO (hilar/Klatskin)	✖	⚠ (not preferred)	✓
Benign strictures	✓	✓ (removable only)	✖
Biliary leak	✓	✖	✖

Other Considerations

- MRI compatibility: Nitinol stents are MRI-safe.
- Patency monitoring: Periodic imaging and liver function tests.
- Cost-effectiveness: SEMS cost more initially, but reduce need for re-interventions.

When selecting a Nitinol self-expanding biliary stent, it is essential to consider the nature of the biliary obstruction (malignant versus benign), anatomical location, patient-specific factors, and the stent's specific design features such as coverage (covered versus uncovered), radial force, flexibility, and potential for migration (Fig. 5.13).

Summary of Nitinol Biliary Self-expanding stents and their characteristics currently available on the market are presented in Table 5.4.

S.M.A.R.T. biliary stent from Cordis is constructed by laser cutting of a Nitinol tubing, ensuring a smooth, sharp edge-free surface. It is available in various diameters (6–8 mm) and lengths (120–150 mm). It is designed for palliation of malignant biliary strictures.

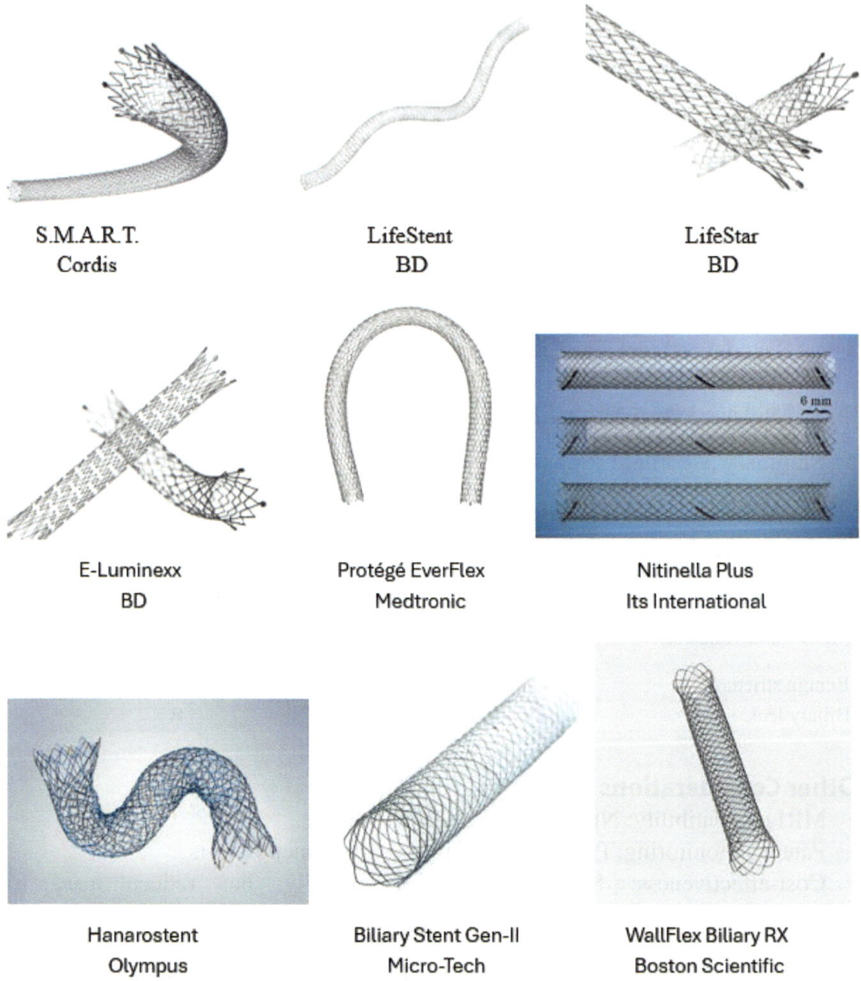

Fig. 5.13 Dedicated Biliary Nitinol Self-Expanding stents available on the market

LifeStent and LifeStent XL Biliary Stent System by BD is made from laser cutting of a Nitinol tubing, features of a unique helical design engineered to accommodate bending, compression, and torsion. Aims and approved for maintaining luminal patency in the biliary tree affected by malignant neoplasm.

LifeStar Biliary Stent System by BD is laser cut from the Nitinol tubing offers a range of stent sizes, from 6 mm to 14 mm in diameter and lengths up to 120 mm. Designed for flexibility and conformability within the biliary anatomy. Intended for the treatment of biliary strictures, providing options to match patient-specific anatomical requirements. It has an optimized pin-and-pull delivery system for simple, easy, and precise deployment.

Table 5.4 Comparison chart of the commercially available dedicated Biliary Nitinol Stents

Brand	Company	Construction	Coverage		
			Uncovered	Partially	Fully
S.M.A.R.T	Cordis	Laser cut	X		
LifeStent LifeStent XL	BD	Laser cut	X		
LifeStar	BD	Laser cut	X		
E-Luminex Biliary	BD	Laser cut			
Protégé EverFlex	Medtronic	Laser cut	X		
Nitinella Plus	Its Interventional	Woven	X	X	X
Hanarostent	Olympus	Woven	X		
Biliary-Stent Gen-II	Micro-Tach	Woven	X	X	X
WallFlex Biliary RX	BSC	Woven	X	X	X

Protégé EverFlex Self-Expanding Biliary Stent System by Medtronic is laser cut from Nitinol tubing and comes in various diameter and length options. Used for the palliative treatment of malignant biliary strictures, offering flexibility and ease of deployment.

Nitinella Plus Biliary Stent by Its Interventional is a self-expanding design constructed by woven Nitinol wire and can be implanted endoscopically or transhepatically. It has variable weave at distal and proximal ends to minimize migration. It is available in different versions, as uncovered or partially covered or fully covered with silicone. It is indicated for palliative treatment of biliary strictures caused by malignant neoplasms.

Hanarostent Biliary by Olympus is a woven Nitinol stent with large flare ends, designed to prevent migration. It is an uncovered stent designed to be used for palliative treatment of bile duct strictures caused by malignant tumors. Can be recaptured, retrieved, or repositioned when partially deployed from the delivery system.

Biliary-Stent Gen-II by Micro-Tech is a woven Nitinol stent with atraumatic ends, which is preloaded on the delivery system for endoscopic or percutaneous transhepatic deployment. It is available in fully, partially, and uncovered versions. The delivery system has a "point-of-no-return" feature in uncovered and partially covered variants that allows partial recapture and repositioning.

WallFlex Biliary RX Stent by Boston Scientific Corporation is constructed with a closed loop platinum cored Nitinol wire mesh with looped and flared ends, designed to be less traumatic than open ends and reduce the risk of epithelial damage without sacrificing radial force. It is available in fully covered, partially covered, and uncovered versions to accommodate various clinical scenarios.

E-Luminexx Biliary Stent by BD is a laser-cut Nitinol stent with high-radial strength and flexibility, facilitating effective deployment and conformability within the biliary ducts.

Majority of the woven Nitinol Biliary stents are available as uncovered, partially, or fully covered, which gives more diversification for their use in specific clinical scenarios. The downside of the woven stent design is that they shorten substantially during release, which make their deployment a little more tricky and potentially less accurate.

On the other hand, all laser-cut Nitinol Biliary stents come as bare-metal uncovered devices, which have less tendency to migrate. Their long-term patency is not as good as with covered stents, but they provide adequate drainage in the properly selected patients and clinical settings.

Gastrointestinal Nitinol Self-Expanding Stents

Self-expanding metal stents (SEMS), particularly those made of Nitinol, have revolutionized the palliative management of malignant and benign strictures in the gastrointestinal (GI) tract. Nitinol, an alloy of nickel and titanium, offers unique properties, such as superelasticity and thermal shape memory, making it an ideal material for stent construction. In the GI tract, Nitinol self-expanding stents are most commonly deployed in the esophagus and duodenum to relieve obstruction, facilitate oral intake, and improve quality of life in patients with luminal narrowing.

Nitinol and Self-Expanding Stent Technology in the GI Tract

Properties of Nitinol

Nitinol's distinctive characteristics include:

- Superelasticity: Enables the stent to return to its original shape after compression.
- Thermal memory: Activates shape restoration at body temperature.
- Biocompatibility: Minimizes tissue reaction and encrustation.
- Corrosion resistance: Ensures durability within the acidic GI environment.
  These properties allow for safe, atraumatic deployment, and sustained radial force, essential for maintaining luminal patency.

Nitinol self-expanding esophageal stents are now the cornerstone of endoscopic and radiologic management of upper gastrointestinal (GI) tract obstruction and leaks, particularly in the palliative setting for malignant dysphagia and in selected benign conditions such as refractory strictures and post-surgical perforations or anastomotic leaks.

Early esophageal stents were rigid plastic tubes or stainless-steel/elgiloy devices adapted from vascular practice, but these had substantial limitations in deliverability, patient comfort, and long-term patency. The introduction of Nitinol, with its shape memory and superelastic properties, allowed stents to be manufactured at a target diameter, compressed into relatively low-profile delivery systems, and then reliably expand at body temperature with sustained radial force. Early series in obstructing esophageal cancer demonstrated that self-expanding Nitinol stents could be deployed safely, rapidly alleviate severe dysphagia, and maintain patency long enough to provide meaningful palliation in patients with limited life expectancy [62]. These foundational data, combined with better tolerability than rigid plastic tubes, established Nitinol self-expanding metal stents (SEMS) as the default technology for malignant esophageal obstruction.

Today, the main indication for Nitinol SEMS remains palliation of malignant dysphagia in patients with inoperable or incurable esophageal cancer or extrinsic compression from mediastinal malignancy. Modern guidelines from the European Society of Gastrointestinal Endoscopy (ESGE) explicitly recommend partially or fully covered self-expanding metal stents over laser therapy, photodynamic therapy, or surgical bypass for palliative treatment of malignant dysphagia, reflecting high-quality evidence that SEMS offer rapid, durable relief of swallowing difficulty with acceptable safety [63]. Large observational cohorts and more recent prospective studies confirm that stent placement leads to immediate improvement in dysphagia scores and restoration of oral intake in the vast majority of patients, with median stent patency often exceeding the patient's remaining survival time [64]. A recent 2025 series again showed that self-expanding metallic stents remain highly effective for palliation, improving nutritional status and quality of life with low procedure-related mortality in appropriately selected patients [64]. These data have cemented Nitinol SEMS as the standard palliative intervention for malignant esophageal obstruction worldwide, with brachytherapy reserved as an adjunct or alternative in patients with longer anticipated survival and access to specialized oncologic facilities [63].

Modern esophageal Nitinol stents are almost invariably covered devices, built on a braided or laser-cut Nitinol framework with a thin polymer membrane of silicone, polyurethane, or PTFE. The Nitinol scaffold provides flexible yet strong radial force, allowing the stent to conform to the esophageal lumen and maintain patency against tumor compression, while the covering creates a smooth inner surface designed to resist tumor ingrowth and reduce food impaction. Early experience with bare metal stents showed that tumor tissue readily proliferated through the mesh, causing recurrent obstruction despite otherwise intact scaffolding. A landmark prospective randomized trial by Vakil and colleagues compared a membrane-covered expandable metal stent to conventional bare-metal prostheses and found that covered stents provided significantly better palliation, largely because of reduced tumor ingrowth and fewer reinterventions [65]. As a result, fully uncovered Nitinol stents are now rarely used in malignant disease, and the main design debates concern the extent and configuration of coverage rather than whether to cover at all.

Two broad categories of covered Nitinol SEMS are now in common use: fully covered and partially covered stents. Fully covered self-expanding metallic stents (FCSEMS) have a continuous membrane over the entire length of the device, preventing tissue ingrowth anywhere along the stent and facilitating later removal if needed. Partially covered SEMS (PCSEMS) typically have a central covered segment across the tumor with bare proximal and distal flares, promoting tissue embedding at the ends to reduce migration while still protecting the stricture from tumor ingrowth. Multiple comparative studies and at least one randomized trial have evaluated the relative performance of fully versus partially covered Nitinol SEMS in malignant dysphagia. A large multicenter randomized study by Didden and co-workers showed no significant difference in overall stent dysfunction between fully and partially covered SEMS, but the mechanisms of failure differed: fully covered stents had more migration, whereas partially covered stents were more prone to tumor ingrowth at the uncovered ends [66]. A subsequent prospective comparison from Asia and a 2020 meta-analysis reported similar findings, namely that both designs offer comparable overall patency and survival, but fully covered stents trade a lower risk of ingrowth for a higher risk of migration, while partially covered stents do the opposite [67]. Contemporary practice therefore individualizes the choice based on tumor location, length, expected survival, and the perceived risk of migration; for example, partially covered stents are favored in very short strictures or at the gastroesophageal junction, where migration into the stomach is problematic, whereas fully covered stents may be preferred when future removal is contemplated or when ingrowth risk is high.

Beyond simple cylindrical designs, Nitinol's flexibility has allowed development of specialized esophageal stents with anti-reflux valves, hourglass shapes, or multi-segmented architecture. Anti-reflux valves at the distal end are intended to reduce gastroesophageal reflux when stents traverse the lower esophageal sphincter, though clinical data on their superiority over non-valved stents are mixed. Multisegmented fully covered Nitinol stents, designed to improve conformability and reduce axial stiffness, have been tested in malignant dysphagia with good technical success, but a recent 2024 study had to be prematurely terminated because of stent-related complications, highlighting the delicate balance between mechanical sophistication and safety [68]. Overall, standard cylindrical covered Nitinol SEMS remain the workhorse devices, with niche roles for more exotic designs.

In addition to their established place in malignant dysphagia, Nitinol esophageal stents are widely used in benign conditions, though here the goals and risk tolerance are very different. For refractory benign esophageal strictures (RBES) caused by radiation, caustic injury, anastomotic scarring, or eosinophilic esophagitis, temporary placement of fully covered Nitinol SEMS is now an accepted if still somewhat controversial option after failure of repeated balloon or bougie dilatation [69]. ESGE guidelines recognize that FCSEMS can be used in RBES but stress that they should be fully covered and removed within a maximum of about 3 months to limit tissue reaction and difficult extraction [63]. Reviews of benign strictures emphasize that stent therapy yields stricture resolution in roughly 30–60% of cases, depending on etiology, but is limited by a high incidence of migration and recurrent dysphagia, so a careful risk–benefit assessment and patient counselling are mandatory [70]. Long-term cohort studies, such as those by Bakken, Buscaglia, and Wilson, have shown that temporary FCSEMS can achieve durable symptom relief in a subset of patients with benign disease, but also document frequent complications including migration, pain, bleeding, and the need for repeat procedures; their experience supports the notion that FCSEMS are best reserved for truly refractory cases and managed by experienced centers [71].

Nitinol SEMS play a particularly important role in the management of esophageal perforations and post-surgical anastomotic leaks. The shift toward endoscopic sealing of leaks using covered metal stents, often combined with drainage of associated collections, has dramatically reduced the need for reoperation in many patients. A comprehensive review of endoscopic management of esophageal leaks notes that fully covered self-expanding metal stents have become a mainstay for acute iatrogenic perforations and post-esophagectomy or post-gastrectomy anastomotic leaks, with closure rates routinely above 80% when stents are properly positioned and associated sepsis is controlled [72]. Studies from thoracic surgery cohorts confirm that esophageal stent placement is a safe and effective treatment for acute perforation, with most leaks sealing after one stent and survival driven primarily by the severity of underlying sepsis and comorbidities [73]. The question of optimal dwell time has been addressed in series such as Mahidhara's, which suggested removal at around 2–3 weeks for acute perforation and somewhat shorter times for anastomotic leaks, balancing the need for tissue healing against the growing risk of tissue overgrowth and stent-related complications with longer dwell [74]. Recent work focusing specifically on fully covered Nitinol stents for perforations, including a 2025 surgical series, shows high rates of leak closure, a mean removal time of about 6 weeks, and successful retrieval in most patients, reinforcing FCSEMS as the preferred device in this high-stakes setting [75].

Complications of Nitinol esophageal SEMS are well described and shape both device design and clinical indications. Migration is the most frequent problem, particularly with fully covered stents in benign disease or short malignant strictures. Reported migration rates vary widely but can exceed 30% in some benign-series, leading to recurrent dysphagia, risk of gastric or intestinal obstruction, and additional procedures to reposition or remove the stent [71]. Technical and endoscopic strategies have been developed to mitigate migration, including longer stents with generous proximal and distal margins, flared ends, hourglass shapes that harness esophageal contour for anchoring, and endoscopic fixation techniques. A large 2021 analysis of partially and fully covered SEMS demonstrated that prophylactic endoscopic suturing of FCSEMS significantly reduced migration rates without adding major complications, and this technique is now increasingly used in high-risk situations such as benign strictures or short malignant lesions [76]. Other adverse events include retrosternal pain, bleeding, food impaction, stent-induced ulceration, and, rarely, perforation during placement or as a late event in friable tumors. Long-dwelling stents can provoke hyperplastic tissue at the edges, leading to new strictures and making removal difficult; this is one reason why guidelines insist on strict time limits for SEMS in benign indications [63].

From a materials and innovation perspective, Nitinol remains the dominant metal for esophageal SEMS, but there is active exploration of alternatives and adjuncts. One area of rapid development is biodegradable esophageal stents, which aim to provide temporary support without the need for removal and without leaving permanent metal in benign disease. Polymer-based and magnesium alloy biodegradable stents have been tested in refractory benign strictures, with early studies suggesting reasonable safety and efficacy, though with issues such as unpredictable degradation, early collapse, and inflammation [77]. A recent comprehensive review of biodegradable esophageal stent materials concluded that, while these devices show promise for benign strictures and even palliative malignant strictures, they are not yet ready to replace Nitinol SEMS in routine practice because of limited long-term data and variable mechanical performance [77]. At the same time, research into functional coatings for Nitinol stents—such as drug-eluting membranes or anti-biofilm surfaces—seeks to reduce granulation tissue, bacterial colonization, and sludge formation, mirroring trends already seen in vascular and biliary stents, although these remain largely experimental in the esophageal field.

Taken together, the current status of esophageal Nitinol self-expanding stents is that of a mature yet still evolving technology. In malignant dysphagia, they are firmly established as first-line palliative therapy, delivering rapid and reliable relief of obstruction and allowing patients to eat and drink with acceptable quality of life until death. Fully and partially covered Nitinol SEMS are considered equivalent in overall efficacy, with differences in migration versus ingrowth patterns guiding individualized selection. In benign disease, fully covered Nitinol stents are powerful but double-edged tools: they can salvage otherwise refractory strictures and seal perforations or anastomotic leaks without surgery, but at the cost of frequent migration, granulation, and the need for meticulous follow-up and timely removal. Guidelines from ESGE and other societies, therefore, emphasize careful patient selection, strict limits on stent dwell time in benign conditions, and the importance of delivering these interventions in experienced centers [63]. Looking ahead, Nitinol SEMS will almost certainly remain the backbone of esophageal stenting for years to come, while incremental advances in segmented designs, fixation methods, valve mechanisms, and biodegradable or drug-eluting alternatives progressively refine how and in whom these devices are used.

Esophageal Nitinol Stents Summary

Indications

- Malignant dysphagia (e.g., esophageal cancer)
- Benign strictures (refractory or recurrent after dilation)
- Esophageal fistulas
- Postoperative anastomotic leaks

Types and Designs

- Covered versus Uncovered:
  - *Covered stents* prevent tumor ingrowth and are preferred for fistulas or leaks.
  - *Uncovered stents* allow tissue embedding for better fixation but risk tumor ingrowth.
- Partially covered stents balance fixation and protection from ingrowth.
- Anti-reflux valves may be integrated in stents placed across the gastroesophageal junction.

Placement and Technique

- Performed under fluoroscopic and/or endoscopic guidance.
- Pre-dilation may be required in severe stenoses.

- Stents are deployed over a guidewire using a delivery system designed to maintain position during deployment.
- Post-deployment imaging ensures proper expansion and placement.

Complications

- Stent migration
- Tumor overgrowth or ingrowth
- Chest pain, bleeding
- Perforation (rare)
- Gastroesophageal reflux

We present a list of commonly available esophageal Nitinol self-expanding stents, along with key characteristics such as design, coverage, special features, and intended clinical use.

Esophageal Nitinol Stents

1. WallFlex™ Esophageal Stent (Boston Scientific)
   - Coverage: Fully covered and partially covered versions (Fig. 5.14)
   - Diameter: 18–23 mm (body); 23–28 mm (flared ends)
   - Lengths: 10–15 cm
   - Features:
     - Progressive flared ends to minimize migration
     - Silicone-based covering (for fully covered)
     - Radiopaque markers for visualization
     - High-radial and recovery force
   - Indications: Malignant strictures, leaks, fistulas

2. Ultraflex™ Esophageal Stent (Boston Scientific)

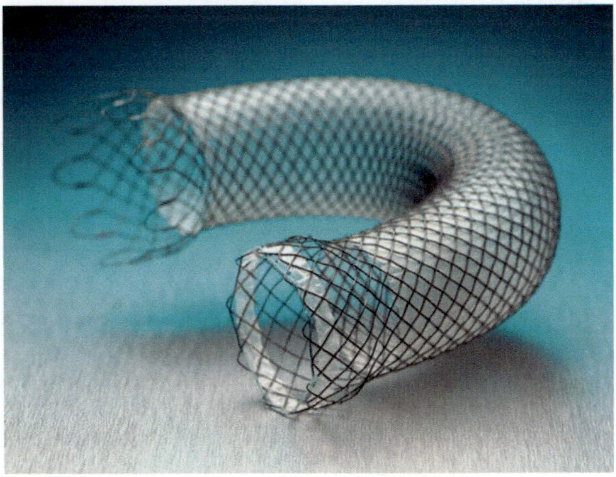

Fig. 5.14 WallFlex partially covered esophageal stent from Boston Scientific

- Coverage: Uncovered and partially covered (Fig. 5.15)
- Diameter: 18–23 mm
- Lengths: 10–15 cm
- Features:
  - Woven Nitinol mesh for flexibility
  - Softer ends for reduced trauma
  - Ideal for tortuous anatomy
- Indications: Malignant or benign strictures

3. Evolution® Controlled-Release Esophageal Stent (Cook Medical)
   - Coverage: Fully and partially covered (Fig. 5.16)
   - Diameter: 18–23 mm
   - Lengths: 6–15 cm
   - Features:

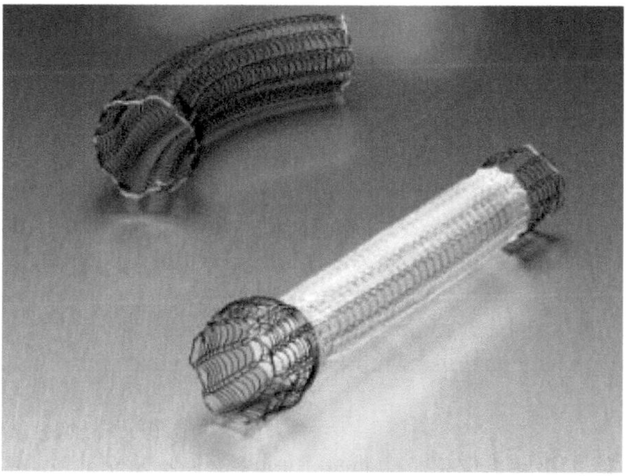

Fig. 5.15 UltraFlex uncovered and partially covered esophageal stent from Boston Scientific

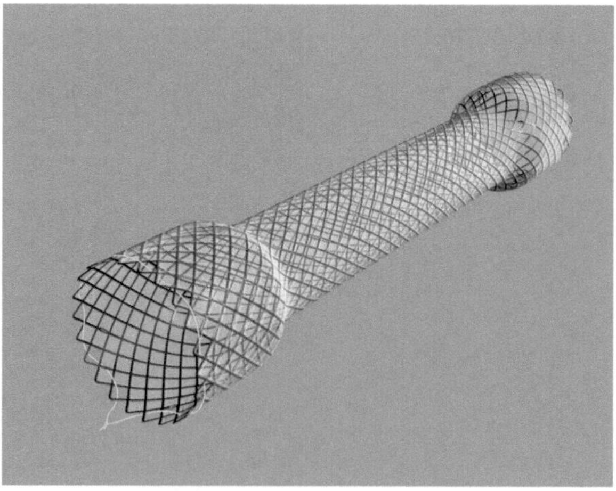

Fig. 5.16 Evolution controlled-release esophageal stent with flared ends and retrieval loop from Cook Medical

  - Controlled-release system (allows repositioning before full deployment)
  - Retrieval loop for repositioning/removal
  - Flared ends for anti-migration
- Indications: Malignant dysphagia, benign strictures, fistulas

4. Niti-S™ Esophageal Stent (TaeWoong Medical)
   - Coverage: Fully covered, partially covered, and uncovered (Fig. 5.17)
   - Diameter: 16–20 mm (body); 20–28 mm (flared ends)
   - Lengths: 6–15 cm
   - Features:
     - Wide variety of stent designs (e.g., anti-reflux valve, segmented)
     - Silicone coating (FC versions)
     - Radiopaque markers
   - Indications: Wide range, including post-surgical leaks, cancer, benign stenosis
5. Bonastent® Esophageal Stent (Standard Sci-Tech)
   - Coverage: Fully covered (Fig. 5.18)
   - Diameter: 18–23 mm
   - Features:
     - Ultra-thin delivery system (reduced esophageal trauma)
     - Resheathable before full deployment
   - Indications: Especially useful in tight strictures due to low-profile delivery

All esophageal Nitinol stents have braded or woven design from Nitinol wire, allowing to preload large in diameter stents in low-profile delivery systems. This design also allows accommodation of stretchable stent coating, like silicone or PTFE, which can still fit in the relatively low-profile delivery systems.

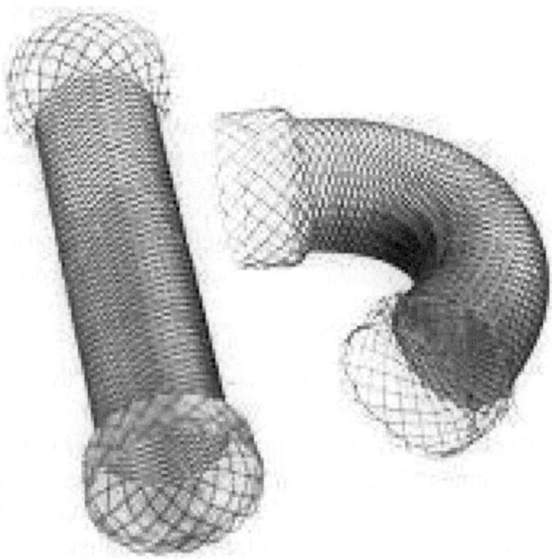

Fig. 5.17 Niti-S partially covered esophageal stent with flared ends from TaeWoong Medical

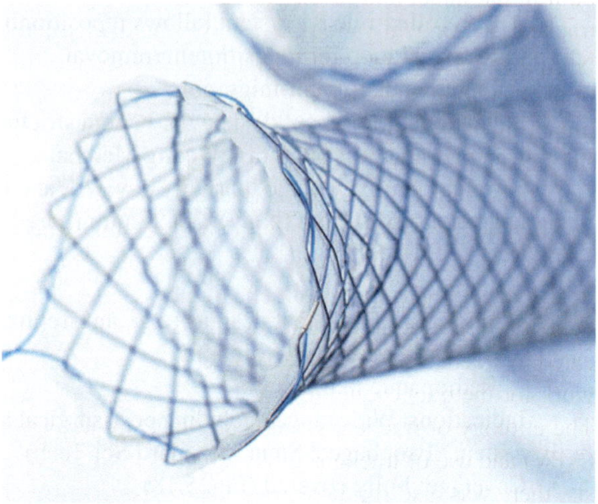

Fig. 5.18 Bonastent fully covered esophageal stent from Standard Sci-Tech

Table 5.5 Side-by-side comparison chart of commercially available Esophageal Nitinol Stents

Stent name	Manufacturer	Coverage	Design features	Indications
WallFlex Esophageal	Boston Scientific	Fully or partially	Flared ends, retrieval loop, silicone covering	Malignant strictures, fistulas
UltraFlex Esophageal NG	Boston Scientific	Uncovered or covered	Flexible braided design, silicone membrane	Malignant/benign strictures
Evolution Esophageal	Cook Medical	Fully or partially covered	Controlled-release, silicone cover, retrieval proximal loop	Malignant dysphagia, leaks
Niti-S Esophageal	TaeWoong Medical	Fully or partially covered	PTFE or silicone membrane, flared ends, anti-reflux valve optional	Malignant and benign esophageal lesions
Bonastent Esophageal	Micro-Tech	Fully or partially covered	Fully radiopaque, minimal shortening, flared ends	Malignant strictures, fistulas
Alimaxx-E Esophageal	Merit Medical	Fully covered	High-radial force, low-axial force	Malignant dysphagia, strictures
Hanarostent Esophageal	M.I. Tech	Fully or partially covered	Braided design, silicone or PTFE covering, flared ends	Malignant strictures, perforations

Side-by-side comparison characteristic of available esophageal Nitinol stents is presented in Table 5.5.

Dedicated self-expanding *Nitinol duodenal stents* are now an established palliative treatment for malignant gastric outlet obstruction and have evolved into a fairly standardized class of "enteral" devices with design features tailored to the peculiar anatomy and biomechanics of the distal stomach, pylorus, and proximal duodenum.

Early work with stainless steel and first-generation metallic stents in the 1990s showed that endoscopic placement could promptly relieve obstruction but was limited by foreshortening, difficult positioning, migration, and tumor ingrowth. Modern Nitinol designs, introduced in the 2000s, addressed many of these problems. They exploit Nitinol's superelasticity and shape memory to provide large-diameter radial force through low-profile delivery systems while preserving flexibility for the sharp gastric–duodenal angulation. Examples include the WallFlex enteral/duodenal stent (Boston Scientific) and Niti-S duodenal stent (Taewoong), which are braided Nitinol mesh devices with diameters around 18–22 mm and lengths typically 6–12 cm, often with flared ends to reduce migration and non-foreshortening designs for accurate placement (bostonscientific.com).

The main contemporary indication for dedicated Nitinol duodenal stents is palliation of malignant gastric outlet obstruction from advanced gastric, pancreatic, duodenal, or periampullary cancers in patients who are not suitable for curative surgery or in whom rapid restoration of oral intake is desired. Large series and multicenter studies have consistently reported high-technical success rates of around 95–100% and clinical success, defined as improved oral intake by gastric outlet obstruction scoring systems, in 80–90% of patients [78]. Symptom relief is usually rapid, with resumption of liquid or soft diet within 1–3 days, much earlier than after surgical gastrojejunostomy. This translates into shorter hospital stays and earlier initiation or continuation of systemic therapy, which is a major advantage in frail oncology patients with limited life expectancy [79].

Device design has become increasingly specialized for duodenal anatomy. Current Nitinol duodenal stents are almost always uncovered to minimize the risk of occluding the papilla or biliary stents and to reduce migration; they rely on a combination of radial force, friction of the mesh against the mucosa and flared or dumbbell-shaped ends for anchoring (bostonscientific.com). The introduction of non-foreshortening Nitinol braids allowed operators to match stent length precisely to the stricture and avoid "shortening away" from the target zone during deployment, a key improvement over early generation devices. A prospective study of a new non-foreshortening Nitinol enteral stent demonstrated safe deployment, durable patency over the typical palliative time frame and meaningful improvements in quality of life in patients with incurable malignant gastric outlet obstruction [80]. More recent high-flexibility designs, such as highly flexible duodenal Nitinol stents, have shown excellent technical success and acceptable rates of re-obstruction in anatomically challenging strictures involving the duodenal C-loop, underscoring the importance of flexibility and conformability in addition to radial force [81].

Despite these advances, long-term patency remains limited, largely because the underlying disease is advanced, and survival is short. Contemporary series and reviews indicate that stent occlusion due to tumor ingrowth, overgrowth, or food impaction typically occurs at 2–4 months, which corresponds roughly to the median survival of this patient population [79]. Re-intervention rates range from 20% to 40% in many cohorts and usually involve placement of a second stent, mechanical cleaning or, increasingly, alternative approaches such as EUS-guided gastroenterostomy in centers with advanced endoscopic expertise [82]. These limitations have shifted the emphasis from maximizing very long patency to optimizing ease of deployment, early symptom relief, and compatibility with other palliative procedures such as biliary stenting or EUS-guided drainage.

Complication profiles of dedicated Nitinol duodenal stents are acceptable and broadly similar across devices. Early adverse events include perforation, bleeding, aspiration, and stent misplacement, each occurring in a small minority of cases; late events include occlusion, migration, biliary obstruction when the papilla is covered, and, rarely, fistula formation [78]. Migration is more frequent with covered stents, so uncovered Nitinol mesh is now standard for duodenum except in experimental settings such as hemostatic-covered stents for bleeding peptic ulcers or malignancies, where short-term placement is intended and anti-reflux properties or hemostatic coverage are desired [83]. MRI safety has been documented for widely used devices like the WallFlex duodenal Nitinol stent, which is classified as MR-conditional or safe at standard field strengths, an important consideration in oncology patients who undergo serial imaging (mrisafety.com).

Guideline statements from major societies now explicitly position Nitinol self-expanding duodenal stents as a first-line palliative option in selected patients. The ASGE guideline on benign and malignant gastroduodenal obstruction and the ESGE guideline on gastric outlet obstruction both recommend endoscopic enteral stenting with self-expanding metal stents as an appropriate alternative to surgical gastrojejunostomy in patients with limited life expectancy or high-surgical risk, emphasizing rapid symptom relief, and shorter hospitalization [84]. At the same time, these documents recognize that in younger, fitter patients with longer expected survival, surgical bypass or, increasingly, EUS-guided gastroenterostomy using lumen-apposing metal stents may provide more durable relief with fewer re-interventions, although randomized data comparing these modalities are still emerging [82]. Thus, dedicated Nitinol duodenal stents are now part of a broader therapeutic algorithm and are chosen based on performance status, prognosis, local expertise, and anatomical considerations rather than being a universal solution.

Comparative data between different duodenal stent brands are limited but suggest some clinically relevant differences. Studies comparing WallFlex and Niti-S Nitinol duodenal stents have shown similarly high-technical success but variable clinical success and re-obstruction rates, with some series reporting higher-clinical success and lower dysfunction rates for Niti-S, possibly related to differences in radial force distribution, flare design, and flexibility [85]. Nevertheless, no device has definitively emerged as superior across all endpoints, and choice is often driven by operator familiarity, availability, and specific features such as delivery system diameter, through-the-scope capability, radiopaque markers, and non-foreshortening behavior. Industry has continued to refine these devices, but there are, as yet, no widely adopted drug-eluting or bioabsorbable Nitinol duodenal stents; research on modifying mesh geometry and surface to limit tumor ingrowth and food impaction is ongoing but remains at an early stage [79].

In summary, dedicated Nitinol self-expanding duodenal stents represent a mature, widely used technology for palliating malignant gastric outlet and proximal duodenal obstruction. Their superelastic Nitinol architecture, large luminal diameter, flexibility, and non-foreshortening deployment provide reliable technical and clinical success in anatomically complex regions, with acceptable complication and re-intervention rates over the limited survival of most candidates. Contemporary practice increasingly integrates these stents into a nuanced treatment strategy that also includes surgical bypass and EUS-guided gastroenterostomy, chosen according to patient prognosis and center expertise. Further advances are likely to focus on prolonging patency, reducing restenosis and migration, and tailoring stent designs to specific stricture locations and coexistence with biliary interventions, but even in their current form Nitinol duodenal stents have become a cornerstone of minimally invasive palliation in upper gastrointestinal oncology.

Duodenal Nitinol Stents Summary

Indications

- Malignant gastric outlet obstruction (e.g., pancreatic, gastric, or duodenal carcinoma)
- Palliative treatment in inoperable cases
- Benign strictures (rare use; usually in select or high-risk surgical candidates)

Types and Features

- Typically uncovered or partially covered
- Designed for flexibility to navigate duodenal curvature
- Larger luminal diameter than esophageal stents
- Anti-migration features such as flared ends or anchoring flaps

Placement and Technique

- Usually performed under fluoroscopic guidance, sometimes with endoscopic assistance.
- Requires careful navigation through the stomach into the duodenum.
- Crosses the stricture with the guidewire, then deploys stent under controlled visualization.
- Enteral nutrition may resume within 24–48 h post-deployment.

Complications

- Stent migration
- Tumor ingrowth or overgrowth
- Obstruction due to food impaction
- Perforation
- Biliary obstruction if the stent compresses the ampulla of Vater

Commercially Available Duodenal Nitinol Stents

1. WallFlex™ Duodenal Stent (Boston Scientific) (Fig. 5.19)
   - Coverage: Uncovered
   - Diameter: 22 mm
   - Lengths: 6, 9, and 12 cm

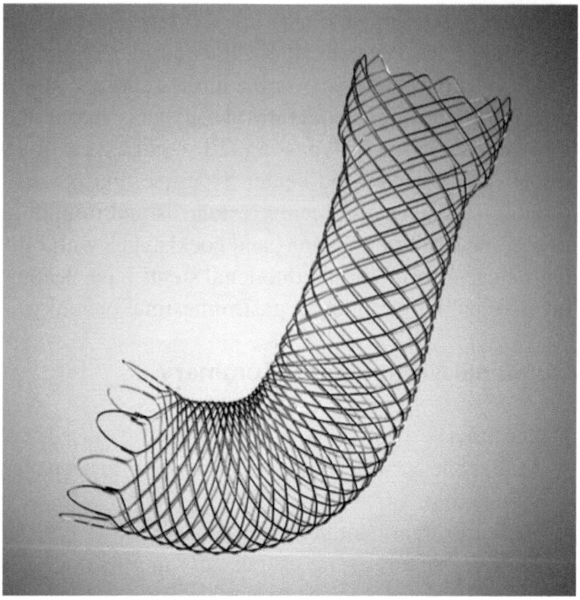

Fig. 5.19 WallFlex Duodenal uncovered stent with flared ends from Boston Scientific

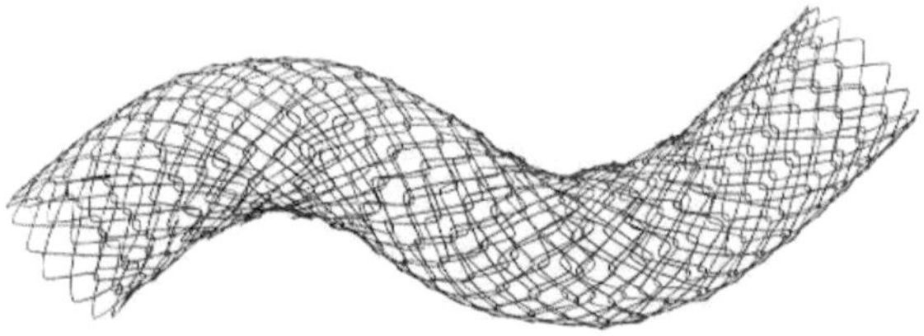

Fig. 5.20 Niti-S uncovered duodenal stent for TaeWoong Medical

- Features:
  - Flared ends to reduce migration
  - Radiopaque markers
  - Braided Nitinol for radial force and flexibility
- Indications: Malignant gastric outlet obstruction (GOO)

2. Niti-S™ Duodenal Stent (Taewoong Medical)
   - Coverage: Uncovered and partially covered versions (Fig. 5.20)
   - Diameter: 20–22 mm
   - Lengths: 6–12 cm
   - Features:
     - Flexible and conformable for duodenal anatomy
     - Optional anchoring flaps
     - Radiopaque for visualization
   - Indications: Palliation of malignant obstruction, some benign cases
3. Evolution® Duodenal Stent (Cook Medical) (Fig. 5.21)
   - Coverage: Uncovered
   - Diameter: 22 mm

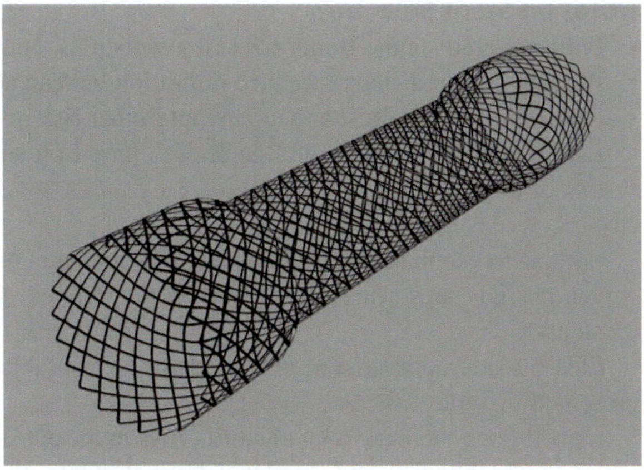

Fig. 5.21 Evolution uncovered duodenal controlled-release stent with flared ends from Cook Medical

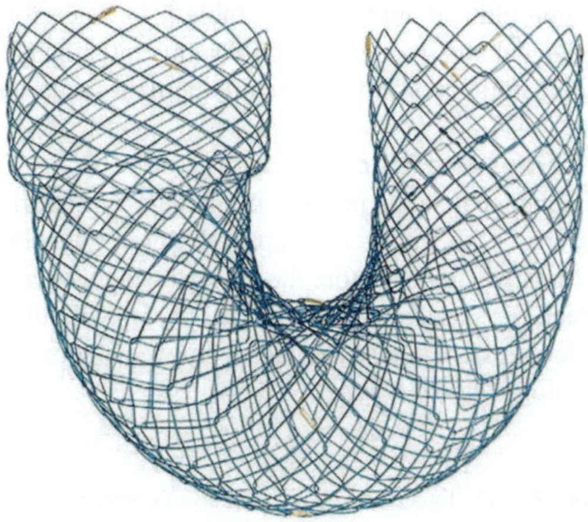

Fig. 5.22 Hanarostent uncovered duodenal stent with one flared end from Olympus Medical

- Lengths: 6, 9, and 12 cm
- Features:
  - Controlled-release delivery system
  - Flared ends
  - Low-profile introducer
- Indications: Gastric outlet obstruction due to malignancy

4. HANAROSTENT® Duodenal/Pyloric (M.I. Tech)
   - Coverage: Uncovered, partially covered (Fig. 5.22)
   - Diameter: 18–22 mm
   - Lengths: 6–12 cm
   - Features:
     - S-shaped or pyloric conforming models
     - High flexibility and strong radial force
     - Anti-migration design
   - Indications: Malignant obstructions of the duodenum or pylorus

Notes on Stent Selection

- Fully covered stents: Better for leaks or fistulas, but higher-migration risk.
- Partially covered stents: Reduce migration but can allow tissue ingrowth.
- Uncovered stents: Best anchorage but higher risk of tumor ingrowth.
- Length and diameter should be chosen based on stricture length, location, and risk of migration.

Similar to esophageal Nitinol stents, all duodenal Nitinol stents have braded or woven design, permitting use of low-profile delivery systems for large in diameter stents.

Side-by-side comparison characteristic of available duodenal Nitinol stents is presented in Table 5.6.

Even though there are a lot of similarities in the construction, features and behavior of the esophageal and duodenal Nitinol stents, there are clear distinguishing characteristics of the devices for intended use in specific anatomic locations and different clinical applications (Table 5.7). Therefore, it is not recommended to use esophageal and duodenal Nitinol stents interchangeably, unless there are no proper suitable options or in very specific clinical scenarios.

Outcomes and Efficacy

- Esophageal stents provide immediate symptom relief, particularly in dysphagia scores, with significant improvement in nutritional intake and quality of life.
- Duodenal stents restore the ability to eat in over 90% of cases, often replacing the need for surgical gastrojejunostomy in palliative settings.
- Median stent patency ranges from weeks to several months, depending on tumor biology and stent type.

Table 5.6 Side-by-side comparison chart of commercially available Duodenal Nitinol Stents

Stent name	Manufacturer	Coverage	Design features	Indications
WallFlex Duodenal	Boston Scientific	Uncovered	Flared ends, high flexibility, radiopaque markers	Gastric outlet obstruction
Niti-S Duodenal	TaeWoong Medical	Uncovered or partially covered	Large, flared ends, flexible design, anti-migration hooks	Malignant duodenal obstruction
Hanarostent Duodenal	M. I. Tech	Uncovered or partially covered	Large flares, flexible body, reduced shortening	Gastric/duodenal obstruction
Evolution Duodenal	Cook Medical	Uncovered	Controlled delivery, enhanced visibility, braided design	Malignant gastric outlet obstruction
Bonastent Duodenal	Micro-Tech	Uncovered	Flared ends, minimal shortening, easy repositioning	Inoperable gastric/duodenal tumors
Alimaxx-D Duodenal	Merit Medical	Uncovered	High-radial force, flexible delivery system	Gastric outlet obstruction

Table 5.7 Key comparison points of the esophageal and duodenal Nitinol stents

Feature	Esophageal stents	Duodenal stents
Coverage	Mostly covered to prevent tumor ingrowth	Usually uncovered to reduce migration
Flexibility	Moderate (less curvature)	High flexibility (for navigating the duodenal loop)
Anti-Migration	Flares, external barbs, anchoring design	Large flares, reduces axial force
Deployment Control	Controlled-release systems common	Fluoroscopic + endoscopic guidance
Removal/ Revision	Easier in fully covered stents	Removal uncommon; often left in situ

Nitinol self-expanding stents represent a vital component of minimally invasive therapy for obstructive gastrointestinal pathologies, particularly in the esophagus and duodenum. Their minimally invasive nature, immediate symptomatic relief, and adaptability to patient anatomy make them indispensable in modern GI interventional practice. Continuous innovation and refinement in stent design promise to further enhance their safety and efficacy in both palliative and potentially curative roles.

Tracheobronchial Nitinol Self-Expanding Stents

Tracheobronchial stents are a vital component in the management of airway obstruction and stenosis. Over the past two decades, advances in materials science and interventional pulmonology have led to the increased use of Nitinol stents due to their favorable biomechanical and biocompatible properties. These stents provide a minimally invasive solution for maintaining airway patency in patients with malignant and benign airway diseases, traumatic injury, or post-surgical complications.

Tracheal and bronchial Nitinol stents are specialized self-expanding metallic stents (SEMS) used to maintain airway patency in patients with central airway obstruction (CAO). Nitinol offers the flexibility, shape memory, and superelastic properties necessary for use in dynamic and anatomically complex airways.

Nitinol self-expanding tracheobronchial stents have become a central tool in interventional pulmonology for the rapid relief of central airway obstruction and management of complex tracheobronchial pathology. Their development followed the earlier use of silicone Dumon stents and stainless-steel or elgiloy metallic stents, but Nitinol's combination of shape memory, superelasticity, and corrosion resistance has made it the dominant metallic platform for modern airway self-expanding metal stents, or SEMS. Nitinol stents can be crimped into relatively small delivery systems, are pliable at room temperature, and then recover a programmed diameter and shape at body temperature with sustained radial force, allowing deployment through rigid or even flexible bronchoscopes while maintaining a stable lumen in a dynamic airway [86].

Clinically, the main indication for Nitinol airway SEMS is palliation of malignant central airway obstruction and sealing of malignant tracheoesophageal or bronchoesophageal fistulas. Patients with lung cancer, esophageal carcinoma, or mediastinal malignancy may develop critical narrowing of the trachea or main bronchi, causing severe dyspnea, post-obstructive pneumonia, and hemoptysis; in these settings, Nitinol SEMS can rapidly restore airway patency, often in conjunction with tumor debulking techniques such as laser, electrocautery, cryotherapy, or mechanical coring. Contemporary reviews and cohort studies consistently show that SEMS placement produces prompt symptomatic relief and improved quality of life in most patients with malignant central airway obstruction, although survival itself is driven mainly by tumor biology rather than the stent [87]. Nitinol SEMS are also used to seal malignant airway–esophageal fistulas, either alone or in combination with esophageal stents, providing protection against life-threatening aspiration and allowing oral intake in selected patients [88].

The role of Nitinol SEMS in benign airway disease is more controversial. In the 1990s and early 2000s, uncovered stainless steel and Nitinol stents were increasingly used for benign post-intubation tracheal stenosis, post-transplant anastomotic strictures, and other non-malignant lesions. Over time, it became clear that long-term implantation in patients with years of life expectancy carried a high burden of complications, including exuberant granulation tissue at the ends and through the mesh, restenosis, mucous impaction, stent fracture, and difficulty or even impossibility of safe removal. In response, the US Food and Drug Administration issued a public health notification in 2005 warning against the routine use of metallic tracheal stents in benign airway disorders and recommending that metallic stents be reserved for cases in which all other options, including surgery and silicone stents, had been exhausted [89]. This advisory has shaped subsequent guidelines and practice patterns; most expert reviews still urge restraint with permanent metallic stents in benign disease and favor silicone stents or surgery whenever feasible, particularly in younger patients and those with transplant-related complications [90].

Despite this caution, Nitinol SEMS have not disappeared from benign indications. Instead, device design and usage philosophy have evolved toward fully covered, retrievable Nitinol stents deployed for limited periods. Early work by Kim and colleagues showed that temporary placement of covered, expandable Nitinol stents could provide effective dilation of benign tracheobronchial strictures with acceptable long-term outcomes if the stent was removed after a finite dwell time [91]. Subsequent series with newer covered Nitinol stents, including long-term cohorts from Asia and Europe, suggest that carefully selected patients with benign strictures, often post-tuberculous or post-intubation, can achieve durable airway patency after a course of temporary SEMS followed by removal, provided that stent-related granulation, infection, and fracture are aggressively managed [92]. A 2025 systematic review and meta-analysis of self-expanding metallic stents for benign tracheobronchial stenosis compiled data from dozens of studies and concluded that SEMS placement can be effective in restoring lumen and symptoms, but also confirmed high rates of complications and reinterventions, underlining that their use must remain cautious and expert-driven [93].

Within the broader airway stent armamentarium, Nitinol SEMS compete and coexist with silicone stents and hybrid stents. Silicone stents, such as the Dumon design and its derivatives, are rigid tubes with external studs that resist migration and can be customized and repositioned relatively easily, but they require rigid bronchoscopy and general anesthesia for placement and may be less suitable in tortuous or small distal airway [90]. Nitinol SEMS, by contrast, can be deployed through smaller, more flexible delivery systems and adapt better to complex airway curvature, and many modern devices can be placed under fluoroscopic and bronchoscopic guidance via flexible bronchoscopy, which partly explains their worldwide popularity. Comparative studies have yielded mixed results. A 2021 prospective study comparing silicone stents with fully covered metallic stents in benign tracheobronchial strictures found that both stent types achieved similar rates of technical success and immediate clinical improvement; overall complication rates rose to nearly 90% in both groups at 6 months, with granulation, migration, and secretion retention being the most frequent events. Interestingly, the risk of complications was somewhat higher for SEMS, but there was no difference in mortality when competing risk analyses were applied [94]. More recently, a 2025 systematic review specifically comparing covered and uncovered self-expanding metal stents for benign airway stenosis concluded that covered SEMS are effective and safe alternatives to uncovered SEMS and silicone stents, with higher-stenting success and less mucosal ingrowth, but the authors still emphasized the need to respect the FDA warning and to use SEMS for benign disease only in carefully selected, closely monitored patients [95].

From a design standpoint, most Nitinol tracheobronchial SEMS are woven or laser-cut tubular meshes, either bare or fully covered with a thin silicone or polyurethane membrane. Uncovered Nitinol stents, typified historically by the Ultraflex design, allow epithelial ingrowth through the mesh, which stabilizes the stent but makes removal difficult and predisposes to late restenosis from granulation and tumor ingrowth [96]. To address this, newer devices are fully covered with a silicone membrane bonded to a Nitinol wire framework, yielding hybrid designs that aim to combine the conformability and self-expansion of Nitinol with a smooth, non-ingrown lumen that can be cleaned and, in principle, removed. Examples include the Aero and AEROmini stents and the Bonastent, which are fully covered Nitinol SEMS approved for malignant tracheobronchial strictures and designed with features such as recapturability when partially deployed, flared ends to reduce migration, and through-the-scope delivery systems allowing flexible bronchoscopic placement [96]. An observational multicenter study published in 2024 showed that Bonastent placement for malignant and selected benign airway stenoses was associated with high-technical success, good short-term safety, and a relatively low rate of serious complications, supporting its use as a mainstream fully covered Nitinol SEMS [97].

Nitinol also enabled the development of complex Y-shaped carinal stents that can be deployed as self-expanding metallic devices. Traditional Y-stents for the trachea and main bronchi were made of silicone and required rigid bronchoscopy and considerable technical expertise. The advent of self-expanding Nitinol Y-carina stents allowed an alternative approach, sometimes deployable partly under fluoroscopic or flexible bronchoscopic guidance, although rigid bronchoscopy remains common. A 2022 single-center series of self-expanding covered Nitinol Y-carina stents for central airway obstruction demonstrated that implantation via rigid bronchoscopy was feasible and safe for both malignant and benign disease, with rapid relief of dyspnea and the possibility of subsequent oncologic therapies in malignant patients [98]. A 2024 multicenter analysis of self-expanding metallic Y stents reported similar conclusions: complication rates were comparable to those reported for silicone Y stents, and SEM Y stents offered the additional advantage of being placeable with flexible bronchoscopy in some settings, thus widening access to carinal stenting outside of high-volume tertiary centers [99].

Notwithstanding their benefits, Nitinol airway SEMS carry a well-characterized profile of complications. Granulation tissue formation at the ends of the stent and through the mesh remains one of the most frequent and clinically relevant problems. Risk factors include longer dwell time, prior or concurrent respiratory infection, and certain stent designs or materials. A large cohort study showed that respiratory infections significantly increase the risk of granulation tissue after airway stenting, and more recent analyses suggest that silicone stents may actually be associated with equal or higher odds of granulation in some contexts compared with metallic devices, complicating simple material-based comparisons [96]. Migration is particularly important for fully covered Nitinol SEMS, especially when undersized, placed across short lesions, or deployed in benign disease where the airway may remodel. Design innovations such as flared ends, barbs, hourglass shapes, and mixed covered–uncovered segments have been introduced to mitigate this, and modern covered Nitinol stents with anti-migration features show lower migration rates than early covered SEMS, though the problem has not been eliminated [96]. Stent fracture, which was a major concern in early metallic airway experience, appears less common with current Nitinol designs than with older stainless steel or repurposed GI stents, but it still occurs, particularly with long-term implantation in benign disease or in high-motion segments, and can complicate removal [88].

Recent reviews emphasize that innovations in tracheobronchial stent design now focus less on proving basic feasibility and more on reducing complications and tailoring stents to complex anatomy. A 2024 design-oriented review highlighted multiple strategies for reducing granulation and migration, including optimizing radial and axial forces, adjusting strut geometry to maintain mucociliary clearance, and adding drug-eluting or bioactive coatings to suppress inflammatory hyperplasia [100]. Another 2024 update on airway stents pointed to emerging technologies such as 3D-printed patient-specific silicone or hybrid stents, biodegradable scaffolds, and drug-eluting metallic stents as potential future directions, though most of these remain in early clinical or preclinical stages [97]. In parallel, interventional pulmonology has become more structured as a discipline; modern guidelines stress careful patient and stent selection, multidisciplinary discussion, and systematic bronchoscopic follow-up to detect and manage complications early, regardless of whether silicone or Nitinol stents are used [86].

Taken together, the current status of tracheobronchial Nitinol self-expanding stents can be summarized as a mature but still evolving technology. In malignant central airway obstruction and malignant fistulas, Nitinol SEMS are firmly established as standard palliative tools that rapidly restore airway patency and improve symptoms when combined with appropriate tumor-directed therapy. In benign disease, their use has shifted from permanent uncovered metallic scaffolds, which clearly carried an unacceptable long-term complication burden, toward carefully selected, time-limited deployment of fully covered, retrievable Nitinol stents, usually when silicone stents or surgery are not feasible or have failed. Ongoing comparative studies and meta-analyses suggest that covered Nitinol SEMS can be as effective as silicone stents in benign disease but at the price of frequent complications and the need for expert management, so the FDA's call for restraint remains relevant. At the engineering level, modern Nitinol SEMS incorporate sophisticated design elements—coverage, anti-migration features, Y-configurations, and flexible delivery systems—that have expanded the range of treatable airway anatomy. Future advances are likely to come from more personalized stent geometry, smarter surfaces, and perhaps bioresorbable or drug-eluting Nitinol platforms, but for now, self-expanding Nitinol stents remain a cornerstone of interventional management for complex tracheobronchial obstruction when deployed in the right patient, by experienced operators, and with meticulous follow-up.

1. Overview of Tracheobronchial Nitinol Stents

   Purpose

   To restore or maintain airway patency in patients with obstructive lesions in the trachea or main bronchi due to:

   - Malignant tumors: From primary bronchogenic carcinoma or metastatic disease compressing the airway.
   - Benign strictures: Secondary to prolonged intubation, tracheostomy, or inflammatory diseases.
   - Tracheomalacia or bronchomalacia: When structural airway collapse occurs during respiration.
   - Fistulas: Tracheoesophageal or bronchoesophageal fistulas.
   - Post-surgical complications: Anastomotic stenosis following lung transplantation or tracheal resection.
2. Material Science of Nitinol
   - Superelasticity: Adapts to changes in airway shape during respiration.
   - Shape memory: Allows compression during delivery and re-expansion once deployed.
   - Biocompatibility: Minimizes local tissue reaction.
   - Corrosion resistance: Suitable for the moist, protein-rich airway environment.
   - Radiopacity: Often includes platinum or tantalum markers for visualization during placement.

3. Design Features

   Nitinol stents are cylindrical mesh structures, designed to exert consistent radial force against airway wall. Key design features include:

   A. Configuration
      - Straight stents: For focal stenosis in the trachea or a single bronchus.
      - Y-shaped stents (bifurcated): For lesions involving the carina, trachea, and both mainstem bronchi.
      - Designed to conform to the tracheobronchial anatomy.

   B. Mesh Structure
      - Open-cell or hybrid designs for flexibility and strength.
      - High-radial force to maintain airway lumen patency against external compression or recoil.
      - Braided design is more flexible and adapt to airway motion.
      - Laser-cut design offers higher-radial force, but less conformable.

   C. Covering Options
      - Covered (silicone or polyurethane layer):
        - Prevent tumor ingrowth or seal fistulas.
        - More prone to migration.
      - Uncovered:
        - Better epithelial integration.
        - May allow tissue ingrowth and restenosis.
      - Partially covered: Balance between integration and protection.

   D. Anti-Migration Features
      - Flaring ends, external ridges, or barbs.
      - Coverage design sometimes aids anchoring.

   E. Sizes
      - Diameter: Typically 10–20 mm (trachea), 8–14 mm (bronchi).
      - Length: Varies from 20 mm to 60+ mm depending on airway segment involved.

4. Delivery and Deployment
   - Typically performed under bronchoscopic (rigid or flexible) and/or fluoroscopic guidance.
   - The general steps include:
     - Pre-procedural planning: Includes high-resolution CT imaging and bronchoscopy to assess the anatomy, location, diameter of the airways, and length of the obstruction.
     - Anesthesia: General anesthesia or moderate sedation depending on patient condition and procedural complexity.
     - Guidewire placement: Under endoscopic or fluoroscopic visualization, a guidewire is advanced beyond the area of obstruction.
     - Stent deployment: The stent, compressed within a delivery catheter, is advanced over the guidewire and released to expand to its preset diameter.
     - Post-deployment assessment: Bronchoscopy confirms stent position, patency, and absence of complications.

5. Clinical Applications (Table 5.8)
6. Advantages of Nitinol Airway Stents
   - Conform to dynamic respiratory movements.
   - Better tolerance in tortuous anatomy.
   - Longer patency than silicone in malignant disease.
   - Easier deployment with smaller delivery systems.
7. Disadvantages and Risks
   - Granulation tissue formation at stent edges (especially with uncovered stents).
   - Mucus plugging due to impaired mucociliary clearance.
   - Migration, especially in fully covered types.
   - Difficulty in removal (especially with uncovered stents in benign disease).
   - Erosion or fistula formation (rare, but serious).
8. Examples of Nitinol Tracheobronchial Stents (Table 5.9)
9. Nitinol versus Silicone Airway Stents (Table 5.10)

Table 5.8 Clinical indications and stent selection

Indication	Preferred stent type
Malignant obstruction	Covered Nitinol SEMS
Benign Strictures	Removable silicone stents; Nitinol SEMS if silicone fails
Tracheomalacia	Uncovered or partially covered Nitinol SEMS
Tracheoesophageal Fistula	Fully covered Nitinol SEMS

Table 5.9 Tracheobronchial Nitinol stents

Stent name	Manufacturer	Scaffold design	Notes
Ultraflex Tracheobronchial Stent	Boston Scientific	Braided	One of the most commonly used, available in straight and Y configuration
AERO Tracheobronchial	Merit Medical	Laser cut	Fully covered, removable
Airway Stent	Micro-Tech	Braided	Available in various configurations and custom shapes
Aerstent	Leufen Medical	Braided	Customizable Y-stents, focus on tracheobronchial anatomy

Table 5.10 Comparison of Nitinol and Silicone tracheobronchial stents

Feature	Nitinol SEMS	Silicone stents
Deployment	Easier (via bronchoscopy or fluoroscopic guidance)	Requires rigid bronchoscopy
Conformability	High	Moderate
Migration risk	Higher in covered SEMS	Lower
Removability	Difficult (especially uncovered)	Easier
Mucostasis risk	Higher	Lower
Granulation formation	More common	Less common
Ideal use	Malignant obstruction	Benign strictures

Guideline Note: The American College of Chest Physicians (ACCP) and European Respiratory Society (ERS) recommend removable silicone stents for benign disease and SEMS for malignant disease, unless silicone stents are not feasible.

In summary, tracheal and bronchial Nitinol stents offer a minimally invasive solution to airway obstruction, with specific applications in malignancy, airway collapse, or fistula management. Tracheobronchial Nitinol stents are a cornerstone of modern interventional pulmonology. Their unique mechanical properties with self-expansion and flexible nature make them well suited for managing complex airway anatomy and pathologies. Despite some limitations, proper patient selection, deployment technique, and follow-up care significantly enhance clinical outcomes. Stent selection must be carefully tailored to the patient's underlying condition, anatomy, and prognosis due to potential complications.

Several bronchial and tracheal Nitinol stents are available, each offering unique features tailored to specific clinical needs. Here's an overview of notable options:

1. BONASTENT® Tracheobronchial Stent (Thoracent) (Fig. 5.23)
   - Material and Design: Woven Nitinol with a patented "hook and cross" structure.
   - Covering: Fully silicone-covered interior to prevent tissue ingrowth and reduce migration.
   - Deployment: Ultra-thin coaxial system; some sizes can be delivered through the working channel of a flexible therapeutic bronchoscope.
   - Repositioning: Can be re-captured up to 70% deployment.
   - Applications: Suitable for both tracheal and bronchial obstructions.
2. AERO and AEROmini® Tracheobronchial Stents (Merit Medical) (Fig. 5.24)
   - Material and Design: Self-expanding Nitinol with proprietary anti-migration struts.

Fig. 5.23 Bonastent fully covered tracheobronchial stent from Thoracent

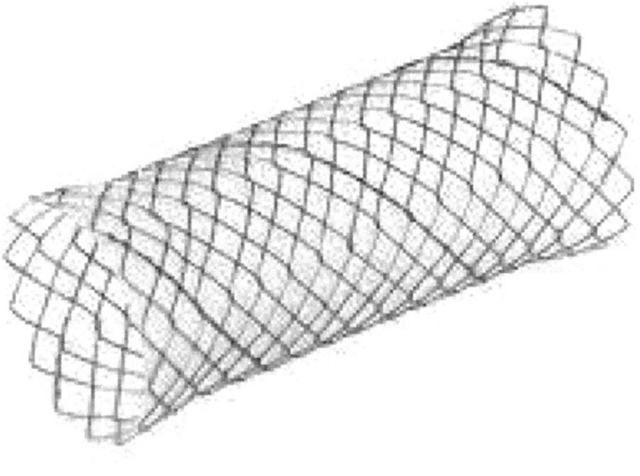

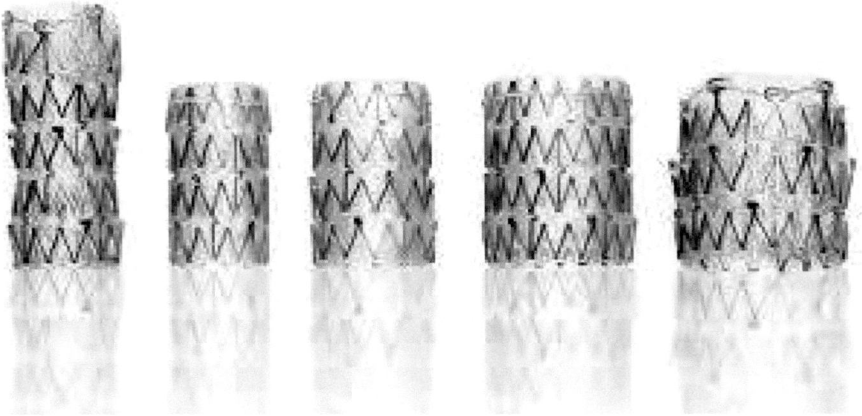

Fig. 5.24 AERO and AEROmini fully covered tracheobronchial stents with laser-cut scaffolding from Merit Medical

- Covering: Fully covered and hydrophilically coated to prevent ingrowth and mucus plugging.
- Deployment: Available in both through-the-scope (TTS) and over-the-wire (OTW) options; TTS stents can be deployed through a 2.8 mm or larger working channel of a therapeutic bronchoscope.
- Sizes: TTS stents available in 6-mm diameter and 10-mm and 15-mm lengths; OTW stents range from 8-mm to 14-mm diameters with a 10-mm length.
- Applications: Designed for treating tracheobronchial strictures produced by malignant neoplasms, especially in small, distal airways.

3. Airway Stent System (Micro-Tech Endoscopy) (Fig. 5.25)
    - Material and Design: Self-expanding Nitinol with a flexible, compliant straight and Y-shape to aid in treating malignant neoplasms at the tracheobronchial carina.
    - Covering: Silicone-covered to restrict tumor ingrowth.
    - Deployment: Low-profile delivery system allows for ventilation and visualization during placement; includes repositioning sutures for adjustment or removal.
    - Applications: Effective for patients with malignant tracheobronchial strictures, particularly at the carina.
4. Ultraflex™ Tracheobronchial Stent (Boston Scientific) (Fig. 5.26)
    - Material and Design: Self-expanding Nitinol with a polyurethane cover to prevent tumor or granulation tissue ingrowth.
    - Deployment: Can be deployed via guide-wire technique or flexible bronchoscopy; some experts also use rigid bronchoscopy.
    - Features: Exhibits "shape memory," self-adjusting to changes in bronchial size without shortening after deployment; deforms at cold temperatures and regains original shape at body temperature.
    - Applications: Used in managing malignant airway obstructions.

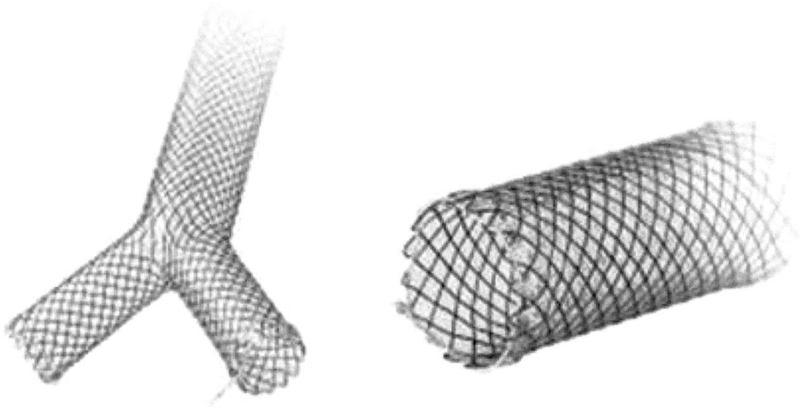

Fig. 5.25 Y-shaped and straight tracheobronchial covered stent from Micro-Tech

Fig. 5.26 Ultraflex tracheobronchial stent covered with Polyurethane from Boston Scientific

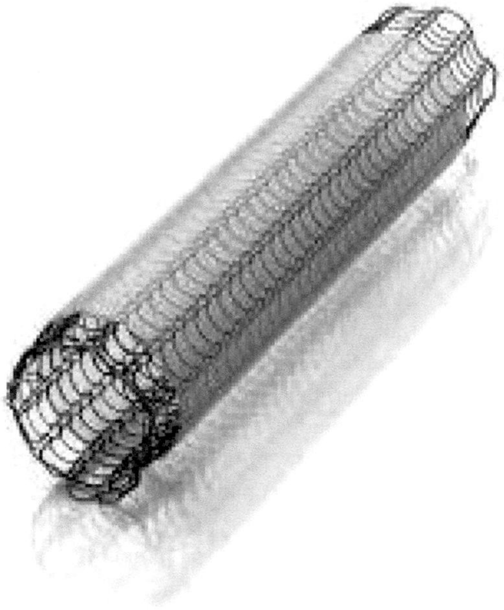

5. MITRA Tracheobronchial Stents (Mitra Industries) (Fig. 5.27)
   - Material and Design: Self-expanding Nitinol stents with natural ductal fitting and adequate radial force.
   - Covering: Fully silicone-covered for enhanced radiopacity and to prevent tissue ingrowth.
   - Applications: Designed for managing strictures and fistulae in the respiratory tract.

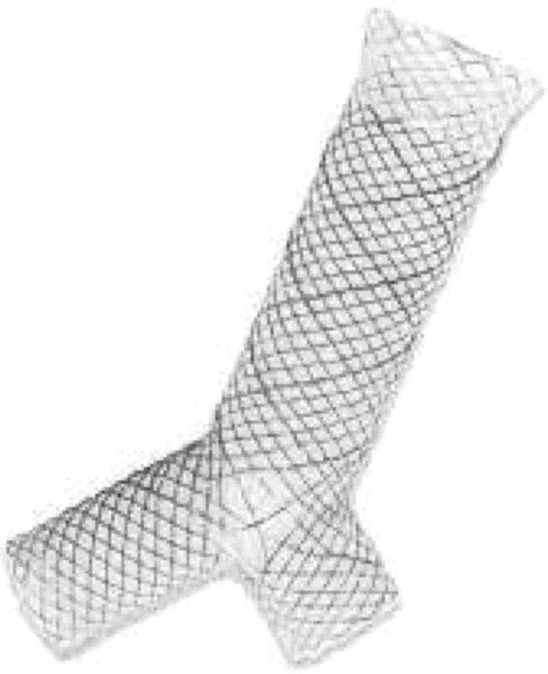

Fig. 5.27 Mitra Y-shaped fully covered tracheobronchial stent from Mitra Industries

6. Aerstent Carina tracheobronchial stent (Leufen Medical) (Fig. 5.28)
   - Material and Design: Self-expanding braded Nitinol stents in Y-configuration.
   - Covering: Durable silicone cover.
   - Applications: Bridging malignant stenoses in the trachea, as well as in the right and left main bronchus.

These stents offer a range of features to address various clinical scenarios in airway management. Selection should be based on specific patient needs, anatomical considerations, and the clinical judgment of the healthcare provider.

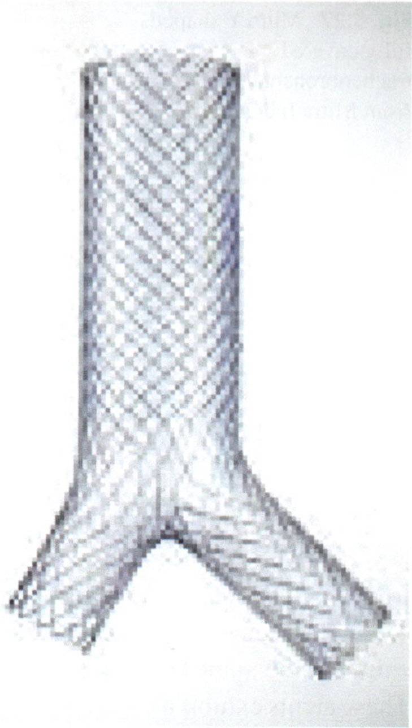

Fig. 5.28 Aerstent Y-Carina from Leufen Medical

Delivery of Nitinol Stents

Nitinol self-expanding stents are delivered to their target location within a blood vessel or other tubular structures, using a specialized catheter system. The entire set up includes an introducer sheath at an access site, a guidewire, and the delivery catheter with preloaded stent, all designed to facilitate navigation, placement, and deployment of the stent. The delivery system is crucial for precise and controlled stent placement, ensuring the device expands and remains in the correct position within the target.

The delivery catheter consists of two coaxial tubular structures. The inner tube provides a lumen for a guidewire. The outer tube covers the inner tube for nearly its entire length and the two are capable of sliding along each other. There is a chamber for stent loading between the inner and the outer tubing at the distal end. Nitinol stents are cooled down, crimped inside this chamber over the inner tube and covered with the outer tubing, keeping the stent restraint.

The delivery catheter is advanced over a wire to the target location under fluoroscopic guidance (Fig. 5.29a, b). Then the outer tubing is slowly manually retracted, while the inner tubing is kept stationary. This maneuver exposes the crimped preloaded Nitinol stent, which starts expanding from being heated to the body

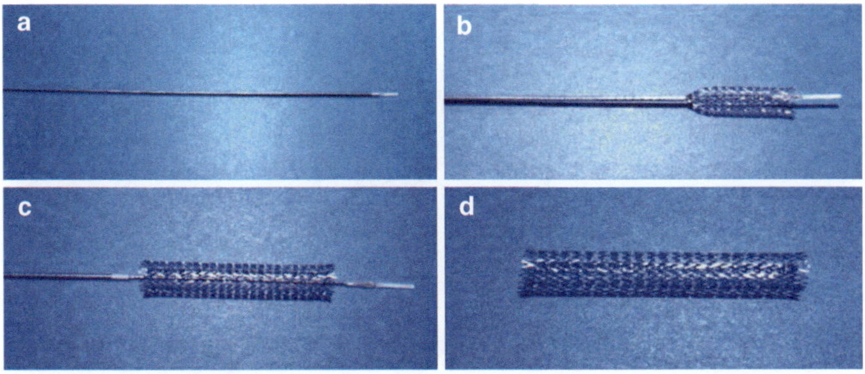

Fig. 5.29 Illustration of the steps involved in Nitinol self-expanding stent delivery and deployment: (**a**) delivery system with loaded compressed stent; (**b**) stent is partially expanded by retracting of the outer sheath of the delivery system; (**c**) stent is completely deployed; and (**d**) delivery system is removed and stent stays in place [101]

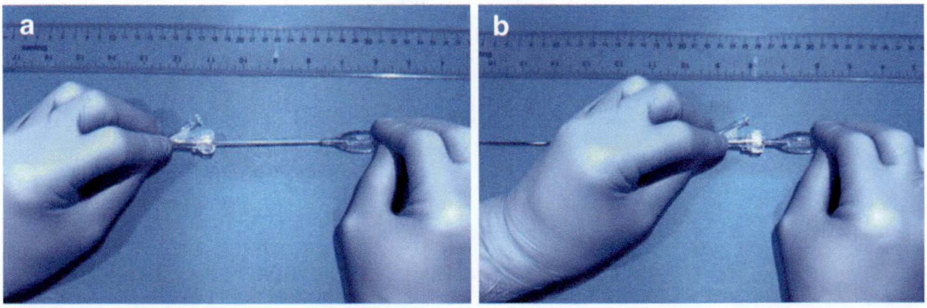

Fig. 5.30 Self-expanding Nitinol stent delivery system with "pin-pull" technique. (**a**) Handling of the proximal end of the delivery system. (**b**) Right hand is fixing ("pin") the hub. Left-hand retracts ("pull") the outer sheath toward the right hand, exposing the stent at the distal end

temperature (Fig. 5.29c). The outer tubing is continued to be retracted back until the entire stent is exposed from the loading chamber and expands completely to its final diameter and shape. The delivery catheter and the guidewire can then be removed, leaving the stent in place at the desired location (Fig. 5.29d).

Retraction of the outer tubing with respect to the inner catheter of the delivery system can be accomplished by manual pull-grip or with a specially designed thumbwheel or trigger activated handles at the proximal end of the system outside the patient (Figs. 5.30, 5.31, and 5.32).

Most current delivery systems for Nitinol self-expanding stents are low profile (some larger for bigger in diameter stents) and flexible, allowing to go through tortuous vessels on the way to the targets.

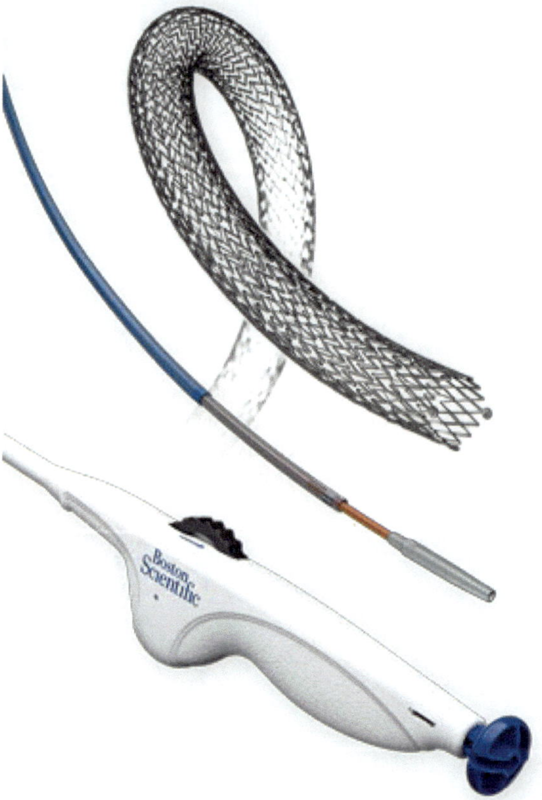

Fig. 5.31 Boston Scientific Innova stent delivery system with a thumbwheel release handle

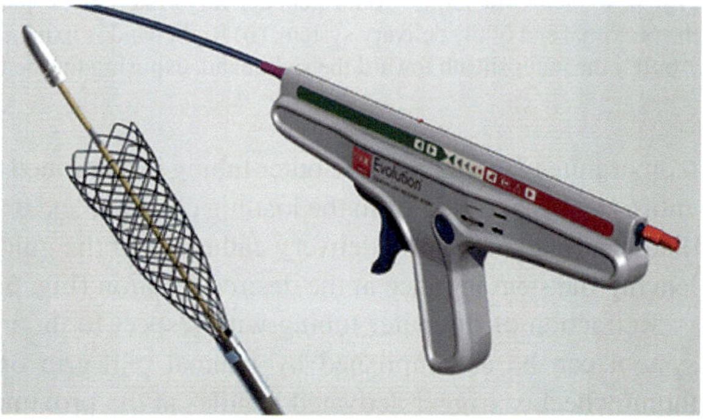

Fig. 5.32 COOK Medical Evolution® Biliary with trigger controlled-release stents

With all clear advantages of the delivery systems for Nitinol self-expanding stents, there are some limitations. Compared to balloon-expandable stents, deployment of self-expanding stents is less precise. Once the outer tubing is being retracted to expose the stent chamber, the inner tubing with preloaded stent not-infrequently inadvertently moves forward, particularly in the setting of tortuous anatomy that the catheter has to go through on the way to the target. If it happens and the front end of the laser-cut Nitinol stent is partially expanded, the stent cannot be resheathed and the system cannot be withdrawn back without causing a significant trauma to the vessel wall by the sharp struts of partially opened laser-cut stent. In this situation the stent has to be deployed completely even in the suboptimal position, sometimes even missing the lesion or only partially covering it, and may require additional stent placement overlapping the first malpositioned one in order to achieve a full adequate coverage of the target lesion.

Some woven Nitinol stents can be resheathed by advancing the outer tubing of the delivery system over partially opened misplaced stent. The entire system can then be pulled back under fluoroscopic guidance and readjusted into the proper position and the process of stent deployment repeated. One example of such system is WallFlex Biliary Stent Rx from Boston Scientific, which allows the stent to be completely restrained back into the loading chamber when it is released from the delivery system for up to 70% of its length.

In order to overcome inaccuracy of placement of laser-cut Nitinol self-expanding stents, we (Dmitry Rabkin, Eyal Morag and Ophir Perelson) came up with several options for improving the precision of self-expanding stents placement [102] (Fig. 5.33). One of the options was to add a third tubing on top of the conventional construction of the delivery system, which would then consist of an inner tubing, intermediate tubing (with the preloaded stent chamber between them at the distal end of the system) and an outer tubing, so-called triaxial system (Fig. 5.34). The purpose of the third layer is to release the built-up tension in the system (Fig. 5.35) and stabilize it when it crosses the tortuous passages on the way to the target location and consequently significantly reducing the undesirable and uncontrolled forward motion of the inner tubing with preloaded stent during its opening, which was described above. This triple-layer design gives better control over navigation, positioning, and release of the stent. The independent movement between the inner shaft, middle catheter, and outer sheath gives very fine control. With the triaxial system the stent is deployed with coordinated control between three layers, reducing the undesired movement of the entire system.

Most of the current newer Nitinol stents, that came to the market in the last few years, are supplied with the triaxial delivery systems (Table 5.11).

We (Dmitry Rabkin, Eyal Morag, Ophir Perelson) have also proposed a completely different delivery system for Nitinol self-expanding stents with bidirectional opening of the chamber with preloaded stent [103] (Fig. 5.36).

A bidirectional-opening delivery system is a special type of stent introducer that allows the stent to be opened from both ends, not just one (Fig. 5.37).

In a normal self-expanding stent system, the outer sheath is pulled back from the front (distal) end, and the stent opens only in one direction. Once the front end is released, you cannot move the stent very much.

In a bidirectional system, the stent is held between two sheath segments—one covering the distal end and one covering the proximal end. We have designed a special handle for controlling the stent opening when operator can pull back either sheath, which means the stent can be opened distally first, proximally first, or gradually from both ends simultaneously (Fig. 5.38).

US007074236B2

(12) **United States Patent**
Rabkin et al.

(10) **Patent No.: US 7,074,236 B2**
(45) **Date of Patent: Jul. 11, 2006**

(54) **STENT DELIVERY SYSTEM**

(75) Inventors: **Dmitry Rabkin**, Framingham, MA (US); **Eyal Morag**, East Hampton, MA (US); **Ophir Perelson**, Beverly Hills, CA (US); **Yoram Hadar**, Netanya (IL)

(73) Assignee: **InTek Technology L.L.C.**, Wilmington, DE (US)

(*) Notice: Subject to any disclaimer, the term of this patent is extended or adjusted under 35 U.S.C. 154(b) by 0 days.

(21) Appl. No.: **10/979,887**

(22) Filed: **Nov. 2, 2004**

(65) **Prior Publication Data**

US 2005/0119721 A1 Jun. 2, 2005

Related U.S. Application Data

(63) Continuation of application No. 10/334,402, filed on Dec. 31, 2002, now Pat. No. 6,849,084.

(51) **Int. Cl.**
A61F 2/06 (2006.01)

(52) **U.S. Cl.** **623/1.12**; 623/1.23

(58) **Field of Classification Search** 623/1.12, 623/1.11, 1.23
See application file for complete search history.

(56) **References Cited**

U.S. PATENT DOCUMENTS

5,201,757	A		4/1993	Heyn et al.	606/198
5,415,664	A		5/1995	Pinchuk	623/1.11
5,580,351	A		12/1996	Helgren et al.	604/411
5,690,644	A		11/1997	Yurek et al.	623/1.11
5,800,517	A	*	9/1998	Anderson et al.	623/1.11
5,906,619	A		5/1999	Olson et al.	606/108
5,980,280	A		11/1999	Zatenauer et al.	623/1.1
6,030,413	A		2/2000	Lazarus	623/1.11
6,063,112	A		5/2000	Sgro	623/1.12
6,203,550	B1		3/2001	Olson	606/108
6,224,609	B1		5/2001	Ressemann et al.	606/108
6,254,609	B1	*	7/2001	Vrba et al.	606/108
6,380,457	B1	*	4/2002	Yurek et al.	623/1.11
6,440,937	B1		8/2002	Bosche et al.	514/19
6,506,179	B1		1/2003	Tiefenthal et al.	604/103.06
6,517,553	B1		2/2003	Klein et al.	606/144
6,530,947	B1	*	3/2003	Euteneuer et al.	623/1.11
6,696,121	B1		2/2004	Jung, Jr. et al.	428/35.7
6,699,275	B1	*	3/2004	Knudson et al.	623/1.12
6,755,856	B1		6/2004	Fierens et al.	623/1.15
2002/0111666	A1		8/2002	Hart et al.	623/1.11
2002/0165554	A1		11/2002	Dworschak et al.	606/108
2003/0051735	A1		3/2003	Pavcnik et al.	128/831
2003/0163189	A1		8/2003	Thompson et al.	623/1.11
2004/0117000	A1		6/2004	Ruetsch	623/1.15

* cited by examiner

Primary Examiner—Corrine McDermott
Assistant Examiner—Thomas J. Sweet
(74) *Attorney, Agent, or Firm*—Wolf Block Schorr & Solis-Cohen LLP

(57) **ABSTRACT**

A first stent delivery system provided with a sheath for covering the stent, the sheath including proximal sheath portion adapted to be movable in a proximal direction and a distal sheath portion adapted to be moveable in a distal direction. A second stent delivery system including an outer and intermediate tubular members covering a chamber with a preloaded stent, the outer tubular member being retractable prior to the retraction of the intermediate sheath and release of the stent. A third stent delivery system including with an inflatable balloon at a distal end of the system for fixing the system in place within the vessel prior to the release of the stent thereby insure accurate stent deployment.

6 Claims, 13 Drawing Sheets

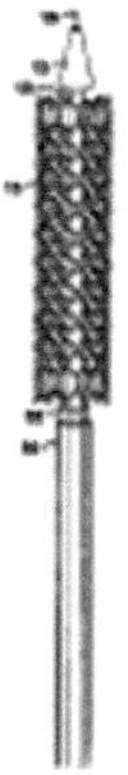

Fig. 5.33 US Patent 7,074,236 B2 stent delivery system

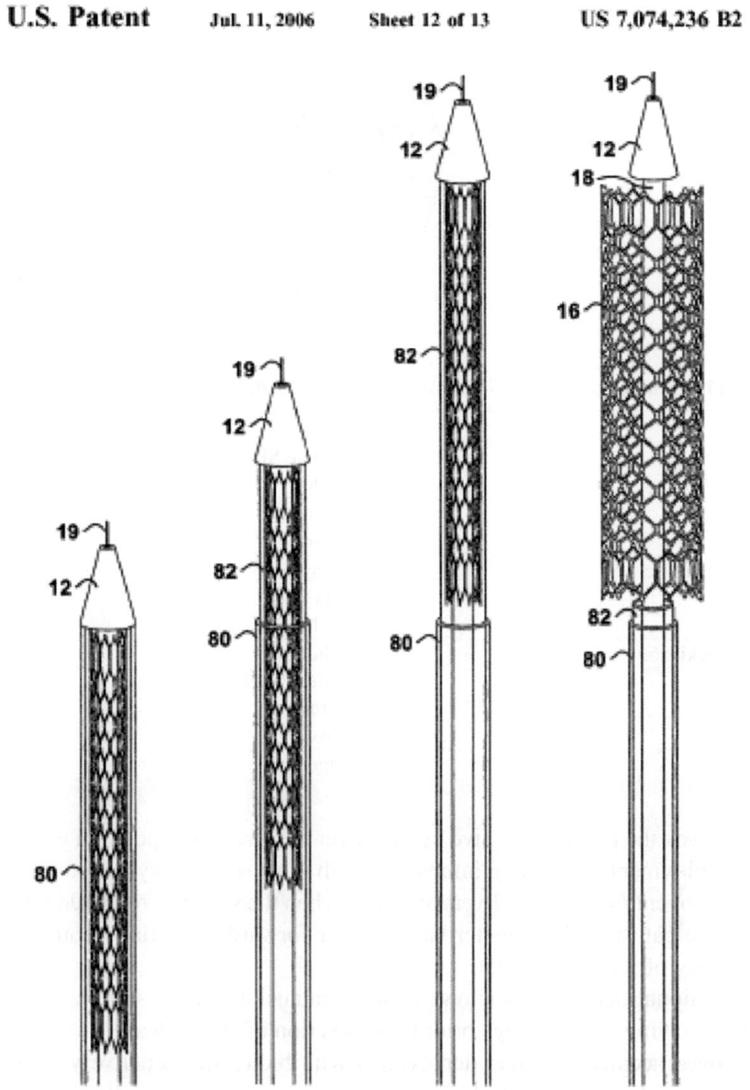

Fig. 5.34 Steps of stent delivery with triaxial system of our design

This gives the operator much more control. If the stent is partially opened in the middle section, but still within the sheath at both ends, it can be repositioned if not placed perfectly, can be re-covered, moved slightly, and redeployed.

The distinguishing feature of this system is that both ends of the stent remain individually controllable during deployment.

The operator can "open distally, adjust, then open proximally," or vice versa, depending on anatomy and accuracy requirements.

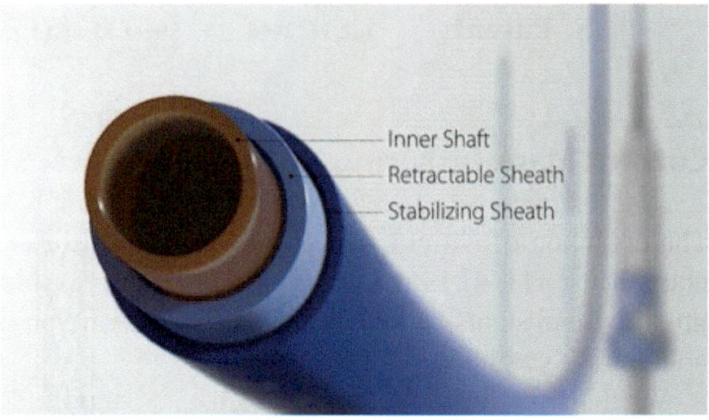

Fig. 5.35 Construction and terminology of triaxial delivery system for self-expanding stents

Table 5.11 Examples of current Nitinol stents with triaxial delivery systems

Company	Product
Medtronic	Complete SE EverFlex
Abbott	Absolute Pro Absolute
Boston Scientific	Innova Eluvia WallFlex
Becton Dickinson	LifeStent LifeStent XL/Solo Covera Venovo
Terumo	Misago Rx

This gives the physician active control over the final stent position even during partial deployment, something impossible with most standard systems.

With conventional stent delivery systems, when the sheath is retracted, the stored radial force can shift the catheter backward or forward, potentially compromising the accuracy of stent placement.

Bidirectional deployment allows counter-balancing forces, stabilizing the system and allowing "fine-tuning" prior to completion of stent release.

Improved accuracy of stent deployment with bidirectional delivery system can be more important in certain clinical scenarios, like iliac bifurcations, subclavian artery origin, carotid bulb, biliary strictures, and complex venous anatomy. Ostial lesions particularly require millimeter-level precision to avoid protrusion into the aorta or missing a portion of the lesion. Bidirectional system allows to first open a proximal end of the stent, final adjustments within the ostium and then complete release of the stent with high accuracy.

By allowing the Nitinol self-expanding stents to open gradually instead of releasing a large radial force all at once, the bidirectional system decreases potential intimal injury, dissection or stretch trauma.

Bidirectional stent delivery systems provide a major upgrade over conventional one-way self-expanding stent systems.

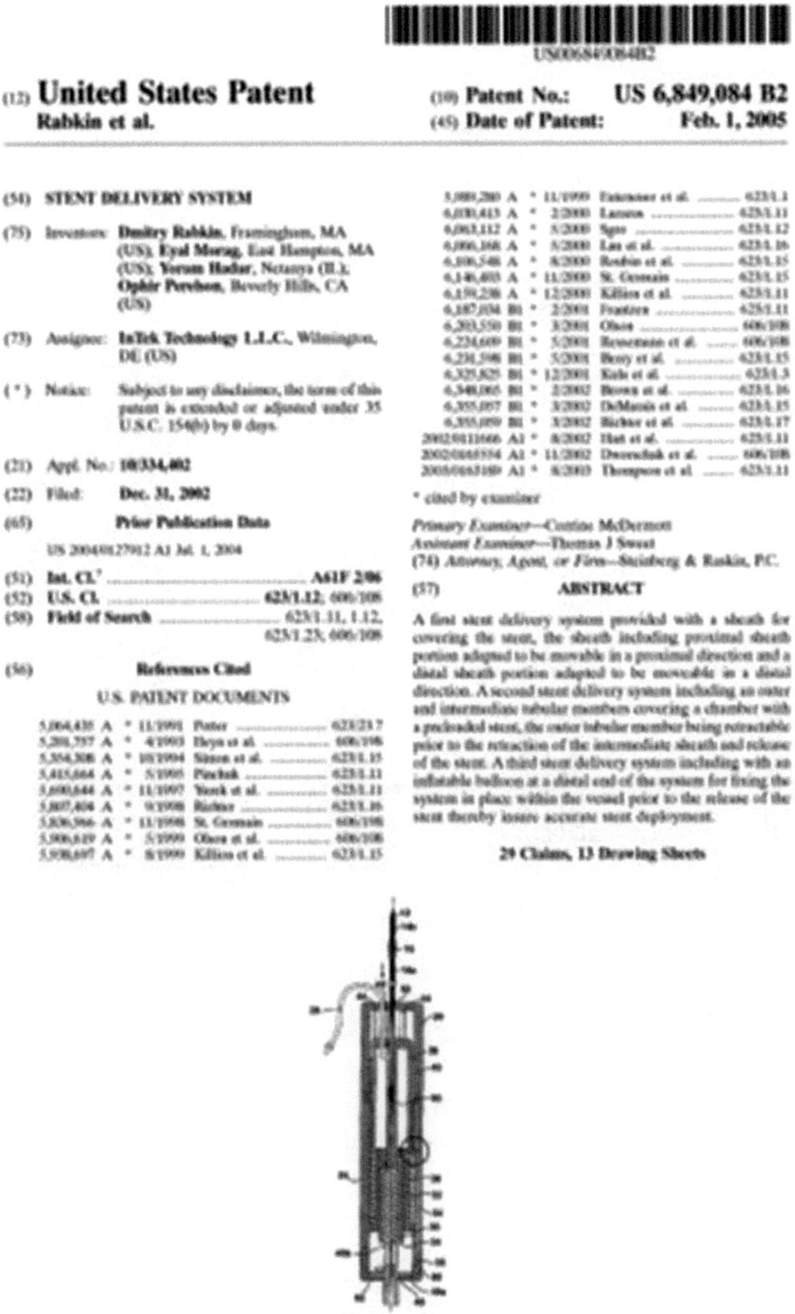

(12) **United States Patent**
Rabkin et al.

(10) **Patent No.: US 6,849,084 B2**
(45) **Date of Patent: Feb. 1, 2005**

(54) **STENT DELIVERY SYSTEM**

(75) Inventors: **Dmitry Rabkin**, Framingham, MA (US); **Eyal Morag**, East Hampton, MA (US); **Yoram Hadar**, Netanya (IL); **Ophir Perelson**, Beverly Hills, CA (US)

(73) Assignee: **InTek Technology L.L.C.**, Wilmington, DE (US)

(*) Notice: Subject to any disclaimer, the term of this patent is extended or adjusted under 35 U.S.C. 154(b) by 0 days.

(21) Appl. No.: **10/334,402**

(22) Filed: **Dec. 31, 2002**

(65) **Prior Publication Data**

(56) **References Cited**

U.S. PATENT DOCUMENTS

* cited by examiner

(57) **ABSTRACT**

A first stent delivery system provided with a sheath for covering the stent, the sheath including proximal sheath portion adapted to be movable in a proximal direction and a distal sheath portion adapted to be moveable in a distal direction. A second stent delivery system including an outer and intermediate tubular members covering a chamber with a preloaded stent, the outer tubular member being retractable prior to the retraction of the intermediate sheath and release of the stent. A third stent delivery system including with an inflatable balloon at a distal end of the system for fixing the system in place within the vessel prior to the release of the stent thereby insure accurate stent deployment.

29 Claims, 13 Drawing Sheets

Fig. 5.36 United States Patent US 6,849,084 B2, featuring the bidirectional delivery system for self-expanding stents

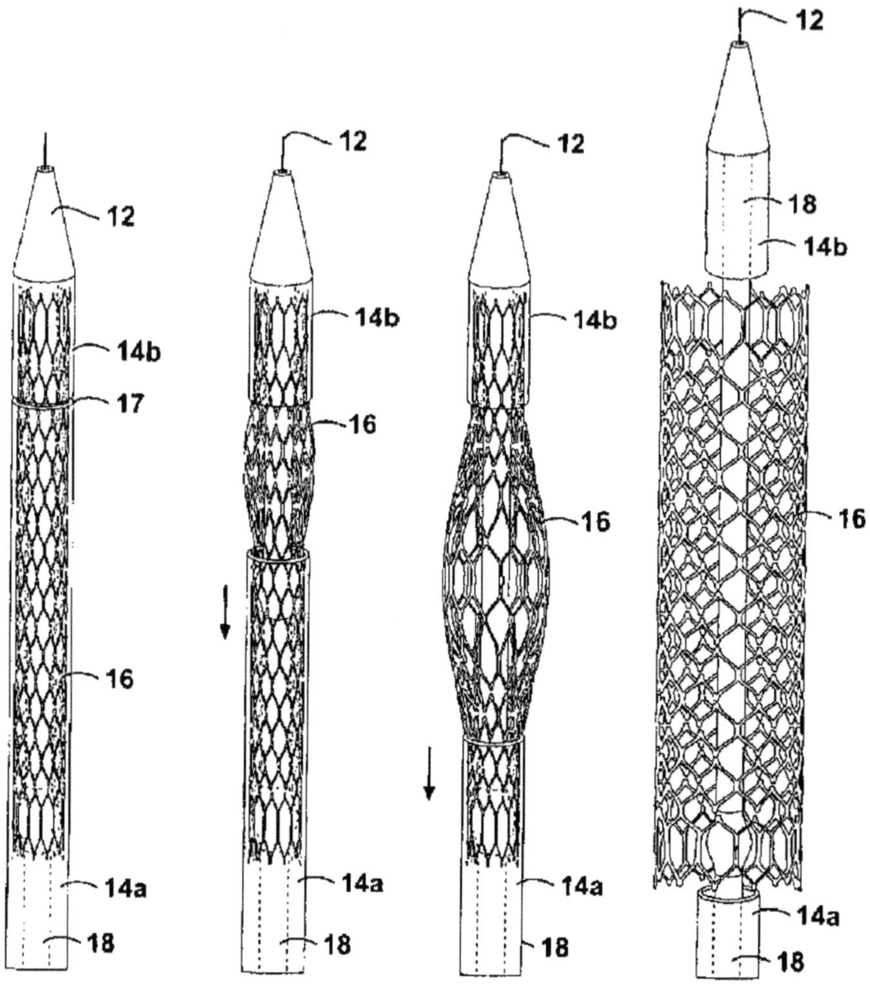

Fig. 5.37 Schematic drawing of the self-expanding stent delivery system with bidirectional opening and steps of stent deployment of our design

They allow deployment from both ends, enabling more precise control, repositioning, and safer placement in complex vascular anatomies.

Key benefits include:

- Superior placement accuracy
- Controlled, gradual deployment
- Ability to recapture and reposition
- Improved safety in tortuous, tapered, or ostial lesions
- Reduced risk of migration or "stent jump"

This technology is especially valuable in delicate or high-precision vascular interventions.

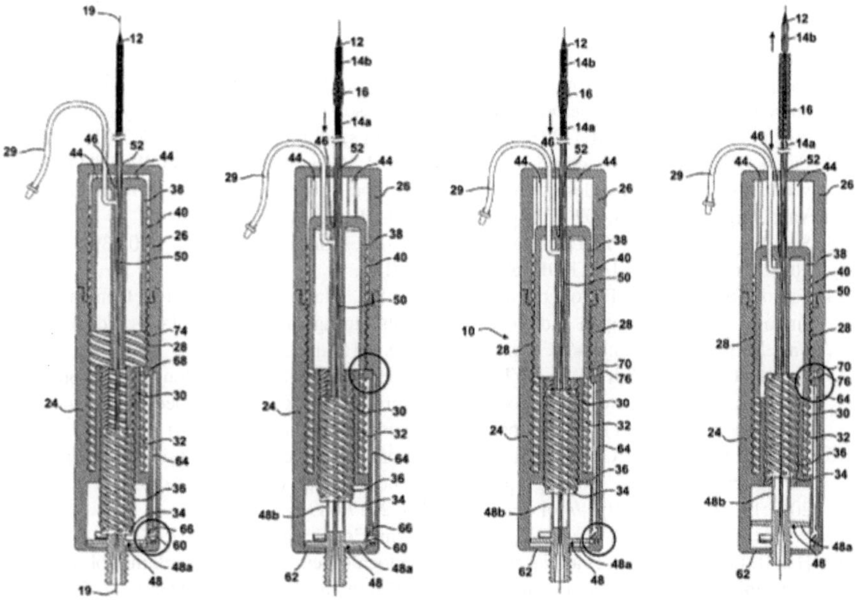

Fig. 5.38 Schematic drawing of the handle controlling bidirectional stent deployment

References

1. Stoeckel D, Pelton A, Duerig T. Self-expanding nitinol stents: material and design considerations. Eur Radiol. 2004;14(2):292–301. https://doi.org/10.1007/s00330-003-2022-5.
2. Mwangi JW, Nguyen LT, Bui VD, Berger T, Zeidler H, Schubert A. Nitinol manufacturing and micromachining: a review of processes and their suitability in processing medical-grade nitinol. J Manuf Process. 2019;38:355–69. https://doi.org/10.1016/j.jmapro.2019.01.003.
3. Vanaei S, Hashemi M, Solouk A, Asghari Ilani M, Amili O, Hefzy MS, et al. Manufacturing, processing, and characterization of self-expanding metallic stents: a comprehensive review. Bioengineering (Basel). 2024;11(10):983. https://doi.org/10.3390/bioengineering11100983.
4. Jiang W, Zhao W, Zhou T, Wang L, Qiu T. A review on manufacturing and post-processing technology of vascular stents. Micromachines (Basel). 2022;13(1):140. https://doi.org/10.3390/mi13010140.
5. Polanec B, Kramberger J, Glodež S. A review of production technologies and materials for manufacturing of cardiovascular stents. Adv Prod Eng Manag. 2020;15(4):390–402. https://doi.org/10.14743/apem2020.4.373.
6. Li Y, Shi Y, Lu Y, Li X, Zhou J, Zadpoor AA, et al. Additive manufacturing of vascular stents. Acta Biomater. 2023;167:16–37. https://doi.org/10.1016/j.actbio.2023.06.014.
7. Palencia-Mercado G, Cedeño-Viveros LD, Elías-Zúñiga A, Vázquez-Lepe EV, Rodríguez-González CA, García-López E. A process chain study for manufacturing nitinol stents. Procedia CIRP. 2024;125:260–5. https://doi.org/10.1016/j.procir.2024.08.045.
8. Kim J, Park JK, Kim HK, Unnithan AR, Kim CS, Park CH. Optimization of electropolishing on NiTi alloy stents and its influence on corrosion behavior. J Nanosci Nanotechnol. 2017;17(4):2333–9. https://doi.org/10.1166/jnn.2017.13324.
9. Udrişte AS, Burduşel AC, Niculescu A-G, Rădulescu M, Grumezescu AM. Coatings for cardiovascular stents—an up-to-date review. Int J Mol Sci. 2024;25(2):1078. https://doi.org/10.3390/ijms25021078.

10. Hoseini SF, Spaggiari A. Design and optimization of a self-expandable NiTi braided stent using MOPSO algorithm. In: X ECCOMAS thematic conference on smart structures and materials (SMART 2023); 2023. p. 454–64.
11. Kang CH, Cho YD, Kim BM, Kim DI, Roh HG, Kim YS, et al. Comparison of open-cell stent and closed-cell stent for carotid artery stenting: assessment of stent geometry and technical outcome. Clin Neuroradiol. 2016;26(2):221–8. https://doi.org/10.1007/s00062-015-0426-1.
12. Pierce DS, Rosero EB, Modrall JG, Adams-Huet B, Valentine RJ, Clagett GP, et al. Open-cell versus closed-cell stent design differences in blood flow velocities after carotid stenting. J Vasc Surg. 2009;49(3):602–6. https://doi.org/10.1016/j.jvs.2008.10.016.
13. Schillinger M, Minar E. Does carotid stent cell design matter? Stroke. 2008;39(3):905–9. https://doi.org/10.1161/STROKEAHA.107.499145.
14. Tadros RO, Spyris CT, Vouyouka AG, Ellozy SH, Marin ML, Faries PL. Comparing the embolic potential of open and closed cell stents during carotid angioplasty and stenting. J Vasc Surg. 2012;56(1):89–95. https://doi.org/10.1016/j.jvs.2012.01.025.
15. Lee HJ, Chen WJ, Shih YT, Tsai YF, Chen CW, Hseu SS. Influence of stenting with open-cell stents vs closed-cell stents on procedure for tortuous vessels: a retrospective study. J Chin Med Assoc. 2019;82(1):44–9. https://doi.org/10.1016/j.jcma.2018.05.001.
16. Tatlı E, Buturak A, Grundüz Y, et al. Comparison of closed-cell vs hybrid-cell stents during carotid artery stenting: procedural and clinical outcomes. Adv Interv Cardiol. 2017;13(2):136–43. https://doi.org/10.5114/aic.2017.68916.
17. Wholey MH, Finol EA. Designing the ideal stent. Endovasc Today. 2007;6:25–34.
18. Han R, Dai W, Wang Y, et al. Fabrication of the locally reinforced open-cell nitinol stents and mechanical properties testing. Int J Precis Eng Manuf Green Technol. 2023;10:47–55. https://doi.org/10.1007/s40684-023-00038-0.
19. Zhang G, Huang Y, Sun Y, et al. Clinical outcomes of carotid artery stenting with open vs closed stent cell design: a large multicenter study. J NeuroIntervent Surg. 2025. Epub ahead of print. https://doi.org/10.1136/jnis-2025-023058.
20. Tadros RO, Malik RK, Vouyouka AG, Ellozy SH, Marin ML, Faries PL. A systematic review of carotid stent design and selection: free-cell area, scaffolding and flexibility. Interv Cardiol. 2013;5(2):207–11. https://doi.org/10.4172/ic.1000145.
21. Hosein F, Bellelli A, Mizzi L, et al. Self-expanding nitinol stents for endovascular peripheral applications: a review. Mater Today Commun. 2024;41:111042.
22. Sabeti S, Schillinger M, Amighi J, et al. Primary patency of femoropopliteal arteries treated with nitinol versus stainless steel self-expanding stents: propensity score–adjusted analysis. Radiology. 2004;232(2):516–21.
23. Yang S, Ni Q, Wang W, et al. Novel self-expanding interwoven nitinol stent for treating femoropopliteal artery disease: 12-month results of a single-center first-in-man study. J Endovasc Ther. 2024;31(5):955–63.
24. Galxerano G, Pasqui E, Anzaldi MG, et al. Use of a self-expanding nitinol stent constructed from two layers of tubular braided nitinol wire mesh in complex femoropopliteal revascularization. J Vasc Surg. 2024;79(4 Suppl):41S.
25. Sullivan T, Zeller T, Nakamura M, et al. Treatment of femoropopliteal lesions with the BioMimics 3D vascular stent system: two-year results from the MIMICS-2 trial. J Endovasc Ther. 2021;28(2):236–45.
26. Balocco S, Rigla J, Andresen R, Wissgott C. One-size-fits-all strategy in carotid artery treatment using the CGuard stent: feasibility and clinical pilot study. CVIR Endovasc. 2025;8:86.
27. Müller-Hülsbeck S, Vajda Z, Odrowaz-Pieniazek P, et al. Contemporary carotid artery stenting practices and peri-procedural outcomes in different European countries: ROADSAVER study multicentric insights. CVIR Endovasc. 2025;8:29.
28. Kluckner M, Nierlich P, Hitzl W, et al. Long-term results of endovascular treatment with nitinol stents for femoropopliteal TASC II C and D lesions. Medicina (Kaunas). 2022;58(9):1225.
29. Tannu M, Jones WS, Swaminathan R, et al. Femoropopliteal endovascular intervention: a review of the current landscape. Circ Cardiovasc Interv. 2025;18(5):e014024.

30. American College of Phlebology. Practice guidelines: management of obstruction of the femoroiliocaval venous system. American College of Phlebology; 2015:1–8.
31. Murphy E. Venous stenting: a behind-the-scenes look at the trial data. Endovasc Today. 2022;21(11):37–42.
32. Ah Taha M, Busutti A, Davies A, et al. Clinical outcomes and overview of dedicated venous stents for management of chronic iliocaval and femoral deep venous system. Phlebology. 2024;30(2):320–30.
33. Morris R, Jackson N, Khan T, et al. Performance of open and closed-cell laser-cut nitinol stents for the treatment of chronic iliofemoral venous outflow obstruction in patients treated at a single centre. Eur J Vasc Endovasc Surg. 2022;63(4):613–21.
34. Williams Z, Dillavou E. A systematic review of venous stents for iliac and venacaval occlusive disease. J Vasc Surg Venous Lymphat Disord. 2020;8(1):145–53.
35. Razavi M, Black S, Gagne P, et al. Pivotal study of endovenous stent placement for symptomatic iliofemoral venous obstruction. Circ Cardiovasc Interv. 2019;12(12):e008268.
36. Murphy E, Gibson K, Sapoval M, et al. Pivotal study evaluating the safety and effectiveness of the Abre venous self-expanding stent system in patients with symptomatic iliofemoral venous outflow obstruction. Circ Cardiovasc Interv. 2022;15(2):e010960.
37. Hoffman L, Gagne P, Brown J, et al. Twelve-month end-point results from the evaluation of the Zilver Vena venous stent in the treatment of symptomatic iliofemoral venous outflow obstruction (VIVO clinical study). J Vasc Surg Venous Lymphat Disord. 2023;11(3):532–41.
38. Dake M, Sullivan G, Shammas N, et al. Three-year results from the Venovo venous stent study for the treatment of iliac and femoral vein obstruction. Cardiovasc Intervent Radiol. 2021;44(12):1918–29.
39. De Wolf M, de Graaf R, Kurstjens R, et al. Short-term clinical experience with a dedicated venous nitinol stent: initial results with the Sinus-Venous stent. Eur J Vasc Endovasc Surg. 2015;50(4):518–26.
40. Bai H, Kibrik P, Shaydakov M, et al. Indications, technical aspects and outcomes of stent placement in chronic iliofemoral venous obstruction. J Vasc Surg Venous Lymphat Disord. 2024;12(5):101904.
41. Sheng C, Lu XW, Shi HT, et al. One-year outcomes of a novel venous stent for symptomatic iliofemoral venous obstruction: prospective cohort study. BMC Med. 2024;22:324.
42. Morris R, Jackson N, Smith A, Black S. A systematic review of the safety and efficacy of inferior vena cava stenting. Eur J Vasc Endovasc Surg. 2023;65(2):298–308.
43. Badesha A, Black S, Khan G, Harper A, et al. A meta-analysis of the medium- to long-term outcomes in patients with chronic deep venous disease treated with dedicated venous stents. J Vasc Surg Venous Lymphat Disord. 2024;12:101722.
44. Gwozdz A, Doyle A, Hunt B, et al. Effect of thrombophilia on clinical outcomes of chronic post-thrombotic patients after iliofemoral stenting with nitinol venous stents. J Vasc Surg Venous Lymphat Disord. 2021;9(4):888–94.
45. Morris R, Khan T, Black S. Complications of deep venous stenting and their management. Cardiovasc Intervent Radiol. 2024;47:1669–76.
46. Mohan B, Adler D. Stents… stents… stents! Biliary and pancreatic stents for ERCP. Pract Gastroenterol. 2023;47(7):27–41.
47. Bezzi M, Orsi F, Salvatori F, et al. Self-expanding nitinol stent for the management of biliary obstruction: long-term clinical results. J Vasc Interv Radiol. 1994;5(1):287–93.
48. Nam HS, Kang DH. Current status of biliary metal stents. Clin Endosc. 2016;49(2):124–30.
49. Jang S, Stevens T, Parsi M, et al. Superiority of self-expanding metallic stents over plastic stents in treatment of malignant biliary strictures. Clin Gastroenterol Hepatol. 2022;20(2):e182–95.
50. Luangsukrerk T. Mechanical property and problems of the self-expandable metal stent in pancreaticobiliary cancer. J Dig Cancer Res. 2022;10(2):92–8.
51. Isayama H, Komatsu Y, Tsujino T, et al. A prospective randomized study of covered versus uncovered diamond stents for management of distal malignant biliary obstruction. Gut. 2004;53(5):729–34.

52. Kullman E, Frozanpor F, Söderlund C, et al. Covered versus uncovered self-expandable nitinol stents in the palliative treatment of malignant distal biliary obstruction: results from a randomized, multicenter study. Gastrointest Endosc. 2010;72(5):915–23.
53. Almadi M, Barkun A, Martel M. No benefit of covered vs uncovered self-expandable metal stents in patients with malignant distal biliary obstruction: a meta-analysis. Clin Gastroenterol Hepatol. 2013;11(1):27–37.
54. Yang MJ, Kim JH, Yoo BM, et al. Partially covered versus uncovered self-expandable nitinol stents with anti-migration properties for the palliation of malignant distal biliary obstruction: a randomized controlled trial. Scand J Gastroenterol. 2015;50(12):1490–9.
55. Elkilany A, Allwarraky M, Denecke T, et al. Stent performance in palliative transhepatic treatment of malignant biliary obstruction: a randomized study comparing covered versus uncovered stents. Acta Radiol. 2020;61(12):1591–9.
56. Han YM, Kwak HS, Jin GY, et al. Treatment of malignant biliary obstruction with a PTFE-covered self-expandable nitinol stent. Korean J Radiol. 2007;8(5):410–7.
57. Wu CH, Wang SF, Lee MH, et al. Efficacy of fully covered self-expandable metal stents for distal biliary obstruction caused by pancreatic ductal adenocarcinoma: primary metal stent vs metal stent following plastic stent. Cancers (Basel). 2023;15(11):3001.
58. Chun JW, Paik WH, Woo SM, et al. Prevention of stent migration of covered self-expandable metal stents in distal malignant biliary obstruction: a review of literature. Gastroenterol Rep. 2025;13:goaf058.
59. Li Y, Yuan K, Deng C, et al. Biliary stents for active materials and surface modification: recent advances and future perspectives. Bioact Mater. 2024;42:587–612.
60. Song G, Zhao H, Liu Q, et al. A review on biodegradable biliary stents: materials and future trends. Bioact Mater. 2022;17:488–95.
61. Gonzalez-Abos C, Lorenzo C, Ausania F. Biodegradable biliary stents in pancreaticoduodenectomy for mitigating biliary complications in high-risk anastomoses. Surg Endosc. 2025;39:4872–80.
62. Winkelbauer FW, Schöfl R, Niederle B, et al. Palliative treatment of obstructing esophageal cancer with nitinol stents: value, safety, and long-term results. AJR Am J Roentgenol. 1996;166(1):79–84.
63. Spaander M, van der Bogt R, Baron T, et al. Esophageal stenting for benign and malignant disease: ESGE guideline 2021. Endoscopy. 2021;53(7):751–62.
64. Hatayama Y, Ishigami H, Kamezaki H, et al. Efficacy of palliative stenting in patients with esophageal obstruction attributable to malignancy. Den Open. 2025;5(1):e70120.
65. Vakil N, Morris A, Marcon N, et al. A prospective, randomized, controlled trial of covered expandable metal stents in the palliation of malignant esophageal obstruction at the gastroesophageal junction. Am J Gastroenterol. 2001;96(6):1791–6.
66. Didden P, Reijm A, Erler N, et al. Fully vs partially covered self-expandable metal stent for palliation of malignant esophageal strictures: a randomized trial (the COPAC study). Endoscopy. 2018;50(10):961–71.
67. Wang C, Wei H, Li H, et al. Comparison of fully covered vs partially covered self-expanding metallic stents for palliative treatment of inoperable esophageal malignancy: a systematic review and meta-analysis. BMC Cancer. 2020;20:73.
68. Kogel L, Reijm A, Lantinga M, et al. Multisegmented esophageal fully covered self-expandable metal stent for palliation of malignant dysphagia: a prospective, multicenter feasibility and safety study. Gastrointest Endosc. 2024;99(6):1027–31.
69. van Halsema E, van Hooft J. Clinical outcomes of self-expandable stent placement for benign esophageal diseases: a pooled analysis of the literature. World J Gastrointest Endosc. 2015;7(2):135–53.
70. van der Bogt R, Nikkessen S, Bruno M, et al. Stents for benign esophageal strictures. Tech Innov Gastrointest Endosc. 2020;22(4):200–4.
71. Bakken J, Wong Kee Song LM, de Groen PC, et al. Use of a fully covered self-expandable metal stent for the treatment of benign esophageal diseases. Gastrointest Endosc. 2010;72(4):712–20.

72. Ong G, Freeman R. Endoscopic management of esophageal leaks. J Thorac Dis. 2017;9(Suppl 2):S135–45.
73. Ong G, Freeman R, Ascioti A, et al. Patient outcomes after stent failure for the treatment of acute esophageal perforation. Ann Thorac Surg. 2018;106(3):830–5.
74. Freeman R, Ascioti A, Dake M, et al. An assessment of the optimal time for removal of esophageal stents used in the treatment of an esophageal anastomotic leak or perforation. Ann Thorac Surg. 2015;100:422–8.
75. Vadutha V, Bashian E, Cholyway R, et al. Efficacy and outcomes of nitinol covered stents for management of acute iatrogenic and secondary esophageal perforation. J Surg Res. 2025;315:482–7.
76. Das K, Hasak S, Elhanafi S, et al. Performance and predictors of migration of partially and fully covered esophageal self-expanding metal stent for malignant dysphagia. Clin Gastroenterol Hepatol. 2021;19(12):2556–63.
77. Yang Y, Yang Y, Hou Z, et al. Comprehensive review of materials, applications, and future innovations in biodegradable esophageal stents. Front Bioeng Biotechnol. 2023;11:1–22.
78. Kim JH, Song HY, Shin JH. Malignant gastric outlet obstructions: treatment with self-expandable metallic stents. Gut Liver. 2010;4(Suppl 1):S32–8.
79. Masuda S, Ichita C, Koizumi K. Practical guide to duodenal stenting for gastric outlet obstruction: clinical outcomes, selection criteria, placement techniques, and management strategies. World J Gastrointest Endosc. 2025;17(6):107189.
80. van Hooft JE, van Montfoort L, Jeurnink SM, et al. Safety and efficacy of a new non-foreshortening nitinol stent in malignant gastric outlet obstruction (DUONITI study): a prospective, multicenter study. Endoscopy. 2011;43(8):671–5.
81. Miwa H, Sugimori K, Kaneko T, et al. Clinical outcome of a highly flexible duodenal stent for gastric outlet obstruction: a multicenter prospective study. JGH Open. 2020;4(4):729–35.
82. Lim GS, Kim CG. Endoscopic stenting for malignant gastric outlet obstruction: focusing on comparison of endoscopic stenting and surgical gastrojejunostomy. Clin Endosc. 2024;57(5):571–80.
83. Sakamoto Y, Sakamoto T, Ohba A, et al. Efficacy of hemostasis by gastroduodenal covered metal stent placement for hemorrhagic duodenal stenosis due to pancreatobiliary cancer invasion: a retrospective study. Clin Endosc. 2024;57(5):628–36.
84. Jue T, Storm A, Naveed M, et al. ASGE guideline on the role of endoscopy in the management of benign and malignant gastroduodenal obstruction. Gastrointest Endosc. 2021;93(2):309–22.
85. Raina H, Patil P, Mehta S. Technical and clinical success rates of WallFlex duodenal stents in unresectable malignant gastric outlet obstruction: a retrospective observational study from a tertiary cancer hospital in India. Prz Gastroenterol. 2022;17(1):41–6.
86. Bashour SI, Lazarus DR. Airway stents in interventional pulmonology. J Respir. 2024;4(1):62–78.
87. Sabath B, Casal R. Airway stenting for central airway obstruction: a review. Media. 2023;7:18.
88. Sosa AF, Michaud GC. Metallic stents in the airway: should we continue to use them and can we remove them? Curr Respir Care Rep. 2013;2:54–60.
89. US Food and Drug Administration. Public health notification: complications from metallic tracheal stents in patients with benign airway disorders. Silver Spring (MD): U.S. Food and Drug Administration; 2005 July 29.
90. Folch E, Keyes C. Airway stents. Ann Cardiothorac Surg. 2018;7:2.
91. Kim JH, Shin JH, Song HY, et al. Benign tracheobronchial strictures: long-term results and factors affecting airway patency after temporary stent placement. AJR Am J Roentgenol. 2007;188(4):1033–8.
92. Xiong X, Xu L, Cheng D, et al. Long-term follow-up of self-expandable metallic stents in benign tracheobronchial stenosis: a retrospective study. BMC Pulm Med. 2019;19:33.
93. Fan M, Li S, Rao W, et al. Efficacy and safety of self-expandable metallic stent on benign tracheobronchial stenosis: a systematic review and meta-analysis. J Thorac Dis. 2025;17(10):8928–39.

94. Ortiz-Comino RM, Morales A, Lopez-Lisbona R, et al. Silicone stent versus fully covered metallic stent in malignant central airway stenosis. Ann Thorac Surg. 2021;111(1):283–9.
95. Han L, Peck EW, Teo E, See KC. Systematic review comparing the efficacy and safety of covered and uncovered self-expanding metal stents in benign airway stenosis. World J Meta-Anal. 2025;13(1):100176.
96. Liu L, Kong J, George C. Recent advances in airway stenting. Shanghai Chest. 2020;4:6.
97. Aravena C, Gildea T. Advancements in airway stents: a comprehensive update. Curr Opin Pulm Med. 2024;30(1):75–83.
98. Schulze AB, Evers G, Tenk FS, et al. Central airway obstruction treatment with self-expanding covered Y-carina nitinol stents: a single center retrospective analysis. Thorac Cancer. 2022;13(7):1040–9.
99. Smith DJ, Vo R, Lachowsky P, et al. Assessing the safety and efficacy of self-expanding metallic Y stents in a community medicine setting. J Respir. 2024;4(4):223–34.
100. Chen S, Du T, Zhang H, et al. Advances in studies on tracheal stent design addressing the related complications. Mater Today Bio. 2024;29:101263.
101. Levy EI, Chaturvedi S. Perforator stroke following intracranial stenting: a sacrifice for the greater good? Neurology. 2006;66:1804.
102. Rabkin D, Morag E, Perelson O, Hadar Y. Stent delivery system. US Patent 7,074,236 B2. 2006 July 11.
103. Rabkin D, Morag E, Hadar Y, Perelson O. Stent delivery system. US Patent application 2005/0038456 A1. 2005 Feb 17.

Mixed Blood

6

Nitinol Stent-Grafts: From Concept to Reality

Background

Nitinol bare-metal stents are intended to use for the purpose of opening up and keeping open the narrowed channels from intrinsic disease, such as atherosclerotic plaque or dissection and from the extrinsic compression by the outside structures, like a tumor or a hematoma. Most of the time the bare-metal self-expanding stents are not helpful in the treatment of vascular aneurysms or vascular injury with ruptured vessels, as the blood can easily go through the openings between the stent struts without sealing an aneurysm or area of extravasation. These are frequently emergent situations and used to be treated with open surgery. In order to treat these conditions with minimally invasive endovascular techniques, new family of devices has been developed by putting together the bare-metal stents and graft materials. Stent-graft is a tubular endoprosthesis combining a metal stent that provides a structural support of the device and serves as a scaffold for attachment of a graft material, usually a synthetic conduit. These devices are most commonly employed in the endovascular aneurysm repair, such as abdominal or thoracic aortic aneurysms, peripheral arterial aneurysms, and vessel injury with internal bleeding.

The first animal implantation of a stent-graft was performed by Dr. Nicolai Volodos in Ukraine in 1986 [1]. In 1991, Dr. Juan C. Parodi, an Argentinian vascular surgeon, performed the first successful human endovascular aneurysm repair using a homemade stent-graft [2]. This was a pivotal moment in vascular surgery.

We (Dmitry Rabkin, Dr. Ducksoo Kim, Dr. Craig Kent, and Stephen Kleshinsky) were one of the first ones exploring this concept and doing extensive research in the development and building multiple prototypes of custom-made stent-grafts. We have designed and built ourselves a series of different Nitinol scaffolds from a single continuous wire in a similar way the prototypes of the Symphony stents were

I. Rabkin, D. J. Rabkin, *Bloodline of Nitinol Stents*,
https://doi.org/10.1007/978-3-032-25697-3_6

made. The handmade frameworks consisted of complex Z-shape or hexagons with varying cell sizes. For some in-vitro experiments we also attached graft material to the commercially available at that time Symphony stents.

For the graft material we have tested different attachments, including Tegaderm Transparent Dressing, Expandable PTFE, Dacron, TecoFlex, Repel Membrane (Figs. 6.1 and 6.2).

Attaching any graft material to a Nitinol metallic scaffold certainly adds overall thickness to the device, particularly when it is compressed inside the delivery system. This makes the delivery catheters more bulky and less flexible. In order to minimize the profile of the devices and their delivery systems we have designed, created, and built Nitinol frameworks with markedly larger cells in their central portions where the graft material is attached. This allowed to have the uniform thickness along the length of the devices when collapsed for loading into the delivery system. A thin layer of the graft material does not add much to overall thickness to

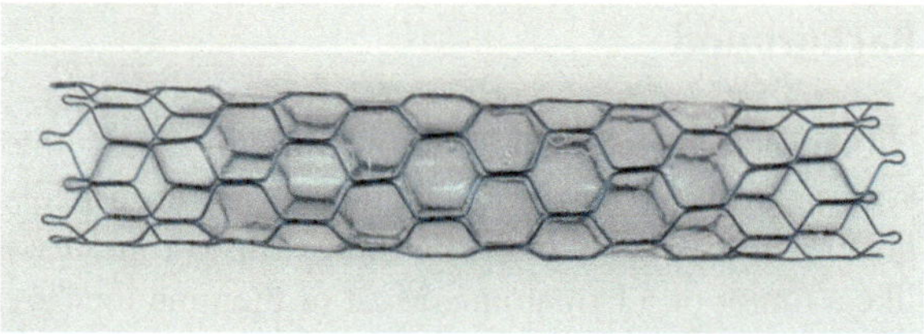

Fig. 6.1 Custom-handmade Nitinol scaffold with uniform cells along its length, covered with TecoFlex in the central portion of the stent-graft

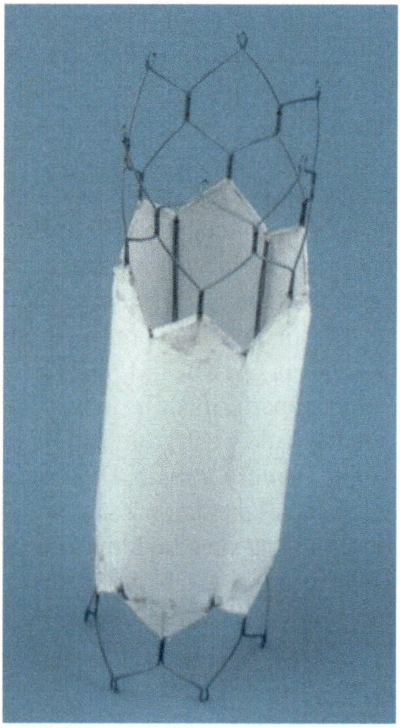

Fig. 6.2 Custom-handmade Nitinol scaffold with Repel Membrane attachment in the central portion of the stent-graft

the device when attached only over the large elongated cell, which can collapse almost into straight wires, making it easier to restrain the device within lowest possible profile delivery catheters. The large elongated cells provide much less radial force, which is not really needed when placed across the aneurysm sack or in the bleeding vessel. At the same time, they offer adequate framework to support the graft material and exhibit sufficient radial force to facilitate the proper opening of the attached graft. The regular configuration cells at the end of the stents provide secure anchoring of the devices in the blood vessels (Fig. 6.3).

We used commercially available and modified vascular sheaths 12–14 Fr to construct the delivery system for our stent-grafts (Fig. 6.4). The size of the delivery catheters was determined by the size of the device and thickness of the attached graft material.

The design of our stent-grafts with adopted elongated large cells in the Nitinol scaffold for the graft attachment allowed to markedly reduce the profile of the delivery catheters (Fig. 6.5) [3].

We have experimented with different patterns of graft material attachments to the Nitinol scaffolds. One version was the straight cut edge of the graft (Fig. 6.6b) and the second version with the zigzag edge, repeating the contour of the Nitinol wire scaffold (Fig. 6.6a). With the straight edge graft, there is a "free floating" fabric crossing the scaffold cells without direct support, while with zigzag pattern the edges of the graft material are in continuous contact with the supporting wires.

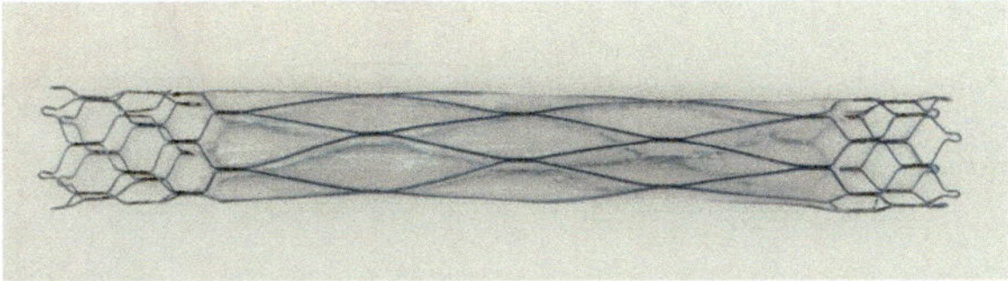

Fig. 6.3 Custom-handmade Nitinol scaffold with central elongated large cells for attachment of the TecoFlex graft material in order to minimize the profile of the collapsed devices for smaller delivery system

Fig. 6.4 Custom-handmade delivery system with partially released stent-graft of our design

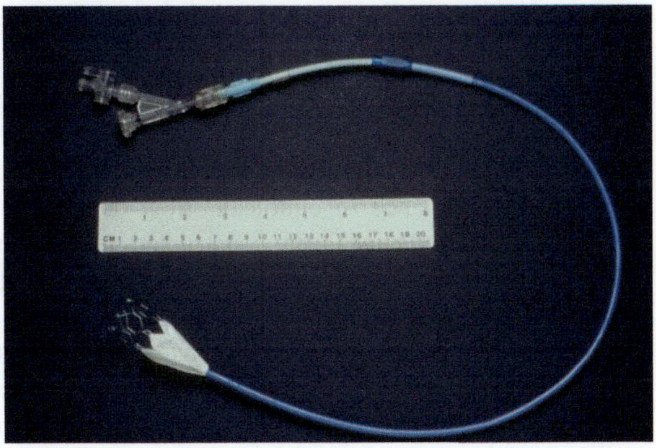

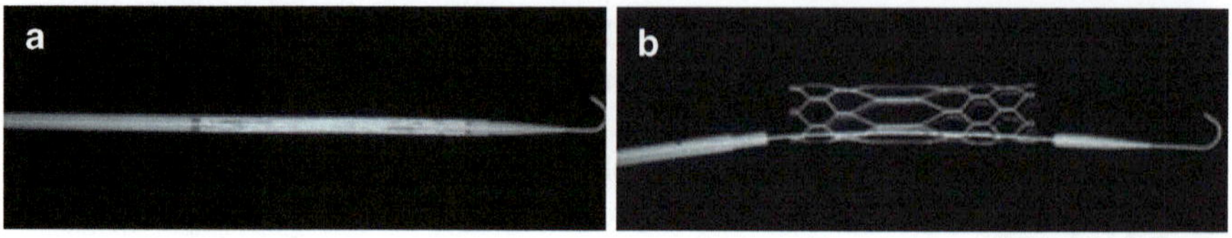

Fig. 6.5 X-rays of the custom-handmade delivery system with loaded stent-graft of our design (**a**) and released stent-graft by retracting the outer sheath (**b**)

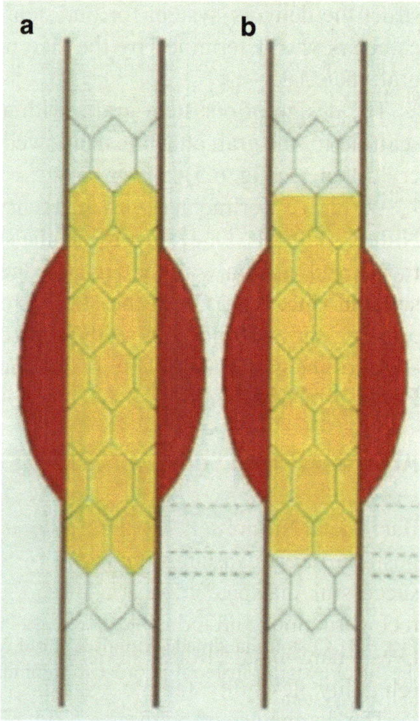

Fig. 6.6 Schematic drawing of two versions of graft material attachment to the Nitinol wire scaffold: (**a**) Zigzag edge, following the course of the wire; (**b**) Straight cut edge, crossing the spaces between the wires

The stent-grafts are always oversized with respect to the diameter of the vessel where they are intended to be placed in order to provide secure fixation, prevent migration, and make a tight seal, so the blood does not go around the graft material, preventing type 1 endoleak. We have tested if the nature of graft material and the pattern of its attachment to the Nitinol scaffold have any influence on the device behavior and incidence of endoleak (flow outside of the graft material in-situ). Custom-handmade devices were constructed with a 30 mm in diameter Nitinol wire scaffold with attached Repel Membrane as a graft material. On one end the graft edges had a zigzag configuration following the pattern of the wire contour. On the other end of the same device the graft had a straight cut border with the free edges crossing in the middle of the frame cells (Fig. 6.7). The devices were placed into a 25 mm in diameter plastic tubing to reproduce the degree of oversize which would

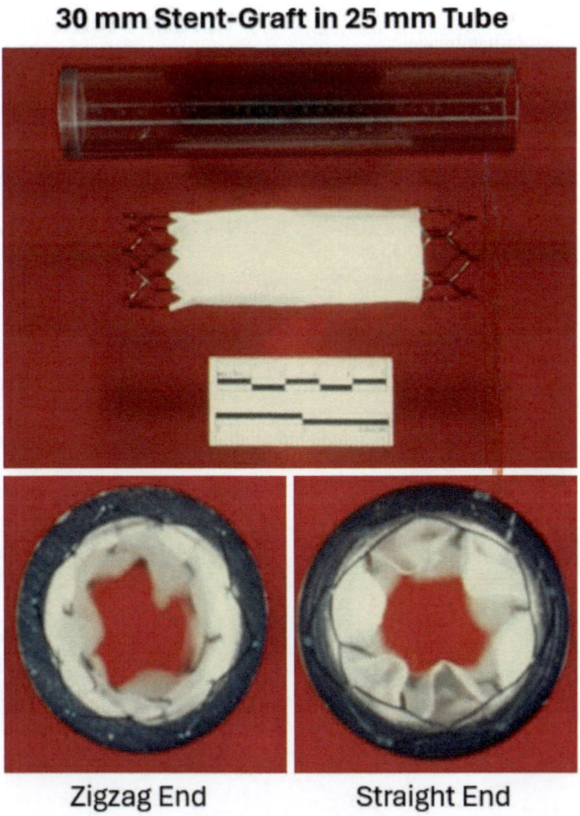

Fig. 6.7 Custom-handmade stent-graft with different pattern of Repel Membrane graft attachment to the Nitinol frame (zigzag on one end and straight on the other end) and cross-sectional views of the device placed into a smaller plastic tube to imitate the blood vessel. There are free flap pockets of graft material with a straight cut pattern and a tight seal with a zigzag attachment

be used in real scenario for this size stent-graft. It demonstrated that with straight edge graft attachment there is an inward protrusion of the free edges of the graft material, creating intraluminal "pockets," when the device is placed into a tube of smaller diameter (Fig. 6.7). With the zigzag edge graft attachment, the graft material is pushed uniformly against the wall of the tube by the wire of the Nitinol frame, eliminating free edges (Fig. 6.7).

We also applied TecoFlex coating to the commercially available Symphony Nitinol stents with two patterns of coating attachments: straight cut and zigzag edges. We tested these devices in similar conditions by placing 14 mm in diameter stent-grafts into 12 mm tubes (Fig. 6.8). It has reproduced the same effect of intraluminal "pockets" of graft material with straight cut attachment, but to a somewhat lesser extent as TecoFlex material is more elastic and stretchable than a Repel Membrane. In our opinion it is beneficial to have a zigzag pattern of graft material attachment to the stent frame, particularly if non-compliant fabrics are used. This would prevent any potential thrombus formation inside the "pockets" and possibly eliminate or decrease the incidence of endoleaks [4].

In order to evaluate if the phenomenon of intraluminal "pockets" of free edges of the straight cut graft material has any influence on degree and occurrence of

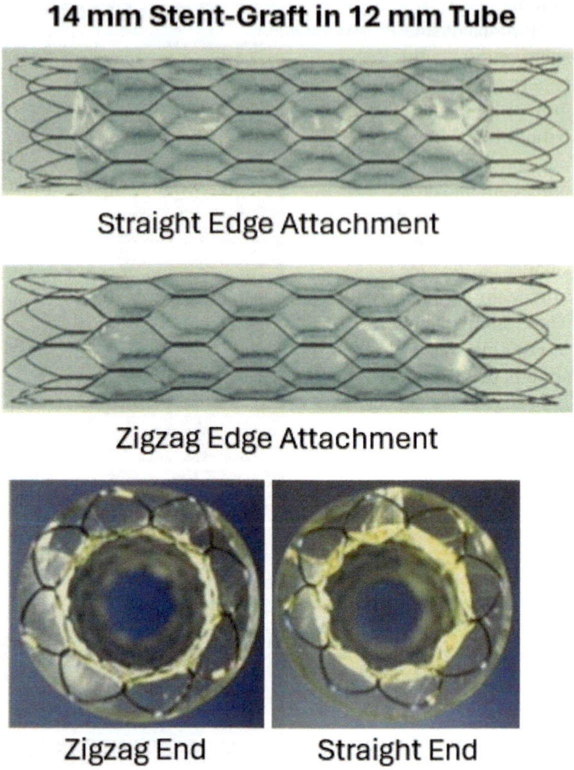

Fig. 6.8 Custom-handmade stent-graft with different pattern of TecoFlex graft attachment to the Nitinol frame and cross-sectional views of the device placed into a smaller plastic tube to imitate the blood vessel. The cross-sections show the zigzag and straight edge designs from an end-on perspective, highlighting the structural differences and effect of graft attachment pattern

endoleak, we have built the in-vitro flow model to test our stent-grafts in the conditions closely imitating the natural environment. It consisted of the Harvard Cardiovascular Pump, heated reservoir for circulating fluid, and the system of tubes with simulated vessel for stent-graft placement (Fig. 6.9).

The pump provided pulsatile flow at 72 beats per minute and the stroke volume of 30 ml. We used 44% Glycerin solution at 37 °C to closely reproduce the specific gravity and viscosity of blood. The pressure in the system was 35/20 mm Hg. The stent-grafts were constructed using commercially available Symphony stents (Boston Scientific), 14 mm in diameter and 60 ml length, with attached Tegaderm transparent dressing as a graft material in two versions, with straight cut edge and zigzag edge. Six conditions were simulated with both versions at different length of the "aneurysm neck." There were 15 stent-graft deliveries per condition and each device was tested for 30 min.

Our experiments demonstrated that adopting the contoured (zigzag) attachment of graft material to Nitinol stent frames minimizes endoleak in-vitro [5].

This effect is more pronounced when the neck of the aneurysm is short. There is an inverse relationship of the neck covered by the stent-graft and degree of endoleak, regardless of graft attachment (Fig. 6.10).

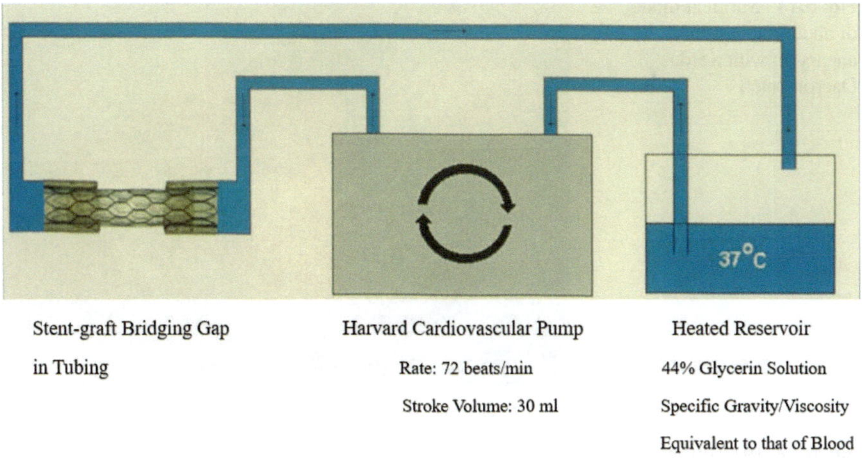

Fig. 6.9 Diagram of In-Vitro Flow Circuit for stent-grafts testing

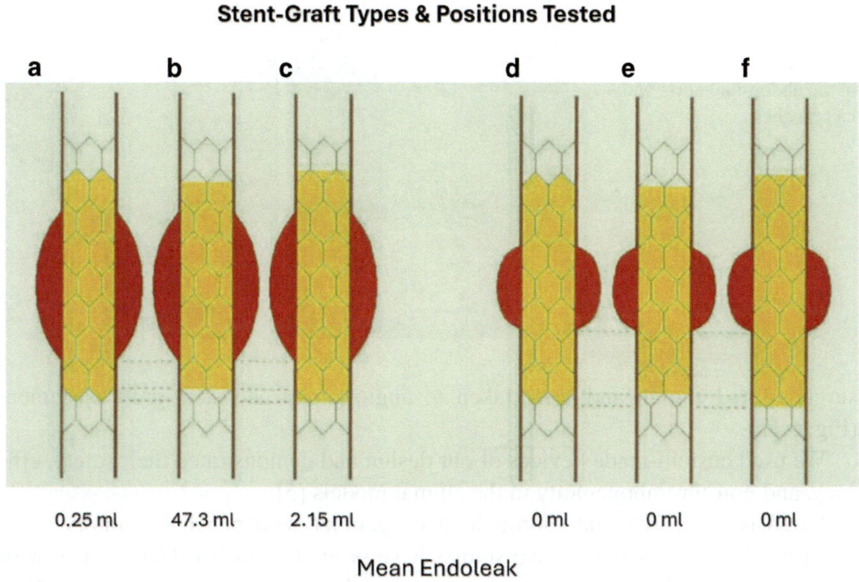

Fig. 6.10 Schematic drawing of the summary of in-vitro flow model experiments

This preliminary work and an in-vitro investigations led us to the animal experiments. We (Dmitry Rabkin, Dr. Ducksoo Kim, and Dr. Craig Kent) have created an animal model of abdominal aortic aneurysm by surgically making a side outpouching with a Dacron material in pigs (Fig. 6.11). The animals were recovered from

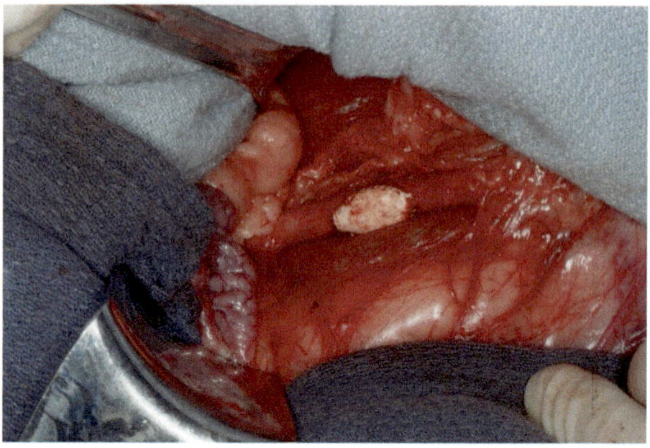

Fig. 6.11 Surgical model of abdominal aortic aneurysm with a side Dacron patch

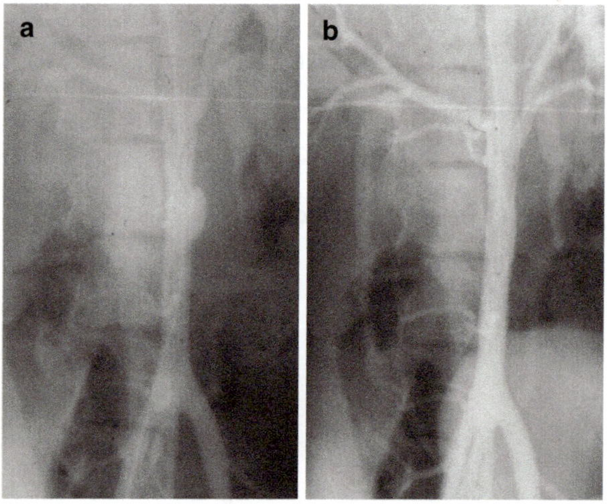

Fig. 6.12 (**a**) Aortogram demonstrates saccular aneurysm of the abdominal aorta. (**b**) Aortogram after endovascular stent-graft placement demonstrates no opacification of the aneurysm and normal flow in the abdominal aorta and its branches

surgery for 1 month and were taken to angiography and stent-graft placement (Fig. 6.12).

We used custom-made devices of our design and demonstrated their safety, efficacy, and non-thrombogenicity in the animal models [5].

Extensive research and thorough investigations with bench laboratory scale experiments, in-vitro and in-vivo studies have promoted further development with fine-tuning of the Nitinol-based stent-grafts and their implementation into the clinical practice.

Current Status

Nitinol stent-grafts are now the dominant platform for endovascular repair of abdominal and thoracic aortic aneurysms and are widely used in selected peripheral vascular beds. In all of these systems, a self-expanding Nitinol scaffold provides radial support and fixation, while an attached graft component made of ePTFE or woven polyester excludes blood flow from the aneurysm sac or diseased segment. Nitinol's superelasticity, fatigue resistance, and corrosion resistance make it particularly suited to these applications, in which devices must be crimped to very small diameters, navigate tortuous anatomy, then recover a stable configuration that can withstand millions of cardiac cycles without fracture [6].

From a design perspective, contemporary aortic stent-grafts use modular constructions with main bodies and iliac limbs or separate thoracic segments, with proximal fixation achieved by bare or partially covered Nitinol rings that incorporate barbs, hooks, or dual-ring configurations. The graft material is typically ePTFE or polyester; despite extensive use of both, there is still no definitive clinical evidence that one fabric is systematically superior, and failures are more often related to anatomy, undersizing, neck degeneration, or fatigue of the metallic scaffold than to the fabric itself [7]. Finite-element and fluid–structure interaction studies have focused on Nitinol strut geometry, crimping strains, sealing pressures at the proximal, and distal landing zones and fatigue safety factors, confirming that superelastic Nitinol can tolerate crimping and cyclic loading better than many alternative alloys, while also highlighting the importance of avoiding excessive plastic strain in hinge regions and at overlap zones [8].

For infrarenal abdominal aortic aneurysms, Nitinol stent-grafts are standard of care in anatomically suitable patients and are also widely used outside classical IFU in "hostile necks" by experienced operators. The Gore Excluder family is a prototypical example of a self-expandable Nitinol–ePTFE stent-graft system; in early series of 72 patients, Nitinol–ePTFE Excluder devices achieved high technical success and acceptable mid-term durability, with low peri-procedural mortality and manageable rates of endoleak and secondary interventions [9]. The Medtronic Endurant AAA stent-graft uses laser-cut suprarenal Nitinol rings with anchoring pins for proximal fixation and a series of Nitinol wire stents sewn to polyester fabric for the body and limbs, specifically engineered to treat short, angulated necks and tortuous iliac arteries without kinking [10]. The Terumo Aortic Anaconda system, composed of ultrathin polyester supported by multiple individual circular Nitinol rings and a distinctive dual-ring proximal configuration, is another example of an entirely Nitinol-based skeleton designed to maximize conformability to difficult infrarenal necks [11].

Large observational series and randomized comparisons of EVAR versus open repair, including devices with Nitinol scaffolds, consistently show reduced perioperative mortality, shorter hospital stay, and improved early quality of life with EVAR, at the cost of higher rates of late reintervention for endoleak, migration, limb occlusion or sac enlargement, and a requirement for lifelong imaging surveillance [12]. Many of the late problems are now recognized as interaction effects between device design and anatomy: short or conical necks, heavy thrombus, severe angulation, and ongoing neck dilatation predispose to proximal type 1 endoleaks or migration, whereas limb kinking and small outflow vessels predispose to limb thrombosis.

Material-focused reviews have pointed out that although Nitinol scaffolds have excellent fatigue performance, repetitive bending and torsion at hinge points, overlap zones and in highly mobile segments of the aorta may still generate microcrack formation over long follow-up; these insights are pushing manufacturers toward smoother strut transitions, more homogeneous ring spacing and more forgiving overlap zones [7].

Nitinol-based fenestrated and branched AAA and thoracoabdominal devices extend these principles into more complex anatomies. Custom and off-the-shelf systems incorporate fenestrations, scallops, and side branches supported by Nitinol rings, with bridging covered stents used to maintain perfusion to the renal, visceral, or arch vessels while still excluding the aneurysm sac. Modern design overviews emphasize how Nitinol's flexibility is crucial for these complex constructs, which must accommodate significant curvature and torsion at the pararenal and visceral segments without kinking or losing seal [13]. Early and mid-term outcomes for fenestrated and branched Nitinol stent-grafts show acceptable target vessel patency and sac regression in high-risk cohorts, but they also underline the cumulative effect of multiple junctions and overlaps on fatigue and the importance of precise planning, oversizing strategy, and landing zone quality.

In the thoracic aorta, self-expanding Nitinol stent-grafts are central to thoracic endovascular aortic repair (TEVAR) for descending thoracic aneurysms, chronic and acute Stanford type B dissections, penetrating ulcers, and traumatic transection. Devices such as the Valiant series pair a polyester graft with a Nitinol exoskeleton and often incorporate a modified proximal bare stent that increases fixation in the arch while minimizing coverage of the left subclavian artery [14]. Historical and contemporary reviews show that TEVAR with Nitinol stent-grafts achieves high technical success and perioperative mortality in the low single digits for elective descending thoracic aneurysm repair, with substantial reductions in early morbidity compared with open thoracotomy and graft replacement [14]. For high-risk indications such as traumatic aortic injury in young patients, specifically curved Nitinol stent-grafts have been developed to conform to the tight curvature of the aortic arch and proximal descending aorta, with small series demonstrating excellent exclusion of injury, rapid stabilization, and low device-related complication rates [15].

Despite these successes, long-term TEVAR follow-up has revealed challenges analogous to infrarenal EVAR but magnified by thoracic biomechanics. The thoracic aorta is subject to greater curvature, motion, and pulsatile strain, so Nitinol rings experience higher cyclic stresses, particularly at the proximal and distal edges near the arch and diaphragm. Device-related complications such as proximal endoleak, retrograde type A dissection triggered by aggressive bare stent fixation, stent-graft infolding or collapse in very small or angulated arches, and distal stent-induced new entry tears in chronic dissections are all recognized issues [14]. Ongoing refinements include lower-profile delivery systems, more gradual proximal flare, optimized radial force distribution, and hybrid constructs that combine Nitinol stent-grafts with surgical debranching or arch reconstruction.

In peripheral arteries, Nitinol stent-grafts occupy a more selective but important niche, primarily in the treatment of superficial femoral and proximal popliteal artery disease, isolated aneurysms, and complex restenotic lesions, as well as selected iliac, tibial, and visceral segments. The Viabahn ePTFE-covered self-expanding Nitinol stent-graft is the best-studied example. In a randomized 4-year comparison of femoropopliteal Viabahn stent-grafts versus prosthetic femoropopliteal bypass, primary patency was somewhat lower in the endovascular arm, but assisted primary and secondary patency and limb salvage were comparable, with the trade-off of more frequent but less invasive reinterventions versus the higher early morbidity of bypass surgery [16]. These findings have supported a "bypass-equivalent" role for Nitinol stent-grafts in selected SFA lesions, especially in patients at higher surgical risk or lacking suitable vein conduit.

More broadly, reviews of peripheral arterial stenting highlight that third-generation self-expanding Nitinol platforms, whether bare or covered, provide greater flexibility and resistance to deformation than earlier stainless steel designs, which is crucial in the femoropopliteal segment subjected to flexion, torsion, and compression during limb movement [17]. Covered Nitinol stent-grafts add the ability to exclude highly calcified plaque, aneurysms or pseudoaneurysms and to seal perforations or dissections, at the cost of higher thrombosis risk if inflow or outflow are inadequate. Contemporary development programs, such as the AGILITY study of a next-generation self-expanding covered stent for advanced PAD, emphasize trackability through tortuous vessels, uniform wall apposition, and long-term flexibility to minimize fracture and edge restenosis [18]. Nitinol-covered stents are also widely used for isolated iliac aneurysms, popliteal aneurysms, visceral and renal artery aneurysms, traumatic arterial injuries, and failing dialysis access, although many of these uses rely on observational rather than randomized data.

On the engineering side, recent work has delved into detailed computational analysis of Nitinol stent-grafts in the aorta, quantifying crimping strains, radial forces, sealing pressures and the impact of thermo-mechanical deployment strategies. Some groups have proposed exploiting Nitinol's temperature-dependent shape recovery to achieve more controlled, gentle deployment by warming or cooling the device, potentially reducing trauma to fragile necks or dissection flaps [8]. New prototype systems for AAA repair using Nitinol frameworks have been optimized through finite-element analysis to balance radial strength and fatigue life, with in-vitro validation confirming that appropriately tuned Nitinol geometries can maintain high fatigue safety factors even under severe pulsatile loading [19]. Experimental work with thin-film Nitinol as a graft covering has shown the feasibility of ultra-low-profile devices with excellent impermeability and flexibility, although these concepts remain investigational and have not yet translated into routine clinical devices [20].

Overall, the current status can be summarized as follows. For abdominal and thoracic aortic aneurysms, Nitinol stent-grafts represent mature, widely adopted technologies that have fundamentally changed the risk profile of aneurysm repair, but they still require careful patient selection and lifelong surveillance because of material–anatomy interactions that can lead to endoleaks, migration, and fatigue-related issues. In peripheral vessels, Nitinol stent-grafts have established roles in femoropopliteal and iliac disease and are increasingly used in complex lesions and aneurysms where plaque exclusion and durable sealing are critical, with performance approaching surgical bypass in selected scenarios but at the cost of higher reintervention rates. Across all territories, future progress is likely to come from further refinement of Nitinol geometry, better understanding of fatigue mechanisms, more sophisticated pre-procedural planning with patient-specific simulations, and possibly new graft materials or bioactive coatings designed to modulate neointimal response at the edges and branch interfaces, while preserving the core advantages of the Nitinol scaffold.

Stent-grafts represent a major advancement in vascular and endovascular medicine, enabling minimally invasive treatment of life-threatening vascular conditions with reduced recovery times. They are now widely used in the management of aortic aneurysm, dissections, and traumatic injuries, and their applications continued to expand as technology advances. Ongoing innovation is addressing limitations in design and applicability, making them increasingly versatile and effective across a wider range of vascular pathologies.

The primary goals of stent-graft use include:

- Preventing aneurysm rupture by excluding the aneurysm sac from blood flow and arterial pressure.
- Restoring vascular integrity in cases of dissection or vessel injury.
- Avoiding the need for open surgery, reducing recovery time, morbidity, and mortality.

Stent-grafts are indicated in a variety of vascular pathologies, particularly:

Aortic Aneurysms
  - Abdominal Aortic Aneurysm (AAA): The most common use. Endovascular Aneurysm Repair (EVAR) involves deploying a stent-graft in the abdominal aorta to exclude the aneurysm.
  - Thoracic Aortic Aneurysm (TAA): Treated with Thoracic Endovascular Aortic Repair (TEVAR), using larger, more flexible stent-grafts.

Aortic Dissections
  - Type B aortic dissections (descending aorta): Stent-grafts can help seal the entry tear and promote false lumen thrombosis.

Traumatic Aortic Injury
  - Especially in young patients with blunt thoracic trauma; stent-grafts are often lifesaving and minimally invasive.

Peripheral Arterial Disease (PAD)
  - Used in arteries such as the iliac, femoral, and popliteal arteries for treating stenosis or aneurysmal disease.

Arteriovenous Fistulas or Grafts
  - For dialysis access, stent-grafts may be used to repair pseudoaneurysms or treat stenoses in the outflow tract.

Other Indications

- Endoleaks after previous EVAR or TEVAR.
- Visceral artery aneurysms (renal, splenic, etc.).
- Venous indications, though less common, such as in treating iliac vein obstructions or endovenous stent-grafting.

Nitinol is the most commonly used metal in self-expanding stent-grafts because it offers a unique combination of mechanical and biological properties that outperform other metals like stainless steel or cobalt-chromium in many vascular applications.

Nitinol can undergo large deformations and return to its original shape without permanent damage. This allows the stent scaffold to compress into a small delivery system and expand to large diameter once deployed, adapting to vessel size, curvature, and movement (important in tortuous vessels like the iliac and SFA). Other metals like stainless steel lack this property and may deform permanently under stress.

Nitinol can "remember" its original shape and return to it when heated to body temperature. This enables precise deployment, which is critical in endovascular procedures where the stent-graft must be compact during insertion and then expand accurately, frequently to much larger size to accommodate the dimensions of thoracic or abdominal aorta.

Nitinol frames of stent-grafts naturally apply constant outward pressure, helping anchor the devices to vessel wall, preventing migration, which is critical for long-term success, particularly in the setting of very high flow like in the thoracic or abdominal aorta. It also reliably expands the graft material and permanently keeps it open to the intended size.

Vast majority of currently available for clinical use stent-grafts utilizes Nitinol scaffolds. Commercially available stent-grafts are produced by several medical device manufacturers and vary by indication (e.g., EVAR, TEVAR, peripheral use) and design (e.g., standard, fenestrated, branched). The choice between the different devices depends on factors such as the location and size of the aneurysm, the patient's anatomy, and operator's preference (Tables 6.1, 6.2, and 6.3).

Table 6.1 Commercially Available Stent-grafts for Endovascular Abdominal Aortic Aneurysm Repair

Device	Manufacturer	Frame Material	Notes
Endurant II/IIs	Medtronic	Nitinol	Highly conformable
AneuRx	Medtronic	Nitinol	Modular device
Talent	Medtronic	Nitinol	Suprarenal uncovered stent
Gore Excluder	Gore Medical	Nitinol	PTFE graft
Incraft	Cordis	Nitinol	Ultra-low profile (13 Fr)
Treovance	Terumo	Nitinol	PET graft
AFX2	Endologix	Cobalt-chromium	Suprarenal version
Ovation	TriVascular	Nitinol	Trimodular design Unique sealing

Table 6.2 Commercially Available Stent-grafts for Thoracic Endovascular Aortic Repair

Device	Manufacturer	Frame Material	Notes
Gore TAG	Gore Medical	Nitinol	Excellent for tortuous anatomy
RelayPlus	Terumo	Nitinol	Woven polyester
RelayPro	Terumo	Nitinol	Low profile
Valiant	Medtronic	Nitinol	Suprarenal uncovered stent, not in USA
E-nside	Artivion	Nitinol	Multibranch system

Table 6.3 Commercially Available Stent-grafts for Peripheral Vascular Indications

Device	Manufacturer	Frame Material	Notes
Viabahn	Gore Medical	Nitinol	e-PTFE graft
Viatorr	Gore Medical	Nitinol	Uncovered portion for TIPS
Viabil	Gore Medical	Nitinol	Biliary strictures
Covera	BD Interventional	Nitinol	Hemodialysis access Venous disease
Fluency Plus	BD Interventional	Nitinol	Arterial and venous disease, AVF

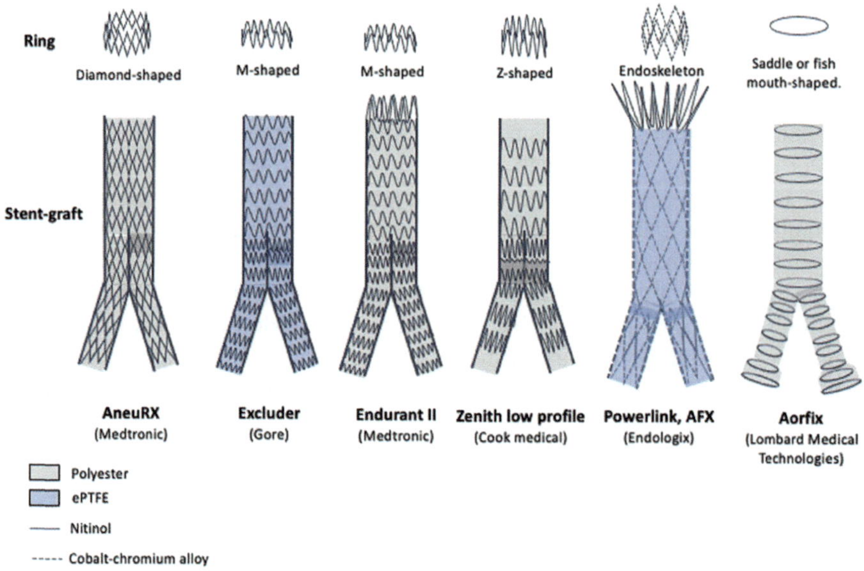

Fig. 6.13 Schematic drawing illustrating the various types of metal frames of commercially available stent-grafts for EVAR [50]

Metallic scaffolds of stent-grafts differ in their constructions from distinctive manufacturers, but all serve the same purpose of secure fixation within the vessels and ensuring proper expansion of the attached graft material with long-term continuous support (Fig. 6.13).

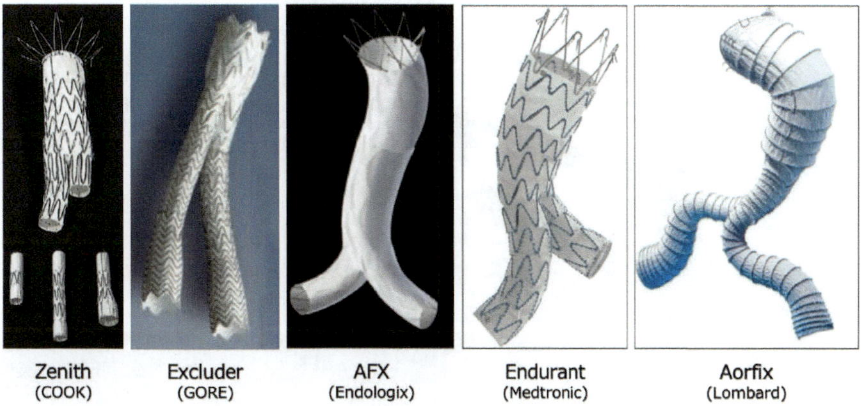

Fig. 6.14 Commercially available stent-grafts for EVAR

Stent-grafts for EVAR are specialized devices used to reinforce the aortic wall in patients with abdominal aortic aneurysms (AAA). EVAR is a minimally invasive alternative to open surgical repair and involves inserting a stent-graft through the femoral arteries and deploying it within the aorta to exclude the aneurysm sac from blood flow, thus preventing rupture. There are different types of stent-grafts used in EVAR: unibody stent-grafts, bifurcated stent-grafts, aorto-uni-iliac devices, fenestrated and branched devices (Fig. 6.14).

Stent-grafts for Thoracic Aortic Aneurysms (TEVAR) are designed to treat aneurysms in the thoracic aorta, particularly in the descending thoracic segment. TEVAR is now the preferred approach for many thoracic aneurysms due to its lower perioperative risk compared to open surgical repair. The procedure is performed from the femoral arterial access with deployment of the devices into the thoracic aorta, across the aneurysm, preventing rupture or dissection, while maintaining the flow to the brachiocephalic branches (Fig. 6.15).

Stent-grafts for the peripheral arterial disease are primarily used in the iliac, femoral, and popliteal arteries to treat occlusive disease. They are more effective than bare-metal stents in long lesions and heavily calcified vessels, as they inhibit intimal hyperplasia and prevent distal embolization. Some of the devices like Gore Viabahn include heparin-bonded layers to reduce incidence of thrombosis. Peripheral arteries (like the SFA and popliteal) are highly mobile and undergo compression, torsion, elongation, and bending. Peripheral stent-grafts are very flexible, allowing them to conform to vessel curvature without kinking or fracturing even when remain in situ long term (Fig. 6.16).

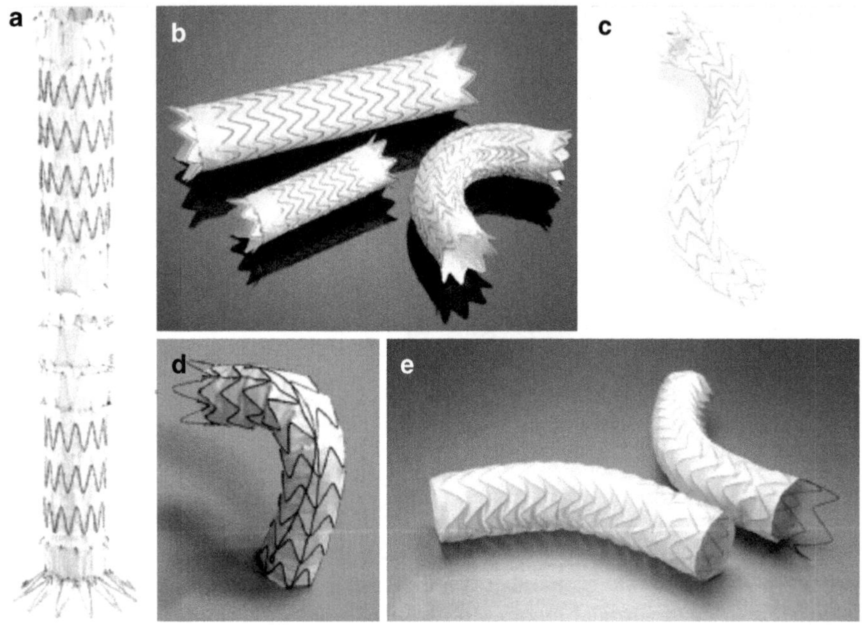

Fig. 6.15 Commercially available thoracic stent-grafts for TEVAR: (**a**) Zenith TX2, (**b**) TAG by Gore Medical, (**c**) Valiant by Medtronic, (**d**) Relay by Terumo, and (**e**) EndoFit by LeMaitre Vascular

Peripheral stent-grafts are also used for aneurysmal disease and in cases of arterial rupture, pseudoaneurysms or arterial perforation. They provide immediate exclusion of aneurysms and sealing of extravasations due to arterial injuries. Stent-grafts are used as a bail-out devices during angioplasty-induced vessel rupture.

Other applications of peripheral stent-grafts include the treatment of hemodialysis patients with arteriovenous access dysfunction, traumatic injuries, pseudoaneurysms, and for embolization prevention.

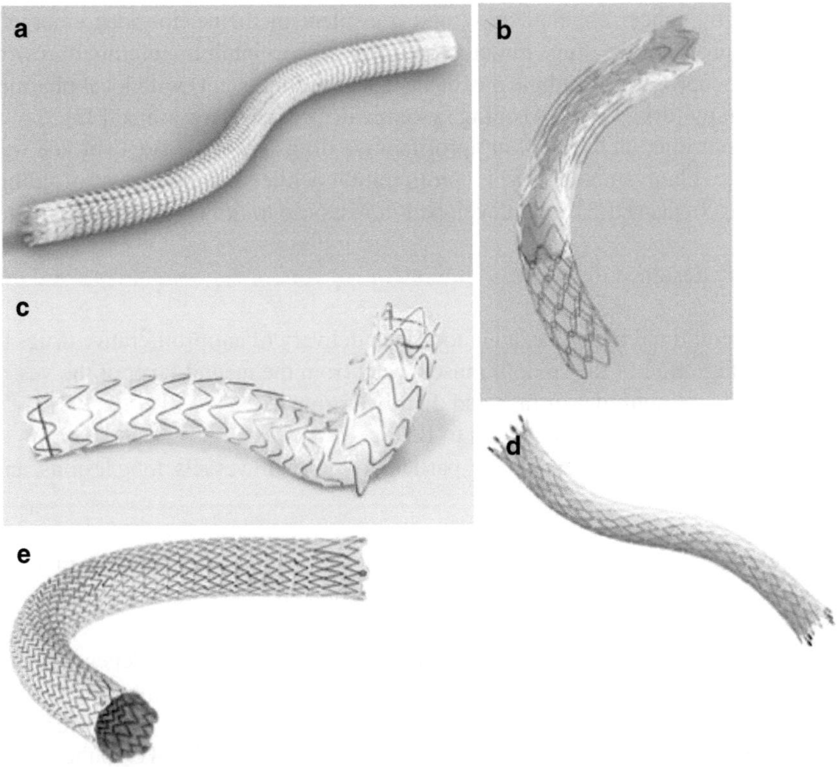

Fig. 6.16 Commercially available stent-grafts for peripheral vascular applications: (**a**) Viabahn by Gore Medical, (**b**) Viatorr by Gore Medical, (**c**) Viabil by Gore Medical, (**d**) Fluency by BD Interventional, and (**e**) Covera by BD Interventional

Nitinol Drug-Eluting Stents

Background

Bare-metal stents (BMS), developed in the 1990s to scaffold arteries and prevent elastic recoil after angioplasty, significantly improved outcomes. However, a major limitation of BMS was in-stent restenosis (ISR)—the re-narrowing of the vessel due to neointimal hyperplasia (excessive smooth muscle cell proliferation and extracellular matrix production). With even most delicate deployment of the stents there is always some degree of trauma to the vessel wall with disruption of the intimal layer. The natural response of the body is to repair these intimal defects by filling them with smooth muscle cells, which migrate from the medial layer of the vessel wall. Sometimes this process goes beyond filling the gaps in the intima and smooth muscle cells continue to proliferate into the lumen of the vessel, causing intimal hyperplasia and in-stent restenosis [21].

Inspired by cancer chemotherapy and transplant medicine, the idea emerged: deliver antiproliferative drugs directly from the stent to inhibit neointimal growth. The key concept was to combine mechanical scaffolding (stent) with local pharmacologic therapy (drug), while keeping systemic drug exposure minimal [22].

Local, controlled delivery of antiproliferative drugs from the stent surface was conceived to blunt smooth-muscle proliferation while maintaining scaffolding. Drug-eluting stents (DES) were developed in response to limitations of bare-metal stents [23].

DES were designed to:

- Inhibit neointimal hyperplasia via localized delivery of antiproliferative drugs to reduce migration of the smooth muscle cells from the medial layer of the vessel wall to the intraluminal surface and their overgrowth.
- Reduce restenosis rates compared to BMS.
- Improve long-term vessel patency, particularly in small vessels, long lesions, and diabetic patients.

Drug-eluting stents provide consistent statistically significant reduction in restenosis and target-lesion revascularization rates compared to bare-metal stents and improved long-term patency [24].

The mechanism of drug release from the stent into the vessel wall depends on the stent's design. There are different concepts and constructions of the drug-eluting stents, which can be divided into two major categories: polymer-based DES and polymer-free DES (Fig. 6.17) [25]. There are also bioabsorbable DES in the development, which are beyond the scope of this manuscript [26].

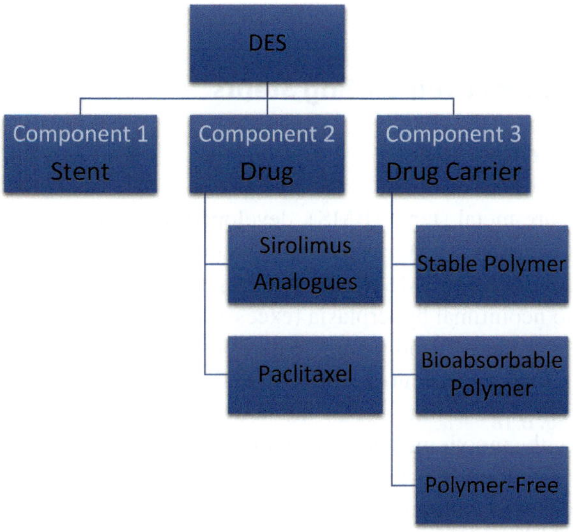

Fig. 6.17 Drug-eluting stent technology

With polymer-based DES, the metallic stents are coated with a polymer that binds and releases the drug over weeks to months. It provides sustained drug release with predictable and controlled kinetics. Polymers influence drug elution timing, local toxicity, and healing response.

Within this category of polymer-based DES, there are different types of coating strategy. The applied polymers can be stable, which remain on the surface of the stents permanently or bioabsorbable, which dissolve over time after drug release [27, 28].

Durable-polymer (DP-DES) Provide long-lasting structure to regulate drug release over weeks to months (Fig. 6.18). Examples include Polyethylene-co-vinyl acetate (PEVA), PBMA. The advantages are that they offer controlled and predictable drug administration. Their performance is proven in the first-generation DES. The disadvantage is that the polymer remains in place after the drug is released and may trigger chronic inflammation, delayed endothelialization, and late stent thrombosis [29].

Bioabsorbable-polymer (BP-DES) The purpose is to deliver drug, then gradually degrade (e.g., into lactic acid) and leave behind a bare-metal scaffold. Examples include Poly-lactic acid (PLA), Polyglycolic acid (PGA), Poly-D,L-lactide-co-glycolide (PLGA). By disappearing over time, they reduce long-term inflammation and improve vessel healing with lower risk of late adverse events [30]. They are

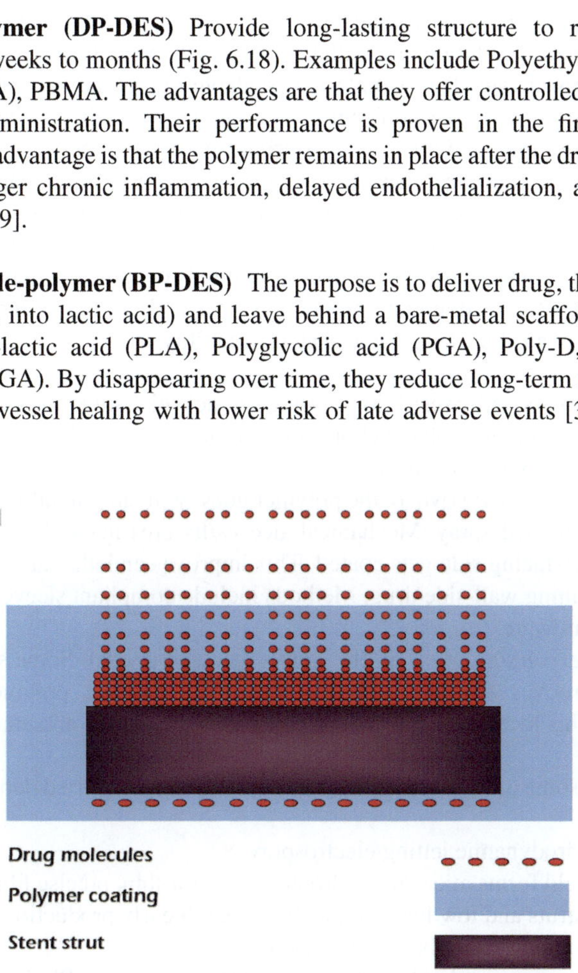

Fig. 6.18 Schematic cross-sectional view of one type of polymer-based drug-eluting stent construction and mechanism of action. A thin polymer layer with a small amount of preloaded drug is facing the vessel lumen. A thick polymer layer with most of drug concentration is in contact with the vessel wall. This particular construction assures very small loss of the drug into the circulation, while majority of it is released into the vessel wall

more complex for manufacturing, polymer degradation timing must match drug-release needs, and some bio-resorption by-products can still provoke inflammation and tissue reaction [31].

Polymer layers act as drug reservoirs/controls, keep drug from washing off during delivery, and can improve biocompatibility; topcoats also tame burst release.

There are several methods how polymers can be applied on the bare-metal stents [32].

Core wet-coating methods (workhorses in industry) involves:

1. Dip coating (immersion + controlled withdrawal), when the stents are dipped in a polymer–drug solution and withdrawn at a set speed; thickness set by viscosity/withdrawal rate. It is simple and scalable but prone to webbing/bridging between struts and non-uniformity on complex geometries; elution can skew toward faster release. Often used for primers or early DES.
2. Spray coating (air, electrostatic, or—most commonly—ultrasonic spray) when atomized droplets are sprayed while the stent rotates/translates on a mandrel. This is the standard for modern DES because it gives uniform thin films, precise dose control, and enables selective (abluminal) coating via masking/fixturing. Ultrasonic systems dominate production lines and are tuned under Quality by Design to control intra- and inter-batch variability.

Process pitfalls and fixes: bridging/ridges/cracks/delamination can occur; mitigated via solids content, solvent choice/evaporation rate, nozzle–part distance, rotation speed, and drying/anneal steps.

Patterning/selectivity (where the polymer goes) with abluminal-only coatings by masking or directed spray. Mechanical sleeves/fixtures mask the luminal side so only the tissue-facing side gets coated. This improves endothelialization luminally while maintaining wall-side drug. Methods include compliant sleeves with internal spray/cure hardware.

Micro-reservoirs/grooves (fill the stent's recessed tracks): Some stents machine abluminal grooves that are filled with a biodegradable polymer–drug (e.g., Firehawk). This localizes payload, reduces polymer volume, and enables low-dose delivery.

There are some other more advanced, but less-commonly used deposition routes:

3. Electrohydrodynamic jetting/electrospray

   High field forms micro/nano-droplets for ultra-thin, precise films—useful for complex struts and low loads; typically research/early production.
4. Electrospinning (nanofiber wraps/mats)

   Creates porous nanofiber meshes carrying drug (e.g., PLGA, chitosan systems). Great surface area and tunable kinetics; mainly preclinical or niche stents/covers.
5. Layer-by-Layer (LbL) polyelectrolyte assembly

   Alternating charged layers (e.g., hyaluronan/chitosan) can embed drug/DNA; thickness at nm resolution; demonstrated on balloon-mounted stents in vivo but not common commercially.

6. Vapor-deposited polymers (parylene CVD; iCVD)
   Gas-phase processes yield conformal ultra-thin films on intricate latticework—ideal as barrier/topcoats or to add functional chemistry (iCVD) without solvents. Parylene has long device history; iCVD enables on-device polymerization of tailored films.
7. Grafting-from (surface-initiated polymerization, e.g., SI-ATRP/RAFT/NMP)
   Grow "polymer brushes" directly from the metal for ultra-thin, covalently anchored layers (anti-fouling, adhesion-promoting, or drug-tethering). Demonstrated on stent alloys; largely research/early translation.
8. Electrophoretic deposition (EPD)
   Electric fields drive charged polymer/drug nanoparticles or micelles onto the struts—useful for room-temperature build-up and complex shapes. Active research for medical devices, including DES prototypes.

Which method is selected for specific product manufacturing depends on multiple different factors.

- For high uniformity, commercial throughput, and complex geometry of stent scaffold—ultrasonic spray (with masking for abluminal-only) is preferred.
- With simple chemistries/primers or low-cost lines—dip coating is selected.
- When ultra-low polymer load/localized delivery is used—groove/reservoir fill or abluminal spray methods are chosen.
- For solvent-sensitive drugs or need for ultra-conformal barrier/topcoat—parylene CVD/iCVD is indicated.
- Research prototypes needing multifunctional, nm-thin films would require LbL or grafted brushes.

The second category of drug-eluting stents is polymer-free [33]. As it stands in its name, there is no polymer coating on the stent surface and the drug is applied directly on the metallic scaffold (Table 6.4).

Polymer-free (PF-DES) There is no polymer matrix, the drug is embedded directly into or on the stent surface (e.g., microporous, nanoporous, or reservoir systems). They have simpler architecture and avoid polymer-related hypersensitivity or chronic inflammation (Fig. 6.19). At the same time, they have less control over drug release kinetics. There is a risk of dose dumping (rapid release), which can potentially reduce long-term efficacy. On the other hand, fast early release may be attractive for high-bleeding risk patients, requiring only a short course of anticoagulation/antiplatelet therapy.

Table 6.4 Comparative overview of the DES platforms

Feature	Durable Polymer	Biodegradable Polymer	Polymer-Free
Drug Control	Excellent	Good	Variable
Chronic Inflammation	Possible	Minimal	None
Late Thrombosis Risk	Higher	Lower	Low
Manufacturing Complexity	Moderate	High	Low
Examples DES	Eluvia	Synergy	Zilver PTX

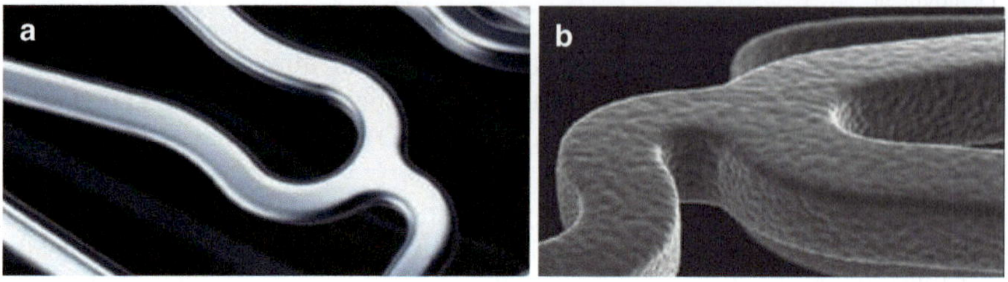

Fig. 6.19 Electron microscopy photographs of the bare-metal stent (**a**) and polymer-coated stent (**b**)

There are different drugs with different mechanisms of action that are used for the purpose of suppressing migration and proliferation of the smooth muscle cells and prevent in-stent restenosis [34, 35]:

- *Sirolimus and analogues (everolimus, zotarolimus, biolimus A9, etc.)* bind FKBP12 and inhibit *mTORC1*, halting the cell cycle in *G1* → strong anti-proliferative and anti-migratory effects on vascular smooth-muscle cells.
- *Paclitaxel* stabilizes microtubules → *mitotic arrest*, with pronounced tissue retention that supports low-dose local therapy (Table 6.5).

With all the advantages that drug-eluting stents provide, there are some risks and trade-offs with the DES:

- Delayed endothelialization (especially with thick coatings in early DES) with increased late and very late stent thrombosis—substantially mitigated with modern thin-strut, biocompatible polymers, and optimized drugs.
- Polymer-related inflammation/hypersensitivity (largely addressed by today's durable fluoropolymers or resorbable polymers).
- Requirement for prolonged dual antiplatelet therapy (DAPT) after PCI; durations now shorter and tailored by bleeding/ischemic risk under current guidelines.
- Cost higher than BMS.

In summary, we present the timetable of the development of the drug-eluting stents:

Origins of Self-Expanding Stents

- 1980s–1990s: Self-expanding stents (SES) were introduced to address the limitations of balloon-expandable stents, particularly in tortuous or mobile vessels, such as in peripheral artery disease (PAD) and neurovascular anatomy.
- Early self-expanding stents were bare-metal, primarily used in femoral, carotid, and neurovascular arteries.

Table 6.5 Comparison of the Drugs Used in Drug-eluting Stents

Drug (class)	Primary purpose	Cellular target/mechanism	Typical use today
Sirolimus (rapamycin)	Suppress neointimal hyperplasia	Potent *mTORC1 inhibitor* → G1 cell-cycle arrest; cytostatic on VSMCs with relative endothelial sparing	Foundation for modern DES (many "sirolimus-eluting" platforms) and ultrathin bioabsorbable-polymer stents.
Everolimus (rapalog)	Suppress neointimal hyperplasia	mTORC1 inhibitor; higher lipophilicity & tissue penetration versus sirolimus	Flagship "second-generation" DES (e.g., XIENCE/Promus) with excellent long-term safety.
Zotarolimus (ABT-578) (rapalog)	Suppress neointimal hyperplasia	mTORC1 inhibitor; designed for controlled elution with durable polymers	Widely used (e.g., Resolute); outcomes comparable to everolimus in all-comers.
Biolimus A9 (umirolimus) (rapalog)	Suppress neointimal hyperplasia	Very *lipophilic sirolimus analogue* (deeper arterial wall uptake)	With *biodegradable* or *polymer-free* coatings; proven in *high-bleeding-risk* (HBR) on 1-month DAPT.
Novolimus (sirolimus metabolite)	Suppress neointimal hyperplasia	mTORC1 inhibitor with lower required tissue concentrations (investigational to widespread outside US)	Used on some platforms (e.g., DESyne); growing real-world evidence.
Paclitaxel (taxane)	Suppress neointimal hyperplasia	*Microtubule stabilization* → mitotic arrest; more cytotoxic & less selective	Largely historical in coronaries; *dominant in peripheral femoropopliteal DES* (e.g., Eluvia, Zilver PTX).

The Need for Drug Elution

- While SES provided good mechanical adaptability, restenosis due to neointimal hyperplasia remained a significant problem.
- Inspired by the success of balloon-expandable drug-eluting stents (DES) in coronary artery disease (2003 FDA approval of Cypher by J&J Cordis; 2004 FDA approval of Taxus by BSC), research moved toward incorporating drug-elution in self-expanding platforms.

First SE-DES

- Early 2000s–2010s: First SE-DES prototypes and trials.
- Zilver PTX™ (Cook Medical) became the first FDA-approved SE-DES for peripheral artery disease in 2012.

Current Status

The most extensive work with drug-eluting stents was done for the coronary applications, but the concept, obtained knowledge, and technology were later introduced, transferred, and applied in the peripheral vascular applications with some required modifications to tailor to the specifics and differences in the peripheral circulation.

Nitinol self-expanding drug-eluting stents represent a specialized, but growing segment of endovascular therapy. Designed to conform to complex vascular anatomies and combined with antiproliferative drug delivery, SE-DES are particularly valuable in long, tortuous, and dynamic vessels—especially in the peripheral vasculature.

Their development marks an important bridge between mechanical adaptability and pharmacological efficacy, with ongoing innovation focused on improving long-term safety, flexibility, and healing.

Nitinol self-expanding drug-eluting stents grew out of the realization that bare nitinol stents, although mechanically well suited to the dynamic superficial femoral and popliteal arteries, were limited by restenosis driven by neointimal hyperplasia, especially in longer lesions and complex morphology. By adding an antiproliferative drug layer to a superelastic Nitinol backbone, the goal has been to combine durable scaffolding with long-term suppression of neointimal growth, while preserving the flexibility, crush resistance, and fatigue performance needed in this biomechanically hostile territory.

Historically, the first true Nitinol self-expanding drug-eluting stents for the superficial femoral artery were sirolimus- and everolimus-eluting adaptations of existing Nitinol platforms such as SMART and Dynalink. The SIROCCO program evaluated a sirolimus-eluting Nitinol stent versus bare Nitinol in SFA disease and showed biological activity with reduced late lumen loss but failed to demonstrate a compelling and consistent advantage in long-term patency or clinical outcomes; edge restenosis and mismatched drug-release kinetics for the large, mobile peripheral vessel were concerns. Everolimus-eluting Nitinol self-expanding stents using the Dynalink platform showed that these devices could be safely implanted, with acceptable primary patency and limb outcomes, but again did not lead to a paradigm shift and remained limited to investigational or niche use [36]. These early experiences highlighted both the feasibility of limus-eluting Nitinol stents in peripheral arteries and the need for more optimized drug, dose, and release systems.

The first widely adopted Nitinol self-expanding drug-eluting stent was Zilver PTX (Cook Medical), a polymer-free paclitaxel-eluting device in which the drug is directly bound to the Nitinol stent surface. In the pivotal randomized Zilver PTX trial, patients with symptomatic femoropopliteal disease were assigned to primary Zilver PTX implantation versus standard care (angioplasty with provisional bare Nitinol stenting), and the study also compared provisional Zilver PTX to provisional bare Nitinol stents. Five-year follow-up showed durable clinical effectiveness: primary patency and freedom from target lesion revascularization were significantly higher in the drug-eluting stent cohorts, with about a 40–50% relative reduction in restenosis and reintervention and no late "catch-up" phenomenon in loss of patency [37]. Subsequent post-market surveillance and Japanese registry data extended these findings into more complex patient populations, including in-stent restenosis, with sustained benefit and acceptable safety. As a result, Zilver PTX became the prototype Nitinol drug-eluting stent for the femoropopliteal segment and remains one of the key platforms worldwide.

A second major step was the introduction of Eluvia (Boston Scientific), a Nitinol self-expanding stent with a thin fluoropolymer coating (PVDF-HFP) that provides controlled, prolonged paclitaxel elution tailored to the time course of peripheral restenosis. Preclinical work demonstrated deeper and more sustained tissue paclitaxel levels compared with polymer-free coatings, and early clinical studies such as MAJESTIC showed very high 1-year patency in SFA–popliteal lesions [38]. The IMPERIAL randomized trial directly compared Eluvia with Zilver PTX in femoropopliteal disease, demonstrating superior primary patency for Eluvia at 12 months and a lower rate of clinically driven target lesion revascularization, with similar safety [39]. Two-year results from IMPERIAL showed that Eluvia maintained numerically higher patency and significantly lower TLR, with no significant difference in all-cause mortality [40]. Real-world series and registries, including complex lesion cohorts, have broadly confirmed favorable 2-year outcomes, although they also reported a non-trivial incidence of vessel wall degeneration or aneurysmal changes adjacent to the stent, prompting continued surveillance and debate about the long-term vascular effects of durable polymers in this location [41].

The relative performance of Zilver PTX and Eluvia has been further clarified by observational comparative studies. Three-year data from the REALDES study found broadly similar primary patency and freedom from clinically driven TLR between the two platforms in real-world femoropopliteal practice, with no statistically significant differences in restenosis severity or limb events, suggesting that lesion complexity, vessel preparation, and operator technique may now be as important as the choice of specific Nitinol drug-eluting stent [42]. A 2024 analysis of US claims data showed that utilization of both Eluvia and Zilver PTX increased after introduction, dipped substantially during the period of regulatory concern around paclitaxel-coated devices, and then partially recovered as updated safety reviews failed to confirm an excess mortality signal, illustrating how macro-level safety debates can strongly influence adoption curves for Nitinol drug-eluting stents [43].

The paclitaxel "mortality signal" controversy, although not unique to Nitinol stents, had direct implications for Zilver PTX and Eluvia because both are self-expanding Nitinol devices eluting paclitaxel. A 2018 meta-analysis of paclitaxel-coated balloons and stents in femoropopliteal disease suggested increased late mortality, leading to regulatory warnings, labeling changes, and a marked decline in use. Subsequent patient-level meta-analyses, inclusion of more complete follow-up, linkage with external datasets, and large real-world studies failed to confirm a causal association between paclitaxel dose and mortality. On the basis of these expanded data, the FDA and other regulators concluded in 2023–2024 that paclitaxel-coated devices, including Nitinol drug-eluting stents, do not appear to increase long-term mortality, though they recommended continued post-market surveillance and shared decision-making with patients [44]. This clarification has stabilized the position of

Nitinol paclitaxel-eluting stents as acceptable and effective options for femoropopliteal revascularization.

In parallel, there has been a deliberate move to develop limus-eluting Nitinol self-expanding stents, aiming to replicate the excellent coronary safety profile of sirolimus and everolimus while avoiding paclitaxel class concerns and potentially improving neointimal control in certain lesion subsets. The NiTiDES stent (Alvimedica) is a prominent example: a self-expanding Nitinol platform with abluminal reservoirs releasing an amphilimus formulation (sirolimus plus fatty acid) in a polymer-free design. The ILLUMINA first-in-human study treated femoropopliteal lesions and reported excellent 12- and 24-month outcomes, with primary patency around 83–84% at 2 years, freedom from clinically driven TLR over 90%, and freedom from device-related major adverse events around 92%, indicating strong efficacy and safety [45]. Extended follow-up presented at major vascular meetings and in peer-reviewed publications has reinforced these results. NiTiDES is marketed in Europe and some other regions and is often framed as the first commercially available sirolimus-eluting Nitinol self-expanding stent for the SFA, but it is not yet widely available in all jurisdictions.

Other limus-based Nitinol drug-eluting stents have been evaluated in smaller trials. Everolimus-eluting self-expanding Nitinol stents, leveraging the Dynalink scaffold and a durable polymer, have been tested in the Superficial Femoral Artery Treatment with Drug-Eluting Stents study, demonstrating procedural feasibility, reasonable patency, and acceptable limb outcomes but without the scale or follow-up needed to displace paclitaxel devices [46]. Newer sirolimus-eluting Nitinol platforms with reservoir-based or abluminal-only drug delivery are in various stages of development, but robust long-term comparative data are still limited. Current reviews of drug-eluting devices for peripheral arterial disease generally regard limus-eluting Nitinol stents as promising but still in an evidence-building phase, while paclitaxel Nitinol stents remain the best-characterized option for most femoropopliteal indications [44].

Below the knee, the role of Nitinol self-expanding drug-eluting stents is more restricted. Most below-the-knee drug-eluting stents in current use are coronary platforms (balloon-expandable cobalt–chromium) deployed off-label in tibial or peroneal arteries for critical limb-threatening ischemia; they are not Nitinol self-expanding devices. Ongoing research into bioresorbable or hybrid scaffolds for infrapopliteal disease includes some Nitinol-based or Nitinol-supported systems, but these are largely investigational. First-in-human and preclinical data on bioresorbable drug-eluting scaffolds, including everolimus-eluting structures for femoropopliteal or tibial arteries, show encouraging patency and the conceptual advantage of "leaving nothing behind," but they still face challenges related to scaffold thickness, deliverability, and fracture risk in the highly mobile peripheral vascular bed [47]. For now, when clinicians speak about Nitinol self-expanding drug-eluting stents, they are usually referring to the femoropopliteal segment rather than infrapopliteal arteries.

From a design and material standpoint, current Nitinol drug-eluting stents incorporate several refinements beyond simply adding a drug coating. The Nitinol

Table 6.6 Approved Peripheral Nitinol DES Devices

Device	Manufacturer	Drug	Polymer	Approval	Artery
Zilver PTX	Cook Medical	Paclitaxel	Polymer-Free	FDA CE	SFA
Eluvia	Boston Scientific	Paclitaxel	Fluoro-polymer	FDA CE	SFA

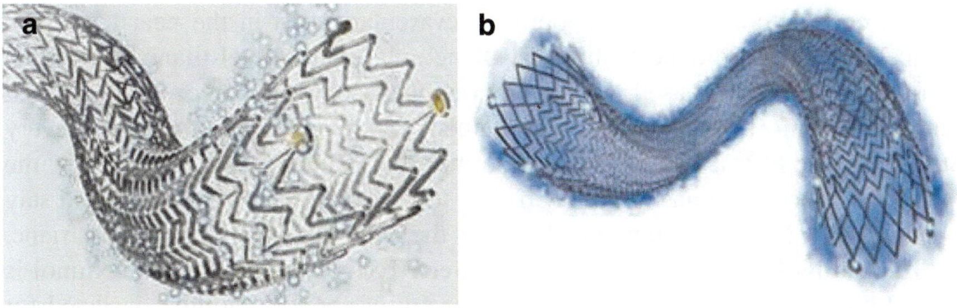

Fig. 6.20 Zilver PTX (**a**) and Eluvia (**b**) drug-eluting Nitinol self-expanding stents

backbone is engineered for high fatigue resistance and flexibility, with specific strut patterns to accommodate flexion, torsion, and compression in the adductor canal and popliteal region. Paclitaxel devices differ not only by polymer strategy (polymer-free surface binding in Zilver PTX versus durable fluoropolymer reservoirs in Eluvia, Table 6.6) but also by total drug dose, elution rate, and the proportion of abluminal versus circumferential coverage, which together influence tissue distribution and duration of the antiproliferative effect [38]. Limus-eluting Nitinol stents such as NiTiDES use abluminal reservoir technology and amphiphilic drug formulations to improve penetration and retention in the arterial wall while limiting luminal exposure, with the aim of reducing thrombogenicity and promoting more physiologic healing [45]. Across all platforms, there is a trend toward thinner struts, more flexible cell geometry, and delivery systems that enable longer single stents to be placed with high precision, reflecting the recognition that mechanical durability and deployment accuracy remain essential even when an effective drug is present.

Clinically, contemporary guidelines and reviews now position Nitinol drug-eluting stents as one of several drug-based technologies used to optimize endovascular treatment of lower-limb peripheral arterial disease. For intermediate-length femoropopliteal lesions, especially when there is significant elastic recoil, flow-limiting dissection, or heavy focal calcification that necessitates a scaffold, a Nitinol drug-eluting stent is often preferred over a bare Nitinol stent because of the clear and durable reduction in restenosis and reintervention rates shown in randomized trials and long-term follow-up [36]. For more diffuse or long-segment disease where metal burden is a concern, drug-coated balloons with or without limited "bailout" stenting remain attractive, and many operators choose between drug-coated balloon-based strategies and Nitinol drug-eluting stents based on lesion length, vessel diameter, runoff quality, and anticipated need for future bypass options. The two leading paclitaxel Nitinol DES platforms (Zilver PTX and Eluvia, Fig. 6.20) have the strongest evidence base and broadest availability, while sirolimus-eluting Nitinol stents such as NiTiDES are gaining a foothold in Europe and other markets but are still accumulating comparative data.

The current status of Nitinol self-expanding drug-eluting stents can be summarized as a balance between consolidation and innovation. On one hand, Zilver PTX and Eluvia represent mature technologies with extensive randomized and real-world data, established indications, and a clarified safety profile, and they will likely remain central tools for femoropopliteal revascularization in the near term. The devices share the same mechanical backbone: a laser-cut nickel-titanium tube that self-expands when released, providing continuous outward force, fracture resistance, and conformability in a vessel segment that bends and shortens with every step. Eluvia's Instructions for Use describe this explicitly and also explain the "shape-memory/superelastic" behavior that lets the stent open on its own and stay open; Zilver PTX's FDA summary describes the same self-expanding Nitinol frame.

Their drug-delivery concepts differ. Zilver PTX is polymer-free: the Nitinol is coated directly with paclitaxel at a dose density of about 3 μg/mm^2, designed for rapid tissue uptake from the stent surface. Eluvia uses a dual-layer durable polymer (a PBMA primer under a PVDF-HFP drug layer) to meter a much lower paclitaxel load (≈0.167 μg/mm^2) over months, aiming to better match the time course of restenosis in the femoropopliteal segment (Fig. 6.21). These design choices—polymer-free "burst" versus polymer-controlled "sustained" release—are the key practical difference in how the drugs are presented to the artery wall.

Mechanistically, both stents work the same two ways: the Nitinol scaffold immediately restores and maintains lumen, while paclitaxel limits smooth-muscle cell proliferation and matrix deposition that would otherwise re-narrow the vessel.

Summary of the clinical trials of SE-DES in femoropopliteal arteries:

- Zilver PTX RCT ($n \approx 476$): versus PTA (with BMS as needed) showed superior patency and freedom from TLR maintained to 5 years. In the *provisional stent* sub-randomization, DES outperformed BMS for 5-year primary patency (72.4% versus 53.0%) and freedom from TLR (84.9% versus 71.6%).

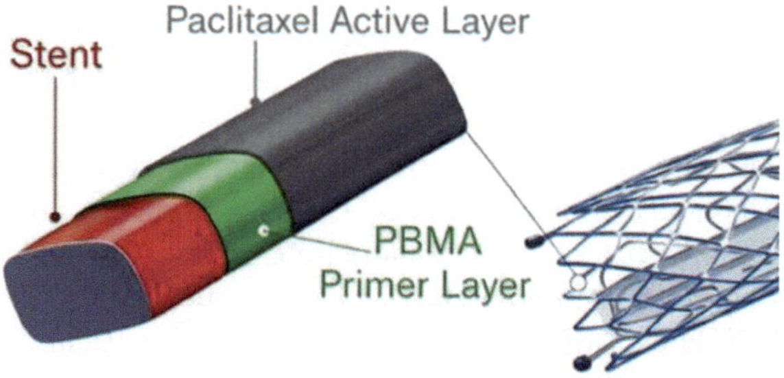

Fig. 6.21 Eluvia coating stent design demonstrating the dual polymer construction. The primer layer promotes adhesion of the active layer to the stent surface, and the active layer provides the controlled release of Paclitaxel [49]

- IMPERIAL RCT (Eluvia versus Zilver PTX): Eluvia achieved higher patency at 12–24 months, and durable outcomes to 5 years with similar freedom from CD-TLR by 5 years (multiple presentations/peer-reviewed reports).
  - 1 year: Eluvia superior in primary patency.
  - 2 years: Eluvia 83% versus Zilver PTX 77% K-M primary patency; lower clinically driven TLR (statistically significant).
  - 5 years: Freedom from CD-TLR numerically higher with Eluvia (70.7% versus 65.8%; $p = 0.35$).
- EMINENT RCT (Eluvia versus BMS): polymer-based paclitaxel DES showed superior 1-year primary patency versus BMS in symptomatic FP lesions.
- Real-world/registries: broader cohorts generally show lower absolute patency than RCTs but consistent benefit trends for Eluvia and Zilver PTX.

On the other hand, limus-eluting Nitinol stents, reservoir-based drug-delivery designs, and bioresorbable or hybrid Nitinol-containing scaffolds are active areas of development aimed at further improving patency, reducing reinterventions, and eventually minimizing permanent implant burden [48]. As evidence accumulates, clinical practice is becoming more individualized, with Nitinol self-expanding drug-eluting stents deployed selectively in patients and lesions where their combination of mechanical support and potent antiproliferative therapy provides a clear advantage within a broader strategy that also includes drug-coated balloons, atherectomy, and, when appropriate, surgical bypass.

Today, operators tend to choose between polymer-free and polymer-based stents based on lesion length, calcification, risk of restenosis, and institutional experience, with both platforms supported by randomized and real-world data. In complex, long, or recoil-prone lesions where scaffolding and sustained drug effect are desired, a self-expanding paclitaxel DES can reduce repeat procedures compared with plain angioplasty or bare metal stents; where scaffolding is less desirable, drug-coated balloons remain an alternative.

Looking ahead, two development tracks are most active. First is pharmacology: renewed efforts with sirolimus-family drugs on Nitinol backbones are ongoing after early sirolimus-eluting Nitinol stents (e.g., the SIROCCO SMART platform) failed to outperform bare stents; newer controlled-release chemistries and micro-reservoir concepts aim to deliver sirolimus more predictably in the leg. Second is engineering: finer struts, improved coatings, and even additive-manufactured Nitinol geometries are being explored to balance fracture resistance with flexibility. The next wave is trying to pair smarter sirolimus-type drugs and smarter Nitinol designs to make results last longer with fewer trade-offs.

Peripheral drug-eluting stents represent a major advancement in PAD treatment, offering improved patency and reduced need for repeat interventions. While paclitaxel-based DES have been the backbone of this field, sirolimus-eluting technologies may shape the future due to safety considerations. Ongoing innovation and long-term data are critical to fully define their role across diverse vascular beds and patient populations.

References

1. Volodos NL, Shekhanin VE, Karporich IP. A self-fixing synthetic endoprosthesis for blood vessel. Vestn Khir. 1986;137:123–5.
2. Parodi JC, Palmaz JC, Barone HD. Transfemoral intraluminal graft implantation for abdominal aortic aneurysms. Ann Vasc Surg. 1991;5:491–9.
3. Rabkin DJ, Lang EV, Kleshinski S, Barnhart W. Miniaturization of the delivery systems for large vessel stent-grafts. In: Annual meeting of the Cardiovascular and Interventional Radiological Society of Europe. Maastricht; 2000.
4. Kim D, Rabkin DJ, Kent KC, Simon M, Kleshinski S, Porter DH, et al. Percutaneous treatment of aortic aneurysms with shape memory alloy stent-grafts. In: Annual meeting of the Cardiovascular and Interventional Radiological Society of Europe. Barcelona; 1992.
5. Rabkin DJ, Kim D, Kent KC, Porter DH, Skillman JJ, Paulin S, et al. Nitinol stent grafts for percutaneous treatment of aortic aneurysms. In: 17th annual scientific meeting of the Society of Cardiovascular and Interventional Radiology. Washington, DC; 1992.
6. Konstantakopoulos A, Kladovasilakis N, Stavroulakis G. Development and mechanical evaluation of stent graft for endovascular aneurysm repair using finite element modeling. Designs. 2025;9(5):103.
7. Hynes N, Acharya Y, Sultan S. The contemporary design of endovascular stent-graft materials: PTFE versus polyester. Front Surg. 2022;9:984727.
8. Jayendiran R, Nour B, Ruimi A. Computational analysis of nitinol stent-graft for endovascular aortic repair (EVAR) of abdominal aortic aneurysm (AAA): crimping, sealing and fluid–structure interaction (FSI). Int J Cardiol. 2020;304:164–71.
9. Cartes-Zumelzu F, Lammer J, Hoelzenbein T, et al. Endovascular placement of nitinol-ePTFE stent-graft for abdominal aortic aneurysms: initial and midterm results. J Vasc Interv Radiol. 2002;13(5):465–73.
10. Arko F, Nussbaum T, Lalka S, et al. The Endurant stent graft. Endovasc Today. 2012 May Suppl:12–18.
11. Pitros C, Mansi P, Kakkos S. Endografts for the treatment of abdominal aortic aneurysms with a hostile neck anatomy: a systematic review. Front Surg. 2022;9:872705.
12. Katzen B, Dake M, MacLean A, Wang D. Endovascular repair of abdominal and thoracic aortic aneurysms. Circulation. 2005;112(11):1663–75.
13. Oderich G, Baumgardt Barbosa Lima G, Schanzer A, et al. Modern complex stent graft designs: a closer look. Endovasc Today. 2021;20(3):67–70.
14. Nation D, Wang G. TEVAR: endovascular repair of the thoracic aorta. Semin Intervent Radiol. 2015;32(3):265–71.
15. Yamaguchi M, Sugimoto K, Tsukube T, et al. Curved nitinol stent-graft placement for treating blunt thoracic aortic injury: an early experience. Ann Thorac Surg. 2008;86(3):780–6.
16. McQuade K, Gable D, Pearl G, et al. Four-year randomized prospective comparison of percutaneous ePTFE/nitinol self-expanding stent graft versus prosthetic femoral–popliteal bypass in the treatment of superficial femoral artery occlusive disease. J Vasc Surg. 2010;52(3):584–91.
17. Litsky J, Chanda A, Stilp E, et al. Critical evaluation of stents in the peripheral arterial disease of the superficial femoral artery—focus on the paclitaxel eluting stent. Med Devices (Auckl). 2014;7:149–56.
18. BD. BD initiates international study to expand treatment options for patients with peripheral arterial disease. BD Newsroom. 2024.
19. Zhou XC, Yang F, Gong XY, et al. New nitinol endovascular stent-graft system for abdominal aortic aneurysm with finite element analysis and experimental verification. Rare Metals. 2019;38:495–502.
20. Rigberg D, Tulloch A, Chun Y. Thin-film nitinol (NiTi): a feasibility study for a novel aortic stent graft material. J Vasc Surg. 2009;50(2):375–80.
21. Buccheri D, Piraino D, Andolina G, Cortese B. Understanding and managing in-stent restenosis: a review of clinical data, from pathogenesis to treatment. J Thorac Dis. 2016;8(10):1150–62.

22. Hill R. Drug-eluting stents: an early systematic review to inform policy. Eur Heart J. 2004;25:902–19.
23. Moliterno DJ. Healing Achilles—sirolimus versus paclitaxel. N Engl J Med. 2005;353:724–7.
24. Kozlik M, Harpula J, Chuchra P, et al. Drug-eluting stents: technical and clinical progress. Biomater Sci. 2023;8(1):72.
25. Wu JJ, Way JA, Kritharides L, et al. Polymer-free versus durable polymer drug-eluting stents in patients with coronary artery disease: a meta-analysis. Ann Med Surg (Lond). 2019;38:13–21.
26. Shen Y, Yu X, Cui J, et al. Development of biodegradable polymeric stents for the treatment of cardiovascular diseases. Biomolecules. 2022;12:1245.
27. Kim HS, Kang J, Hwang D, et al. Durable polymer versus biodegradable polymer drug-eluting stents after percutaneous coronary intervention in patients with acute coronary syndrome: the HOST-REDUCE-POLYTECH-ACS trial. Circulation. 2021;143(11):1081–91.
28. Jang WJ, Park IH, Oh JH, et al. Efficacy and safety of durable vs biodegradable polymer drug-eluting stents in patients with acute myocardial infarction complicated by cardiogenic shock. Sci Rep. 2024;14:6301.
29. Alhara K, Toril S, Nakamura N, et al. Pathological evaluation of predictors for delayed endothelial coverage after currently available drug-eluting stent implantation in coronary arteries: impact of lesions with acute and chronic coronary syndromes. Am Heart J. 2024;277:114–24.
30. Akinapelli A, Chen J, Roy K, et al. Current state of bioabsorbable polymer-coated drug-eluting stents. Curr Cardiol Rev. 2017;13(2):139–54.
31. Rodriguez-Granillo A, Rubilar B, Rodriguez-Granillo G, et al. Advantages and disadvantages of biodegradable platforms in drug eluting stents. World J Cardiol. 2011;3(3):84–92.
32. Livingston M, Tan A. Coating techniques and release kinetics of drug-eluting stents. J Med Devices. 2016;10(1):010111.
33. Colleran R, Byrne R. Polymer-free drug-eluting stents: the importance of the right control. Circulation. 2020;141(25):2064–6.
34. Parker W, Iqbal J. Comparison of contemporary drug-eluting coronary stents—is any stent better than the others? Heart Int. 2020;14(1):34–42.
35. Chen K, Xu L, Liu X. Different drugs in drug-eluting stents for peripheral artery disease: a systematic evaluation and Bayesian meta-analysis. J Thromb Thrombolysis. 2024;57(3):1–11.
36. Laird J, Hong M. Drug-eluting stents in the superficial femoral artery: the long and winding road. Circulation. 2016;133(15):1435–7.
37. Dake M, Ansel G, Jaff M, et al. Durable clinical effectiveness with paclitaxel-eluting stents in the femoropopliteal artery: 5-year results of the Zilver PTX randomized trial. Circulation. 2016;133(15):1472–83.
38. Müller-Hülsbeck S. Eluvia peripheral stent system for the treatment of peripheral lesions above the knee. Expert Opin Drug Deliv. 2016;13(11):1639–44.
39. Gray W, Keirse K, Soga Y, et al. A polymer-coated, paclitaxel-eluting stent (Eluvia) versus polymer-free, paclitaxel-coated stent (Zilver PTX) for endovascular femoropopliteal intervention (IMPERIAL): a randomized, non-inferiority trial. Lancet. 2018;392(10157):1541–51.
40. Müller-Hülsbeck S, et al. Two-year efficacy and safety results from the IMPERIAL randomized study of the Eluvia polymer-coated drug-eluting stent and the Zilver PTX polymer-free drug-coated stent. Cardiovasc Intervent Radiol. 2021;44(3):368–75.
41. Stavroulakis K, Torsello G, Bosiers M, et al. Two-year outcomes of the Eluvia drug-eluting stent for the treatment of complex femoropopliteal lesions. JACC Cardiovasc Interv. 2021;14(6):692–701.
42. Shibata T, Iba Y, Shingaki M, et al. Editor's choice—comparative analysis of three-year results of two paclitaxel-related stents for the management of femoropopliteal disease in a real world setting. Eur J Vasc Endovasc Surg. 2025;69(6):865–73.
43. Kadian-Dodov D, Williams A, Sato R, et al. Trends in the utilization of drug-eluting stents to treat femoropopliteal peripheral artery disease. JVS Vasc Insights. 2024;2(C):100136.

44. Goueffic Y, Brodmann M, Deloose K, et al. Drug-eluting devices for lower limb peripheral arterial disease. EuroIntervention. 2024;20(18):1136–53.
45. Steiner S, Honton B, Langhoff R, et al. Two-year results with a sirolimus-eluting self-expanding stent for femoropopliteal lesions: the first-in-human ILLUMINA study. JACC Cardiovasc Interv. 2022;15(6):618–26.
46. Lammer J, Bosiers M, Zeller T, et al. First clinical trial of nitinol self-expanding everolimus-eluting stent implantation for peripheral arterial occlusive disease. J Vasc Surg. 2011;54(2):394–401.
47. Lammer J, Bosiers M, Deloose K, et al. Bioresorbable everolimus-eluting vascular scaffold for patients with peripheral artery disease (ESPRIT I): 2-year clinical and imaging results. JACC Cardiovasc Interv. 2016;9(11):1178–87.
48. Tannu M, Schuyler Jones W, Swaminathan R, et al. Femoropopliteal endovascular intervention: a review of the current landscape. Circ Cardiovasc Interv. 2025;18(5):e014024.
49. Altit R, Gray W. New innovations in drug-eluting stents for peripheral arterial disease. Curr Cardiol Rep. 2017;19:117.
50. Gozzo C, Caruana G, Cannella R, Farina A, Giambelluca D, Dinoto E, et al. CT angiography for the assessment of EVAR complications: a pictorial review. Insights Imaging. 2022;13:5. https://doi.org/10.1186/s13244-021-01112-4.

From Heritage to Horizon

7

Two-Way Shape Memory Effect of Nitinol

One of the most valuable properties of nitinol is the shape memory effect, when the metal undergoes a reversible phase transformation between the austenite and martensite phases (described in detail in Chap. 1). The atoms of metals are arranged in specific structures, depending on their components, but rarely change structure shape while still solid.

Under high temperatures, the metal enters the austenite phase. In this phase, it achieves maximum stiffness and is spring-like when bent. The metal enters the martensite phase during low temperatures. In this phase, the metal feels rubbery and bends easily. When Nitinol is in its Martensitic form, it can easily deform into a new shape. However, when heated through its transformation temperature, it reverts to austenite and recovers its previous shape.

Slight changes in the alloy composition or heat treatment adjust the temperature at which Nitinol remembers its high-temperature form. The device's use determines which transition temperature you choose. For example, if you were making a medical device, such as a stent, you would select a transition temperature close to or equal to human body temperature.

Nitinol normally shows the one-way shape memory effect: you set a "hot" shape, you can bend it while it is cold (in martensite), and when you heat it above its transformation finish temperature it rebounds back to that set shape. The two-way effect goes a step further, enabling the material to adopt a second, different "trained" shape when cooled. The second-way shape memory effect means the alloy has been trained to remember a pair of shapes without any outside force: a "cold" shape that appears on cooling and a "hot" shape that appears on heating. In the research and manufacturing literature this is almost always called the two-way

I. Rabkin, D. J. Rabkin, *Bloodline of Nitinol Stents*,
https://doi.org/10.1007/978-3-032-25697-3_7

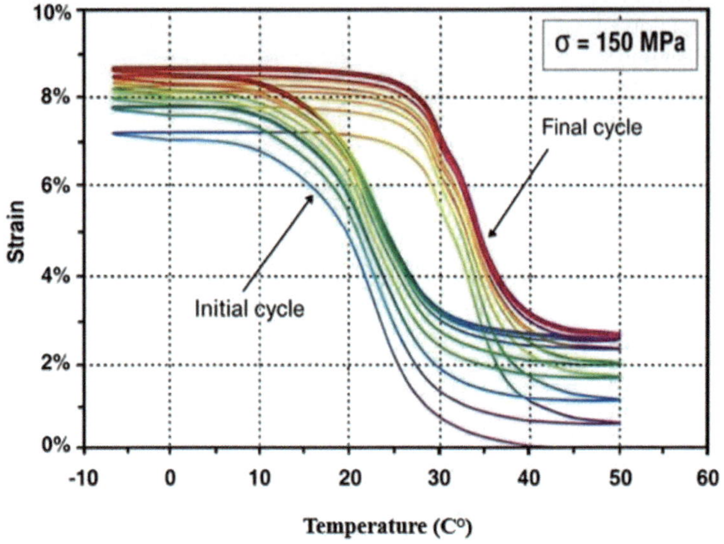

Fig. 7.1 Thermal cycling loading (50 cycles) of a NiTi shape memory alloy wire under constant load of 150 MPa [5]

shape memory effect (TWSME). It does not come "for free"; you have to create internal biases in the metal so, on cooling, the preferred martensite variants form in a way that makes the part adopt the cold shape, and on heating the austenite takes it back to the hot shape [1, 2].

At the microscopic level, Nitinol switches between two solid crystal structures: high-temperature austenite and low-temperature martensite. When you train the material for two-way behavior, you deliberately introduce a pattern of internal stresses and defects (dislocations, fine NiTi precipitates, and sometimes texture) that "steer" which martensite variants appear on cooling. Those variants shear in a preferred direction and the part curls or flexes into its cold shape [3]. Heat removes those variants, austenite returns, and the part recovers the hot shape. This internal bias can be created by thermal cycling under stress, by deforming in martensite and then thermally cycling, or by constrained aging—holding the part in a jig while you age it so the precipitates and residual stresses lock in the bias [4].

With the training process for the second-way shape memory, the material is subjected to repeated heating and cooling cycles, often under a constant stress [2]. During each cycle, it is deformed at the low-temperature martensitic state and then heated to the austenitic state (Fig. 7.1). This process encourages the preferential formation and orientation of martensitic variants, which creates internal stresses that bias the material's shape upon cooling.

A practical recipe has three ingredients: a set hot shape, a set cold shape, and a way to "write" the bias into the metal [6].

1. Heat-set the hot shape. Form the component to the hot shape and heat treat it above the austenite finish temperature (and below the grain-growth/overaging risk) to lock in that geometry.
2. Define the cold shape. Cool to martensite and impose the desired cold geometry (bend/curve) at a strain level the alloy can repeat without damage.
3. Imprint the bias. Either:
   - Thermal cycling under load (keep a constant bending or tensile stress and cycle temperature through the transformation several dozen times),
   - Martensite deformation cycling (deform in martensite, heat to recover, cool, and repeat), or
   - Constrained aging (hold the part in a jig that enforces the cold geometry while aging at an appropriate temperature/time so precipitates form with the right orientation).

All three aim to create stable internal stresses that favor the cold-shaped variants on cooling. Details such as nickel content, prior aging, and exact temperatures strongly affect the result and stability over life [7].

This process has some strength and limitations [8, 9].

Two-way behavior (the second shape) is weaker and less durable than the one-way effect. The achievable stroke on cooling is smaller, it drifts with cycling, and it can fade with time if the internal bias relaxes. Two way is fantastic when you want a self-contained, purely thermal actuator and can tolerate modest strains and careful limits on fatigue.

Retrievable/Repositionable Nitinol Implants

The main reason a stent is used is to prevent the artery from collapsing or narrowing again right after it has been opened, and to give the vessel time to heal and remodel.

The benefits of permanent metallic stents:

- Improved immediate angiographic outcome
- Reduction of acute complications
- Prevention and treatment of dissection
- Freezing recoil
- Reduction of restenosis compared to balloon angioplasty

With all the advantages that the stents demonstrate, they do have certain and clear limitations [10–14]:

- Thrombogenicity
- Require prolonged antiplatelet therapy
- Permanent physical irritation
- Mismatch in mechanical behavior between stented and non-stented areas
- Freezing remodeling
- Long-term endothelial dysfunction
- Inability to adapt to growth
- May preclude later revascularization endovascular or surgical options
- Chronic inflammatory local reaction

The healing period after the stent implantation usually takes several months. Once the vessel has stabilized and new tissue has covered the treated area, the rigid metal structure is no longer essential. At that point, leaving metal behind does not provide new benefits and can actually increase long-term risks such as chronic inflammation, clot formation, or difficulties if future procedures are needed. A metal stent does not necessarily need to stay in place permanently to serve its purpose [15].

The current biological argument is that the stent is only truly needed for a finite period [16]:

1. Immediately after angioplasty, to prevent vessel collapse.
2. For the next several months, to allow healing, remodeling, and re-endothelialization of the vessel.

After ~6–12 months, the vessel has usually stabilized. At this point, a permanent metallic cage provides no further benefit—only persistent foreign-body risk.

In principle, a metallic scaffold is only needed temporarily to allow vessel healing and remodeling. After that, a permanent stent can become a liability.

For this reason, researchers have been working on developing bioresorbable scaffolds that are designed to hold the artery open only during the critical healing phase and then gradually dissolve [17, 18]. They can be made from bioabsorbable polymers or bioabsorbable metals (magnesium).

The potential benefits of bioabsorbable stents:

- Allow physiological repair
- Natural healing process after degradation
- Reconstitution of local vascular compliance
- Temporary limited longitudinal and radial straightening effect
- Possibility for growth

The challenge has been to make these temporary scaffolds as safe and effective as permanent metal stents, but the underlying principle is that long-term support is not required once the remodeling process is complete. However, current technology has not yet delivered a fully reliable, widely adopted resorbable scaffold that matches the long-term safety of metallic drug-eluting stents—but research is moving in that direction.

Some disadvantages of bioabsorbable polymer stents [19]:

- Greater bulk for required mechanical properties
- Extensive recoil
- Intrinsically lower strength
- Exaggerated acute and chronic inflammatory response

Limitations of bioabsorbable metal stents [16, 20–22]:

- Biocorrosion products lead to an inflammatory response and neointimal proliferation
- Local tissue "overload" with degradation products results from accelerated corrosion
- Biocompatibility of degradable biomaterials depends on solubility of released degradation products
- Local toxicity relates to local concentration of the elements over time
- Tissue tolerance for physiologically occurring metals depends on the change in their tissue concentration induced by corrosion
- Elements with high tissue concentration should have better biocompatibility during degradation

As an alternative to bioresorbable stents, we (Dmitry Rabkin, Eyal Morag, and Ophir Perelson) have developed a new concept of retrievable Nitinol stents, which can be removed from the body after they fulfill their mission and no longer needed. The concept is based on the TWSME of Nitinol.

The advantages of retrievable Nitinol stents:

- All benefits of permanent metallic stents
- Allow vessel remodeling
- Do not affect long-term endothelial dysfunction
- Allow ability to adapt to growth
- No interference with later endovascular or surgical revascularization
- Eliminate or minimize chronic inflammation
- Allow physiological repair
- Natural healing process after removal

- No issue with potential negative consequence of bioabsorption process or effect of bioproducts
- Reconstitution of local vascular compliance
- Repositioning of misplaced stents

Retrievable stents can be used for all indications where permanent metallic stents are applicable (atherosclerotic lesions, intimal dissections, vascular perforations, extrinsic compressions), but also markedly widen their applications to different areas, conditions, and purposes.

Retrievable Nitinol implants can be ideal vehicles for:

- Local drug delivery
  - Antirestenotic
  - Antiproliferative
  - Antineoplastic
  - Other
- Regional brachytherapy
- Gene therapy
- Angiogenic therapy
- Nano-technology
- Mictotechnology
  - Monitoring
  - Electrophysiology

Retrievable Nitinol implants can also play a role in individualization of local treatment, provide capability of delivering additional doses of the same or different medications for locoregional therapy, and give a possibility of sequential combination of alternative localized treatments.

With this concept in mind, we have developed a new class of endoluminal devices, made from Nitinol and exhibiting TWSME (Fig. 7.2) [23].

As described above, TWSME provides spontaneous, direct, and reversible change in shape with cooling, without application of the external physical force. It requires training with repetition of deformation cycle and allows restoration of about 30% of "cold" shape. Amplitude of TWSME depends on Nitinol alloy composition.

These devices are adapted to be retrieved or repositioned after their deployment and include an elongated tubular body, similar to a self-expanding Nitinol stent, and at least one "crown" at one or both ends (Fig. 7.3).

The crowns can be different in shape and configuration, but in general are constructed from elongated interconnected elements, resembling leaves (Fig. 7.4).

US008540761B2

(12) **United States Patent**
Rabkin et al.

(10) **Patent No.: US 8,540,761 B2**
(45) **Date of Patent: Sep. 24, 2013**

(54) **TEMPORARY, REPOSITIONABLE OR RETRIEVABLE INTRALUMINAL DEVICES**

(75) Inventors: **Dmitry J. Rabkin**, Framingham, MA (US); **Eval Morag**, East Hampton, MA (US); **Ophir Perelson**, Beverly Hills, CA (US)

(73) Assignee: **Intek Technology LLC**, Wilmington, DE (US)

(*) Notice: Subject to any disclaimer, the term of this patent is extended or adjusted under 35 U.S.C. 154(b) by 569 days.

(21) Appl. No.: **12/573,525**

(22) Filed: **Oct. 5, 2009**

(65) **Prior Publication Data**

US 2010/0087913 A1 Apr. 8, 2010

Related U.S. Application Data

(63) Continuation of application No. 10/333,599, filed as application No. PCT/US02/38374 on Dec. 3, 2002, now abandoned.

(60) Provisional application No. 60/337,060, filed on Dec. 3, 2001.

(51) **Int. Cl.**
A61F 2/82 (2006.01)

(52) **U.S. Cl.**
USPC **623/1.15**; 623/1.16; 623/1.19

(58) **Field of Classification Search**
USPC 623/1.15, 1.16, 1.19
See application file for complete search history.

(56) **References Cited**

U.S. PATENT DOCUMENTS

5,037,427	A *	8/1991	Harada et al.	606/108
5,593,442	A	1/1997	Klein	
5,688,418	A	11/1997	Yoshiyasu et al.	
6,042,606	A	3/2000	Frantzen	
6,296,661	B1	10/2001	Davila et al.	
6,447,478	B1 *	9/2002	Maynard	604/95.05
6,524,335	B1 *	2/2003	Hartley et al.	623/1.13
6,656,215	B1 *	12/2003	Yanez et al.	623/1.13
6,790,218	B2 *	9/2004	Jayaraman	606/191
2001/0011188	A1	8/2001	Berry et al.	

FOREIGN PATENT DOCUMENTS

EP	1036550		9/2000
EP	1138280		1/2004
EP	1294318		12/2004
FR	2745172	A1 *	8/1997
GB	2360456		9/2001
WO	9531945		5/1995

OTHER PUBLICATIONS

Search Report dated Jan. 11, 2005 (5 pages).

* cited by examiner

Primary Examiner — David H Willse
Assistant Examiner — Javier Blanco
(74) *Attorney, Agent, or Firm* — Cozen O'Connor

(57) **ABSTRACT**

A stent formed of a metallic material having a two-way memory adapted to be retrieved or repositioned after delivery includes an elongated tubular body and at least one crown connected to a respective longitudinal end of the body, the crown including a plurality of unconnected leaves, each leaf having a longitudinally extending frame connected at one end to the end of the body. A method of manufacturing the stent so that the crown has a greater two-way memory effect than the body is disclosed.

25 Claims, 18 Drawing Sheets

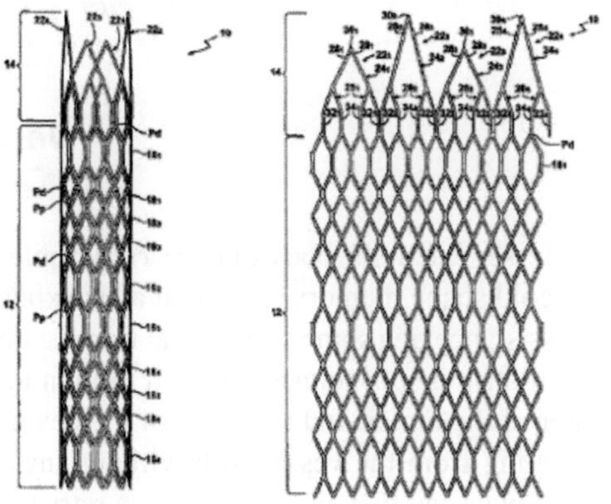

Fig. 7.2 US Patent 8,540,761 B2 temporary, repositionable, or retrievable intraluminal devices

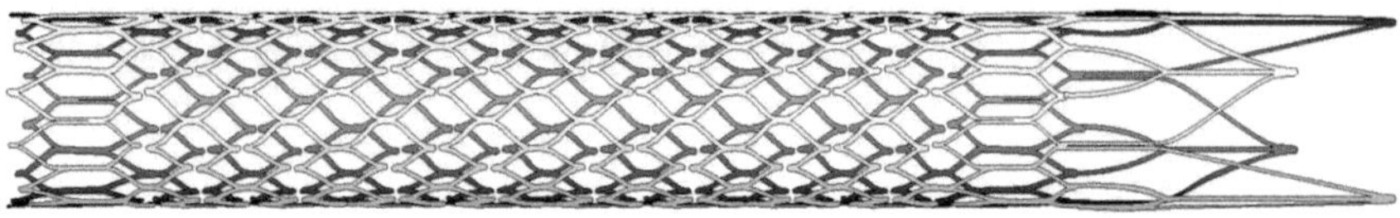

Fig. 7.3 Retrievable Nitinol stent with a crown at one end to facilitate atraumatic separation from the vessel wall and safe efficient retrieval

Fig. 7.4 Different potential versions of crowns of retrievable Nitinol implants

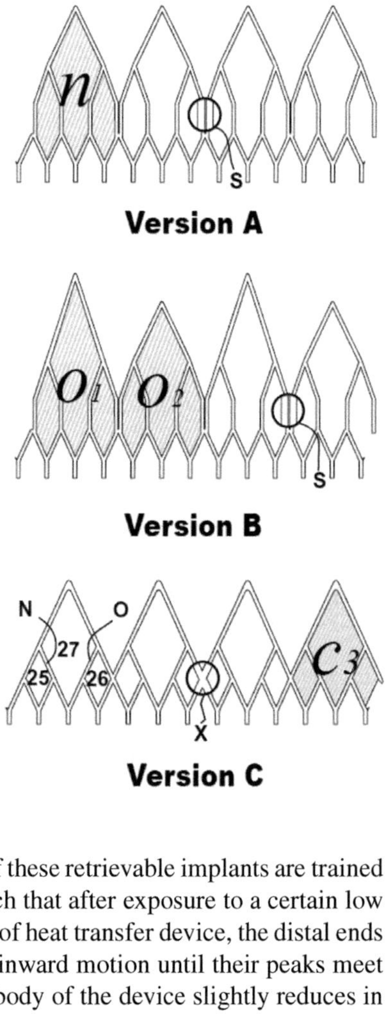

The crown and to a lesser extent the body of these retrievable implants are trained to have a second-way cold shape memory, such that after exposure to a certain low temperature with the assistance of a some sort of heat transfer device, the distal ends of the crown leaves demonstrate pronounced inward motion until their peaks meet each other at the center of the lumen and the body of the device slightly reduces in diameter, gently separating from the vessel wall without any mechanical force or trauma (Fig. 7.5). The device can then be captured by a retrieval system and reversibly engaged for retrieval and/or repositioning.

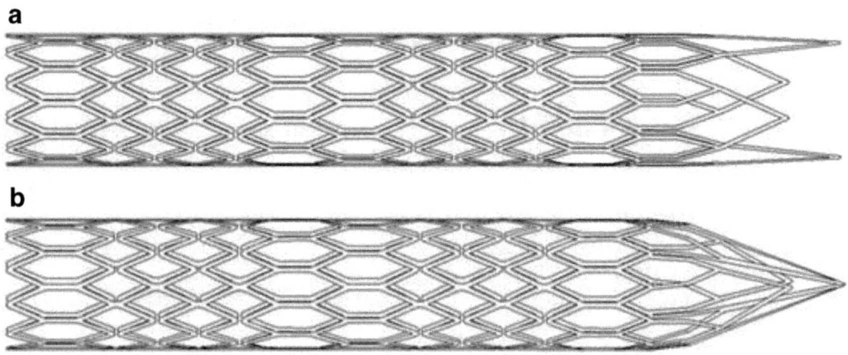

Fig. 7.5 Schematic drawing of the retrievable implant when fully open (**a**) and after cooling with inward motion of the crown leaves and slight reduction in the diameter of the implant body (**b**)

For the purpose of this project, we have partnered with the group of distinguished world-known experts in the field of shape memory materials from the Moscow Institute of Steel and Alloys, Prof. Sergey Prokoshkin, Dr. Elena Ryklina, and Dr. Irina Khmelevskaya. They have developed a practical approach for training of the Nitinol devices of our design to exhibit pronounced second-way cold memory in order to achieve atraumatic separation from the vessel wall and subsequent retrieval (Fig. 7.6). Their extensive work led to the invention of a new and improved process for treating shape memory alloys to induce two-way shape memory effect and a new TWSME training process for retrievable devices, in which the two-way shape memory changes occur within a clinically acceptable temperature range, spanning from about 5°–25 °C to 37 °C [24].

The training cycles for induction of a marked TWSME include repetitive consistent changes in shape of the crown elements and separately the body of the retrievable devices inside the water bath under specific temperatures.

After the training process the achieved cold shape of the crown elements recovers about 30% of its acquired configuration with subsequent heating. Therefore, in order for the crown elements to return from the cold shape to the position where they are aligned longitudinally with the body of the stent after heating, that is, the same circumference, the initial unloaded shape during the training process should face more outward with respect to the body of the stent. This effect is more important for repositioning of the stents, when the crown elements have to return to the same circumferential arrangement as the body of the stent with heating during redeployment, rather than their full retrieval. The cycle of training consists of repetitive deformation of the crown elements from outward position with respect to the body of the stent to exaggerated inward loading over a mandrel, while the entire arrangement is submerged in a water bath with accordingly synchronized changing of the temperature. This is clearly depicted in Fig. 7.7.

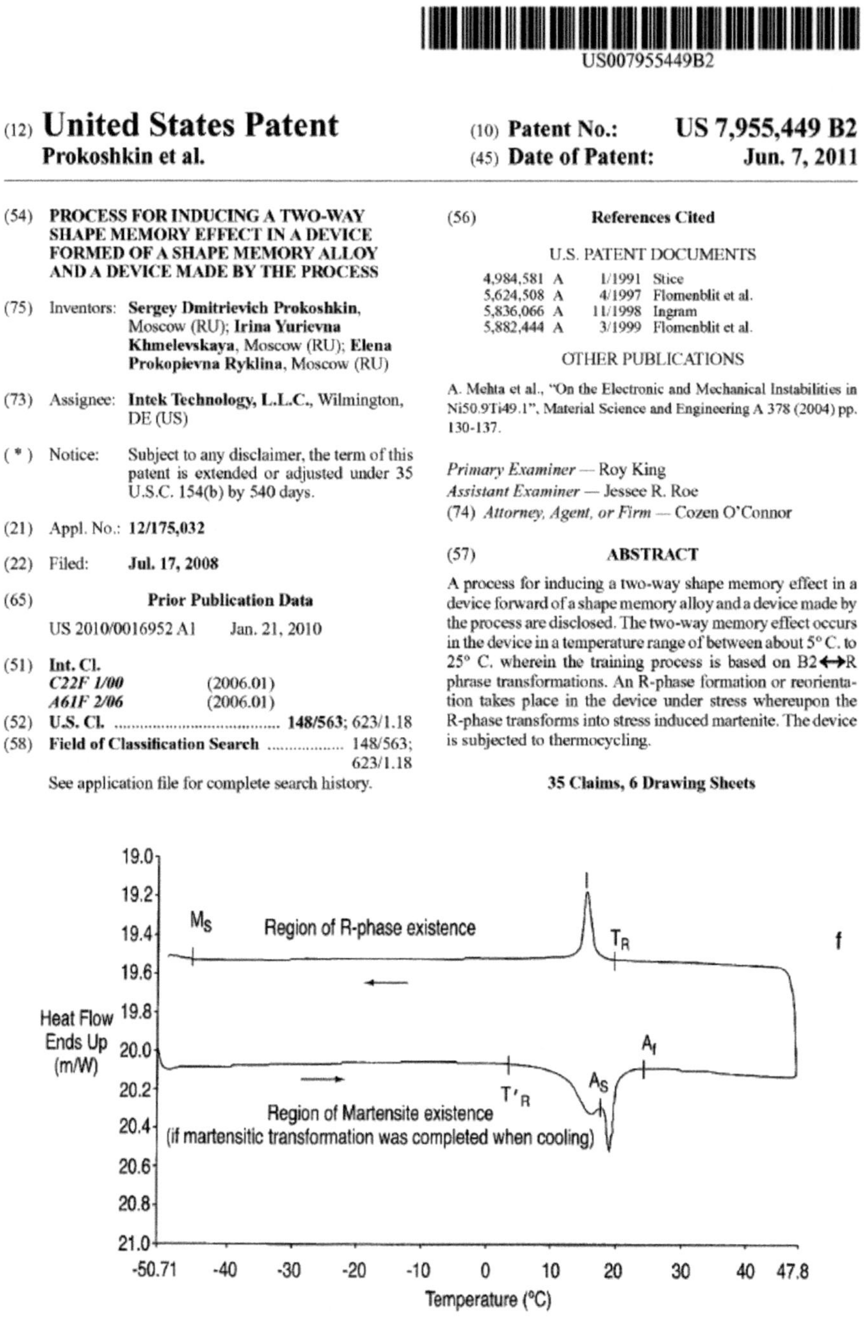

US007955449B2

(12) **United States Patent** (10) **Patent No.: US 7,955,449 B2**

Prokoshkin et al. (45) **Date of Patent: Jun. 7, 2011**

(54) **PROCESS FOR INDUCING A TWO-WAY SHAPE MEMORY EFFECT IN A DEVICE FORMED OF A SHAPE MEMORY ALLOY AND A DEVICE MADE BY THE PROCESS**

(75) Inventors: **Sergey Dmitrievich Prokoshkin**, Moscow (RU); **Irina Yurievna Khmelevskaya**, Moscow (RU); **Elena Prokopievna Ryklina**, Moscow (RU)

(73) Assignee: **Intek Technology, L.L.C.**, Wilmington, DE (US)

(*) Notice: Subject to any disclaimer, the term of this patent is extended or adjusted under 35 U.S.C. 154(b) by 540 days.

(21) Appl. No.: **12/175,032**

(22) Filed: **Jul. 17, 2008**

(65) **Prior Publication Data**

US 2010/0016952 A1 Jan. 21, 2010

(51) **Int. Cl.**
C22F 1/00 (2006.01)
A61F 2/06 (2006.01)

(52) **U.S. Cl.** **148/563**; 623/1.18

(58) **Field of Classification Search** 148/563; 623/1.18

See application file for complete search history.

(56) **References Cited**

U.S. PATENT DOCUMENTS

4,984,581	A	1/1991	Stice
5,624,508	A	4/1997	Flomenblit et al.
5,836,066	A	11/1998	Ingram
5,882,444	A	3/1999	Flomenblit et al.

OTHER PUBLICATIONS

A. Mehta et al., "On the Electronic and Mechanical Instabilities in Ni50.9Ti49.1", Material Science and Engineering A 378 (2004) pp. 130-137.

Primary Examiner — Roy King
Assistant Examiner — Jessee R. Roe
(74) *Attorney, Agent, or Firm* — Cozen O'Connor

(57) **ABSTRACT**

A process for inducing a two-way shape memory effect in a device forward of a shape memory alloy and a device made by the process are disclosed. The two-way memory effect occurs in the device in a temperature range of between about 5° C. to 25° C. wherein the training process is based on B2↔R phrase transformations. An R-phase formation or reorientation takes place in the device under stress whereupon the R-phase transforms into stress induced martenite. The device is subjected to thermocycling.

35 Claims, 6 Drawing Sheets

Fig. 7.6 US Patent No. 7,955,449 B2 process for inducing a TWSME in a device formed of a shape memory alloy and a device made by the process (S. Prokoshkin, I. Khmelevskaya, E. Ryklina)

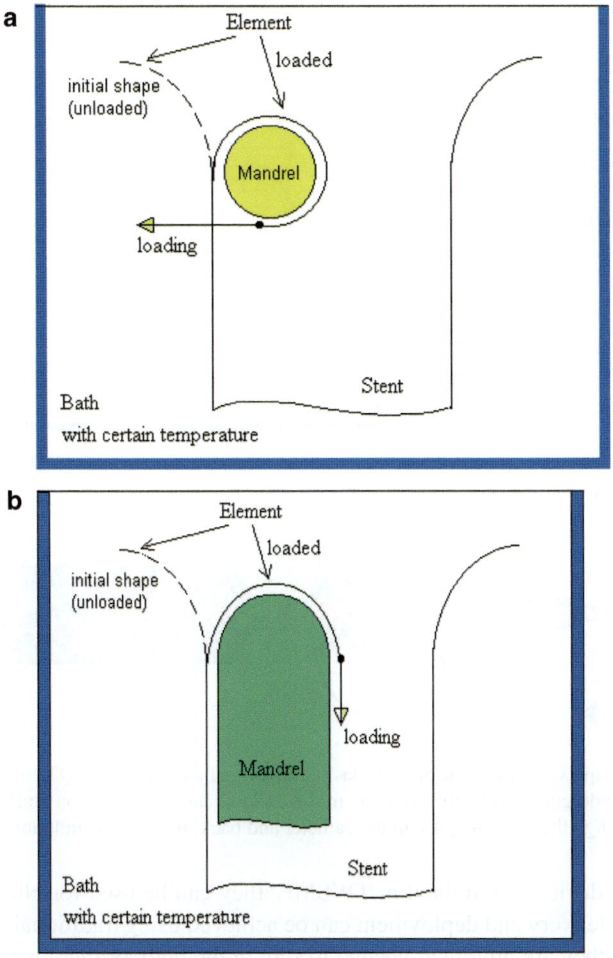

Fig. 7.7 Schematic illustrations showing two arrangements for inducing TWSME in a segment of a crown of a stent by loading the segment around a mandrel

To train the body of the stent to reduce in diameter upon cooling, the stents are placed inside a specially designed sleeve accommodation. The sleeve is repeatedly tightened to a specific diameter and then released to its original position while the stents are submerged in a water bath with synchronized changes in temperature (Fig. 7.8).

These TWSME training processes may sound complicated and time-consuming but can be semi- or completely automated and involve multiple devices at once. In fact, we have already developed a semi-automatic machine for the training of the body of the stents to induce the second-way memory, which was successfully and efficiently used in our practice for this purpose.

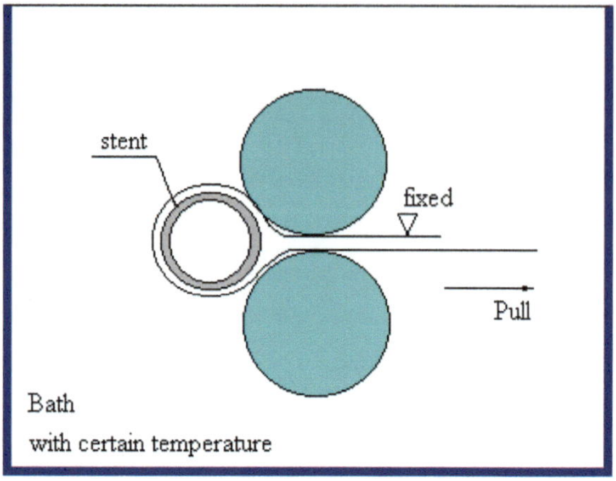

Fig. 7.8 Schematic cross-sectional illustration showing an arrangement for inducing TWSME in a laser-cut tubular body of a stent by controlled reproducible collapsing the body of the stent in a water bath to control the changes of temperature

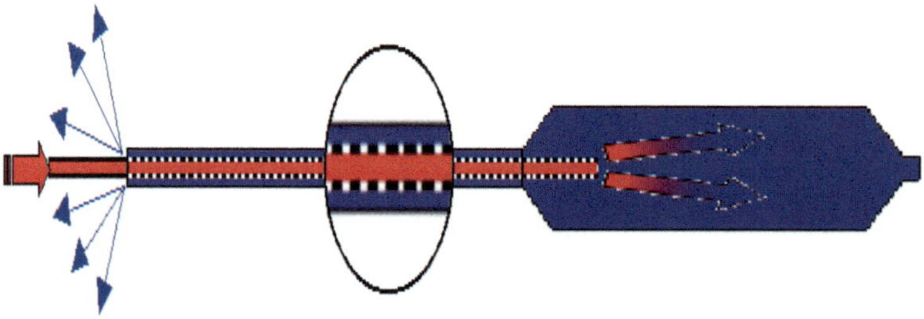

Fig. 7.9 Principles of operation of cryoplasty balloon catheter. Liquid N_2O enters the delivery lumen. N_2O undergoes phase shift to a gas in the balloon causing dilatation and cooling. Gas is exhausted through the annular space in the catheter and back into the cryoinflation device

Once the devices are trained in TWSME, they can be used for clinical applications. Their delivery and deployment can be achieved using traditional delivery systems. When they are no longer needed to stay in the body or there is time for them to come out, they can be retrieved by using specially designed retrieval systems. For targeted localized cooling of the devices, that were previously deployed into their desired locations, we have proposed to adopt a modified cryoplasty balloon catheter supplied with a special capturing mechanism. The technology uses nitrous oxide to fill an angioplasty balloon, cooling the balloon's surface to −10 °C (Fig. 7.9). Example of a cryoplasty device is a PolarCath System from Boston Scientific (Fig. 7.10) [25]. As it is inflated, the cold surface of the balloon gets in contact with the implanted retrievable device, transmitting the cold temperature and effectively cooling it. This triggers the process of restructuring of the Nitinol device into a martensitic configuration and reinstating the cold shape. When the balloon is then deflated, the crown of the implant and to a lesser extent its body, naturally start collapsing over the balloon, separating from the vessel wall without any external mechanical force or additional trauma. The device can then be captured by a special mechanism assembled over the balloon and safely retrieved.

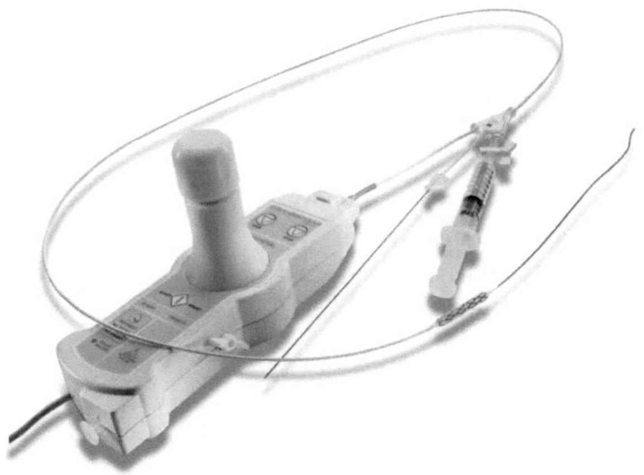

Fig. 7.10 PolarCath cryoplasty balloon system from Boston Scientific Corporation

We (Dmitry Rabkin, Eyal Morag, and Ophir Perelson) have developed multiple versions of the different apparatuses for retrieval/repositioning of the Nitinol implants with TWSME (Fig. 7.11).

The main common principle of all these systems is to combine a way of locally controlling the temperature of the implanted devices with different mechanisms for atraumatic capturing of spontaneously separated from the vessel wall stents [26]. These mechanisms are mounted or built-in into the balloon structure and open or close mechanically with inflation and deflation of the balloon (Fig. 7.12).

When the balloon of the retrieval system is inflated with N_2O, the strategically placed capturing elements automatically open up. After the complete inflation to its desired diameter and transmitting the cold temperature to the previously implanted retrievable device, the stent starts to conform to the balloon and the capturing hooks engage the stent struts and crown. With deflation of the balloon, the stent starts reduce in size and the elements of the crown start converging inward, staying in contact with the balloon surface. The hooks of the retrieval mechanism begin closing over the stent, holding it firmly. The entire assembly of the deflated balloon with the collapsed stent over it is then re-sheathed for repositioning (Fig. 7.13) or complete retrieval (Fig. 7.14).

The concept of retrievable Nitinol implants with TWSME is a promising technology as an alternative to biodegradable implants and beyond. It does have some advantages and unique features, but also has certain limitations and restrictions.

Endothelialization process of the bare metal stents takes about two weeks. Therefore, retrievable bare metal Nitinol stents have to come out within 10–12 days window after their implantation. If an attempt is made to remove them after two weeks being in place, it will cause some neointimal disruption with possible dissections and intimal flaps, increasing risk of thrombogenicity.

On the other hand, drug-eluting Nitinol retrievable stents can stay in place as long as needed, because endothelialization process is markedly delayed or even completely suspended by the eluted drug. These devices can be retrieved at any time after their implantation without any timing restrictions.

US006676692B2

(12) **United States Patent**
Rabkin et al.

(10) **Patent No.: US 6,676,692 B2**
(45) **Date of Patent: Jan. 13, 2004**

(54) **APPARATUS FOR DELIVERING, REPOSITIONING AND/OR RETRIEVING SELF-EXPANDING STENTS**

(75) Inventors: **Dmitry Rabkin**, Chestnut Hill, MA (US); **Eyal Morag**, East Hampton, MA (US); **Ophir Perelson**, Beverly Hills, CA (US)

(73) Assignee: **InTek Technology L.L.C.**, Wilmington, DE (US)

(*) Notice: Subject to any disclaimer, the term of this patent is extended or adjusted under 35 U.S.C. 154(b) by 0 days.

(21) Appl. No.: **09/845,098**

(22) Filed: **Apr. 27, 2001**

(65) **Prior Publication Data**

US 2002/0161377 A1 Oct. 31, 2002

(51) **Int. Cl.**[7] **A61F 2/06**; A61M 29/00
(52) **U.S. Cl.** **623/1.11**; 606/191; 604/104
(58) **Field of Search** 623/1.11; 606/198, 606/195, 194, 192, 108; 604/93.01, 96.01, 97.01, 103.08, 113, 104

(56) **References Cited**

U.S. PATENT DOCUMENTS

5,002,556 A	*	3/1991	Ishida et al.	606/191
5,569,295 A	*	10/1996	Lam	606/198
5,616,149 A	*	4/1997	Barath	606/159
5,776,141 A	*	7/1998	Klein et al.	606/108
5,902,268 A	*	5/1999	Saab	604/96
5,910,144 A	*	6/1999	Hayashi	606/108
6,217,585 B1	*	4/2001	Houser et al.	606/108
6,319,251 B1	*	11/2001	Tu et al.	606/41

FOREIGN PATENT DOCUMENTS

EP	0778010	6/1997

* cited by examiner

Primary Examiner—Corrine McDermott
Assistant Examiner—Alvin Stewart
(74) *Attorney, Agent, or Firm*—Steinberg & Raskin, P.C.

(57) **ABSTRACT**

Apparatus for delivering and deploying a stent formed of a shape memory alloy to a desired position in a tubular area of the body, and/or for repositioning and/or retrieving a stent formed of a two-way shape memory alloy. An arrangement is provided by which the temperature of the stent is locally adjusted during delivery, repositioning and/or retrieval in a safe and controlled manner by engagement with an expandable and collapsible thermal transfer member situated on a catheter assembly.

25 Claims, 48 Drawing Sheets

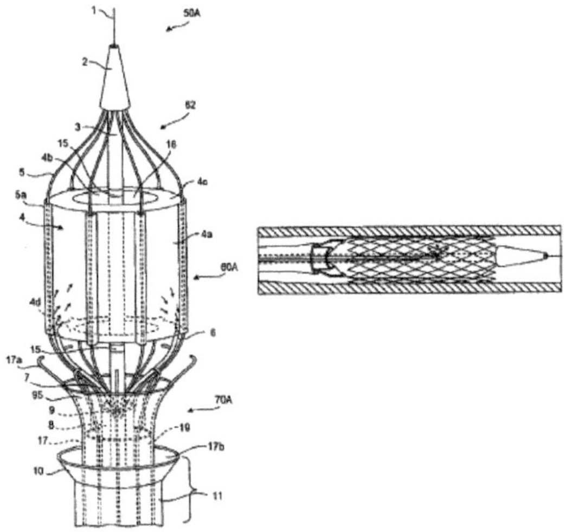

Fig. 7.11 US Patent 6,676,692 apparatus for delivering, repositioning, and/or retrieving self-expanding stents

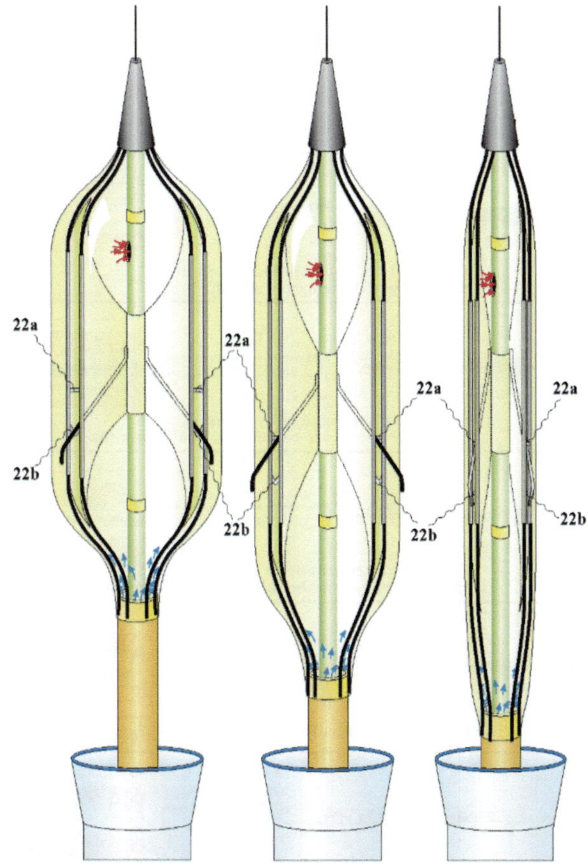

Fig. 7.12 One of the embodiments of the system for stent retrieval and mechanism of action. The system combines a cryoballoon and a built-in capturing mechanism activated by inflation and deflation of the balloon for capturing collapsing stent during cooling

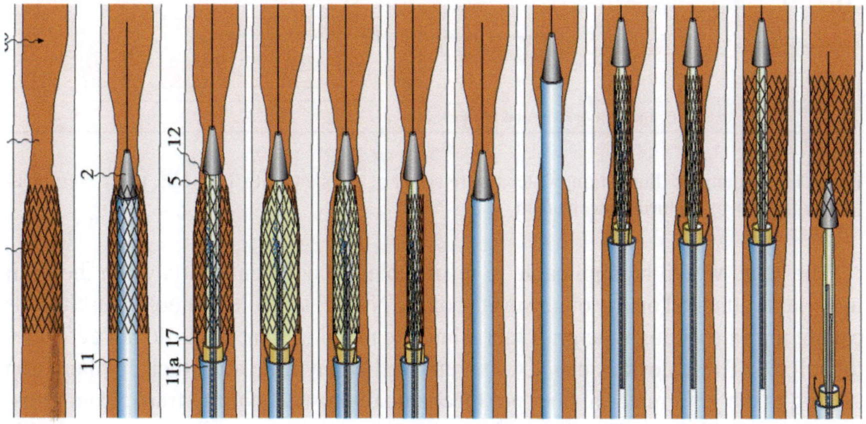

Fig. 7.13 Schematic illustration of steps of repositioning of the stent with TWSME, using a cryoballoon

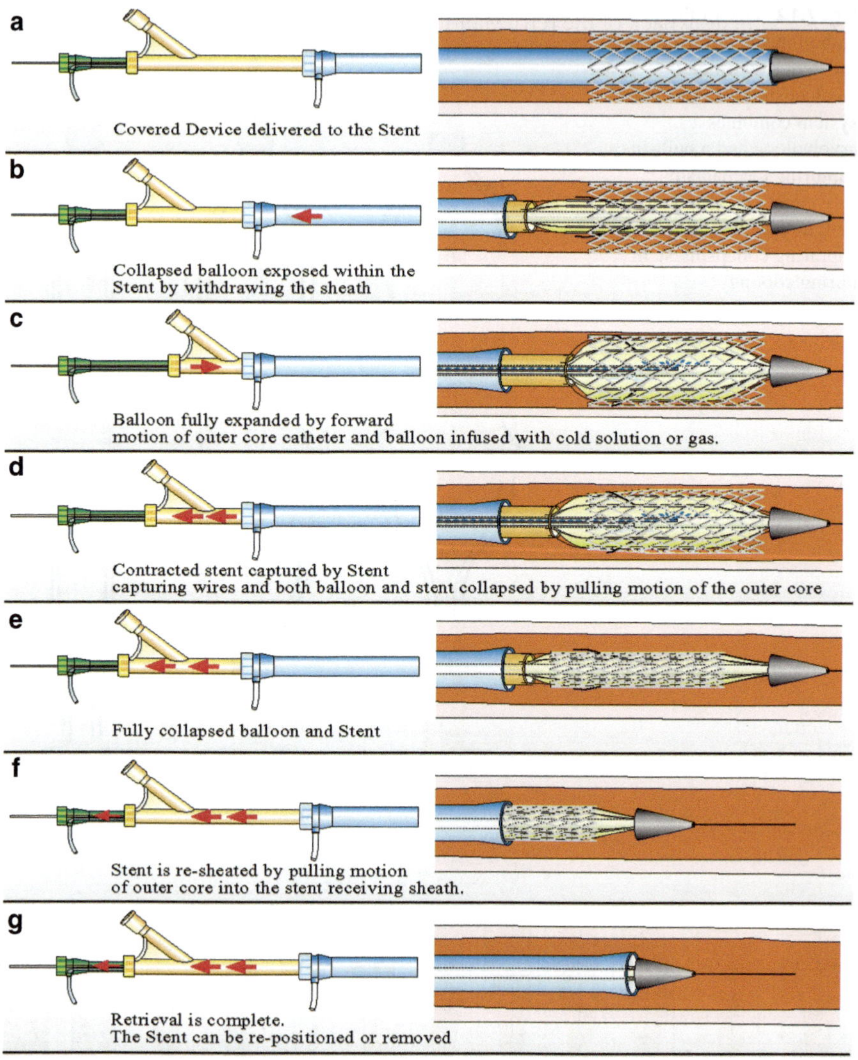

Fig. 7.14 Schematic illustration of steps of retrieval of the stent with TWSME, using a cryoballoon with built-in capturing mechanism

The same would be applicable to retrievable Nitinol stent grafts when the graft material is attached on the outer surface of the Nitinol scaffold. Smooth muscle cells cannot migrate through the graft fabric and the metallic stent struts do not get endothelialized. These devices can also be removed at any time after their implantation as long as the graft material does not mechanically restrict Nitinol frame from transferring to a cold shape. The force of transitioning of Nitinol scaffold to a collapsible state should overcome the strength of the fabric, which is easily achievable by selecting the proper graft material.

The main drawback of the retrievable Nitinol implants with TWSME is that their retrieval requires an additional procedure, even though minimally invasive. All the potential benefits that these devices may bring likely surpass the negative aspect of another procedure for their retrieval.

In conclusion, retrievable Nitinol implants based on TWSME provide a new exciting innovative approach in the management of cardiovascular and other disorders. They can play a role as a primary treatment or supplementary to conventional methods, with high potential in local and regional therapy. These devices can also find promising applications in monitoring and electrophysiology.

References

1. Lahoz R, Puértolas JA. Training and two-way shape memory in NiTi alloys: influence on thermal parameters. J Alloys Compd. 2004;381(1–2):130–6.
2. Yoo YI, Lee JJ. Two-way shape memory effect of NiTi under compressive loading cycles. Phys Procedia. 2011;22:449–54.
3. Yoo YI, Lee JJ. Study on the two-way shape memory characteristics induced by compressive loading cycles. Adv Mater Res. 2010;123:1023–6.
4. Omer O, et al. Experimental study on two-way shape memory effect training procedure for NiTiNOL shape memory alloy. Int J Eng Appl Sci. 2015;9(9):1840–6.
5. Lagoudas DC, editor. Shape memory alloys: modeling and engineering applications. New York: Springer; 2008.
6. Lahoz R, Gracia-Villa L, Puértolas JA. Training of the two-way shape memory effect by bending in NiTi alloys. J Eng Mater Technol. 2002;124(4):397–402.
7. Liu Y, Xiang H. Factors influencing the development of two-way shape memory behaviour in NiTi. J Phys IV (France). 1991;1(C4):599–604.
8. Wada K, Liu Y. Thermomechanical training and the shape recovery characteristics of NiTi alloys. Mater Sci Eng A. 2008;481–482:166–9.
9. Lexcellent C, Leclercq B, Bourbon G. The two-way shape memory effect of shape memory alloys: an experimental study and a phenomenological model. Int J Plast. 2000;16(10–11):1155–68.
10. Duda SH, Bosiers M, Lammer J, et al. Drug-eluting and bare nitinol stents for the superficial femoral artery: long-term results. J Endovasc Ther. 2006;13(5):701–10.
11. Hoffmann R, Mintz GS, Dussaillant GR, et al. Patterns and mechanisms of in-stent restenosis. Circulation. 1996;94(6):1247–54.
12. Finn AV, Nakazawa G, Joner M, et al. Vascular responses to drug-eluting stents: importance of delayed healing. Arterioscler Thromb Vasc Biol. 2007;27(7):1500–10.
13. Inoue T, Croce K, Morooka T, et al. Vascular inflammation and repair: implications for restenosis after stenting. Thromb Haemost. 2011;105(3):435–41.
14. Jeong U, Ahn C, Hwang SY, et al. Stent-induced hemodynamic disturbances and vascular injury: mechanisms of restenosis. Ann Biomed Eng. 2018;46(3):396–409.
15. Colombo A, Karvounis E. Biodegradable stents: "fulfilling the mission and fading away". Circulation. 2000;102(4):371–3.
16. Iqbal J, Onuma Y, Ormiston J, et al. Bioresorbable scaffolds: rationale, current status, challenges, and future. Eur Heart J. 2014;35(12):765–76.
17. Hou LD, Li Z, Pan Y, et al. A review on biodegradable materials for cardiovascular stent application. Front Mater Sci. 2016;10(3):238–59.
18. Bowen PK, Shearier ER, Zhao S, et al. Biodegradable metals for cardiovascular stents. Adv Healthc Mater. 2016;5(10):1121–40.

19. Giacchi G, Omedè P, Benedetto S, et al. Bioresorbable scaffolds: current technologies and potential disadvantages. Int J Cardiol. 2016;207:22–9.
20. Puricel S, Cuculi F, Weissner M, et al. Bioresorbable coronary scaffold thrombosis: multicenter registry. J Am Coll Cardiol. 2016;67(8):921–31.
21. Kereiakes DJ, Ellis SG, Metzger C, et al. Three-year results of the ABSORB III trial. Circulation. 2017;135(2):208–17.
22. Bowen PK, Drelich J, Goldman J. Biodegradable metals for cardiovascular stents: mechanical challenges and failure modes. Adv Mater. 2013;25(18):2577–98.
23. Rabkin DJ, Morag E, Perelson O. Temporary, repositionable or retrievable intraluminal devices. US Patent 8,540,761 B2. 2013.
24. Prokoshkin SD, Khmelevskaya I, Ryklina E. Process for inducing a two-way shape memory effect in a device formed of a shape memory alloy and a device made by the process. US Patent 7,995,449 B2. 2011.
25. Elder M. The next-generation PolarCath system. Endovasc Today. 2018;17(1 Suppl):2–5.
26. Rabkin DJ, Morag E, Perelson O. Apparatus for delivering, repositioning and/or retrieving self-expanding stents. US Patent 6,676,692 B2. 2004.

Legacy in Bloom

8

Current Global Market of Nitinol-Based Stents and Future Projections

The Global Nitinol Self-Expanding Stents Market is witnessing strong expansion, growing from USD 5903.85 million in 2024 to an estimated USD 11,883.84 million by 2033, at a compound annual growth rate (CAGR) of 8.0%. The market growth is being propelled by rising prevalence of cardiovascular, peripheral artery, and gastrointestinal disorders, alongside increasing adoption of minimally invasive procedures across both developed and emerging healthcare systems. Nitinol will remain the default material for SES. Nitinol, with its superior biocompatibility, elasticity, and durability, has become the material of choice for self-expanding stents, reinforcing its adoption across multiple clinical applications. Virtually all modern self-expanding designs across peripheral, carotid, venous, and GI are built from Nitinol because of its superelasticity and shape memory, which give crush resistance, conformability, and trackability that other alloys struggle to match. That's been true historically and is reaffirmed in recent reviews focused specifically on Nitinol SES.

The analysis, statistics, and projections on Global Nitinol Self-Expanding Stents Market are based on the most recent report from STRAITS RESEARCH, which was specifically prepared for the purpose of this manuscript and quoted in this chapter with their exclusive permission [1].

Straits Research is a market intelligence company providing global business information report and services. Their exclusive blend of quantities forecasting, and trends analysis provides forward-looking insight. Their business reports represent the latest and the most reliable information indispensable for businesses to sustain a competitive edge.

Each syndicated research report covers a different sector, such as pharmaceuticals, chemical, energy, food and beverages, contraction, med devices, consumer

I. Rabkin, D. J. Rabkin, *Bloodline of Nitinol Stents*,
https://doi.org/10.1007/978-3-032-25697-3_8

goods, and technology. These reports provide in-depth analysis and deep segmentation to possible micro-levels, with wider scope and stratified research methodology, these syndicated reports strive to serve the overall research requirement.

Independent market snapshots suggest the global self-expanding stents category grows in the low- to mid-single digits through 2030, with segment outliers. One widely cited analysis pegs SES at ~$3.22B in 2022 with ~4% CAGR to 2030. Venous stents, however, are the fastest-growing SES niche, typically modeled at ~8–10% CAGR into the early 2030s as post-thrombotic and non-thrombotic iliac vein lesions are treated more routinely.

GI (esophageal/biliary/colonic) SEMS market expands more modestly (~5% CAGR). These figures vary by methodology, but the relative pattern—venous fastest, GI moderate, peripheral steady—has been consistent across reports.

Why venous is surging: Dedicated Nitinol venous platforms are now mainstream and keep improving. After the first FDA-approved dedicated devices (Vici, Venovo) opened the US market in 2019–2020, subsequent approvals and launches (e.g., Medtronic Abre; Philips Duo PMA in May 2024 with first implants soon after) broadened options and indications, and should sustain higher procedure growth. Expect continued competition around crush resistance, radial force, and flexibility tailored to iliofemoral biomechanics.

Peripheral femoropopliteal SES will stay large but competitive with drug-coated balloons. Two macro forces shape share here. First, the 2023 FDA update concluding paclitaxel-coated devices are unlikely to increase mortality effectively removed the biggest cloud over drug-eluting modalities, supporting durable use of paclitaxel-eluting Nitinol SES (e.g., Eluvia). Second, drug-coated balloons (DCB) keep expanding indications, creating "DCB first" strategies in many labs; that caps SES share growth, but does not eliminate it—especially in longer, calcified, or dissected segments where scaffolding is helpful.

Clinical data continue to favor modern DES over BMS when scaffolding is chosen. Five-year and extension readouts from the IMPERIAL program consistently show strong long-term patency and low reintervention with Eluvia versus alternatives, bolstering the case for polymer-controlled paclitaxel release in SFA disease. That evidence base tends to stabilize DES share inside the peripheral SES sector.

GI SEMS (biliary, esophageal, colonic) grows steadily off a smaller base, driven by malignant obstruction palliation and incremental design tweaks (antimigration features, covering/anti-tumor ingrowth strategies). Forecasts generally sit around mid-single digit CAGR through 2030.

What is new in the tech pipeline (and what it implies for share):

- Venous: "Differential" or zone-specific architecture (hybrid cell patterns and braided/laser-cut combinations) to balance flexibility across the iliac curve with crush resistance at the inguinal ligament—typified by the 2024 PMA-cleared Philips Duo system. This design direction should keep venous SES in a high-growth lane and gradually redistribute share toward newer platforms that document fewer fractures and reinterventions.
- Peripheral biomechanics: Biomimetic geometries (helical centerline stents like BioMimics 3D, Varyan) seek to induce swirling flow and reduce neointimal

hyperplasia. Innovative technology is used to improve the performance of vascular stents by adopting the principle of biomimicry; developing structures that imitate those occurring naturally. Three-year registry data in complex disease are encouraging and may nudge BMS-style niches toward these designs when drug therapy is not selected.

- Drug delivery: Expect continued dominance of paclitaxel-eluting SES where scaffolding is needed, while sirolimus remains more active on the DCB side for now; early hybrid concepts (temporary or retrievable scaffolds paired with sirolimus delivery) are being studied and could open a middle-ground tactic for long lesions or in-stent restenosis—potentially limiting permanent SES use in some anatomies if outcomes hold.
- Delivery systems: Triaxial SES delivery (outer stabilization + protective middle sheath + inner shaft) is now a de-facto standard for precise placement in long, tortuous segments and will persist as a design baseline; improvements here mainly shift share within brands by enabling longer stents, lower profiles, and better pushability, not by changing overall SES dynamics.

Putting that together as a practical market-share picture for the next five to seven years: the SES category should keep a stable foothold in peripheral PAD, expand materially in venous as dedicated designs proliferate and long-term data mature, and climb slowly in GI. Because nearly all SES are Nitinol, Nitinol's share inside the SES category remains overwhelming. Directionally, most analysts expect overall SES dollars to grow modestly (low-single digit CAGR) while venous grows the fastest (high-single to low-double digits), shifting the internal mix of Nitinol SES toward venous over time.

Regionally, North America remains the largest market, projected to reach USD 4.73 billion by 2033, driven by high procedure volumes, advanced healthcare infrastructure, and rapid uptake of next generation coated stents. Europe follows closely with USD 2.99 billion, benefiting from strong regulatory support for minimally invasive vascular interventions. However, Asia Pacific stands out with the fastest CAGR of 9.6%, fueled by a rapidly aging population, increasing burden of cardiovascular and gastrointestinal disorders, and significant expansion in healthcare access, particularly in China, India, and Southeast Asia. Latin America and the Middle East and Africa represent smaller shares, though both are expected to see steady adoption as awareness and healthcare investment rise.

From a product perspective, Peripheral Nitinol Self-Expanding Stents dominate, contributing nearly one-third of the global market by 2033, reflecting their critical role in treating peripheral artery disease (PAD). Carotid and Drug-Eluting Nitinol Self-Expanding Stents collectively represent another significant portion, driven by advancements in stroke prevention and restenosis reduction technologies. Gastrointestinal stents are also expanding in demand, supported by higher incidence of gastrointestinal cancers and obstructions requiring minimally invasive solutions. Emerging applications such as bronchial and venous stents, while smaller in size, are gaining clinical recognition and showing healthy CAGR growth above 7% (Table 8.1).

Table 8.1 Global Nitinol self-expanding stents market share by product type 2025–2033 (USD Million)

Product Type	2025	2026	2027	2028	2029	2030	2031	2032	2033	CAGR (%)
Peripheral	2107.17	2274.48	2458.46	2631.05	2852.58	3080.74	3331.64	3590.40	3883.56	7.9
Carotid	1100.35	1194.97	1299.05	1397.20	1523.11	1653.66	1798.99	1949.65	2120.15	8.5
GI	769.18	827.77	891.75	950.50	1026.67	1104.65	1190.28	1277.96	1376.71	7.5
Bronchial	386.33	419.12	455.42	489.98	533.94	579.53	628.89	680.10	738.26	8.4
DES	1166.45	1253.57	1348.60	1435.55	1548.48	1663.86	1790.71	1920.35	2066.25	7.4
Stent-grafts	516.26	559.49	606.94	651.59	708.81	767.97	833.48	901.23	977.89	8.3
Venous	393.82	425.58	460.22	493.53	535.23	576.86	622.88	668.68	721.02	7.9
Total	6439.56	6954.97	7520.45	8049.39	8728.82	9427.25	10,196.87	10,988.37	11,883.84	8.0

Peripheral Nitinol Self-Expanding Stents

Key Market Trends, Growth Factors, and Opportunities

Peripheral Nitinol self-expanding stents are primarily deployed in the treatment of peripheral artery disease (PAD), where arteries outside the heart, particularly in the legs, become narrowed due to atherosclerosis. These stents provide the dual benefit of radial strength and flexibility, making them suitable for arteries in dynamic regions such as the superficial femoral artery and iliac arteries, where external forces like bending, twisting, and compression are common. The self-expanding property of Nitinol, a nickel–titanium alloy, ensures that the stent conforms to the vessel's anatomy and maintains lumen patency even under biomechanical stress. Growing incidence of PAD, driven by rising rates of diabetes, hypertension, obesity, and smoking, significantly fuels demand. Additionally, aging populations across the US, Europe, and Asia-Pacific regions are pushing the adoption of peripheral stents as vascular diseases become more prevalent. The market is also witnessing technological improvements such as low-profile delivery systems, drug-coated stents, and hybrid stents that enhance long-term outcomes and reduce restenosis. Technological innovation—longer single-piece Nitinol scaffolds, refined cell geometries to reduce restenosis, drug-coated stent platforms, and improved delivery systems—addresses historical failure modes such as in-stent restenosis and fracture. Favorable reimbursement structures in developed economies and expanding minimally invasive endovascular procedures in emerging countries further strengthen the outlook. However, challenges remain in terms of in-stent restenosis, thrombosis risks, and the need for frequent follow-up interventions. Despite these limitations, the shift from open surgery to endovascular stenting, coupled with rising hospital infrastructure in emerging markets, positions peripheral Nitinol self-expanding stents as one of the largest and fastest-growing subsegments in the overall market (Fig. 8.1).

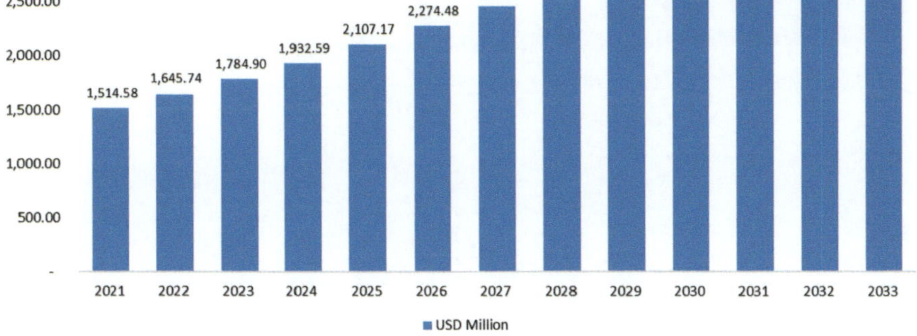

Fig. 8.1 Global Nitinol self-expanding stents market, by peripheral self-expanding stents 2021–2033 (USD Million)

Carotid Nitinol Self-Expanding Stents

Key Market Trends, Growth Factors, and Opportunities

Carotid Nitinol self-expanding stents are specifically designed for the treatment of carotid artery stenosis, a condition characterized by the narrowing of the carotid arteries that supply blood to the brain. These stents play a critical role in reducing the risk of ischemic strokes, which are often caused by reduced or obstructed blood flow. Carotid stenting, as an alternative to carotid endarterectomy (surgical removal of plaque), has gained clinical acceptance due to its minimally invasive approach and reduced recovery time. Nitinol's unique properties of shape memory and superelasticity are highly advantageous in carotid applications, as the stent must adapt to the dynamic vessel structure of the neck and provide reliable long-term patency. Carotid stents are also designed with embolic protection devices to minimize the risk of stroke during implantation, making them safer and more effective. The growing prevalence of atherosclerosis, hypertension, diabetes, and lifestyle-related cardiovascular conditions is fueling the demand for these stents globally. Moreover, increasing adoption of advanced stent designs with drug-eluting properties, improved scaffolding, and thinner struts is enhancing patient outcomes. Market growth is further supported by favorable reimbursement policies in developed healthcare systems, rising awareness of stroke prevention, and the expanding geriatric population, which is more susceptible to carotid artery disease. Additionally, clinical evidence supporting the non-inferiority of carotid stenting compared to surgical interventions is influencing physician adoption. However, challenges such as procedural risks in high-surgical risk patients, regulatory hurdles, and cost constraints in developing economies remain significant factors. Nonetheless, continuous advancements in stent technology and expanding indications for carotid stenting are expected to sustain growth in this segment (Fig. 8.2).

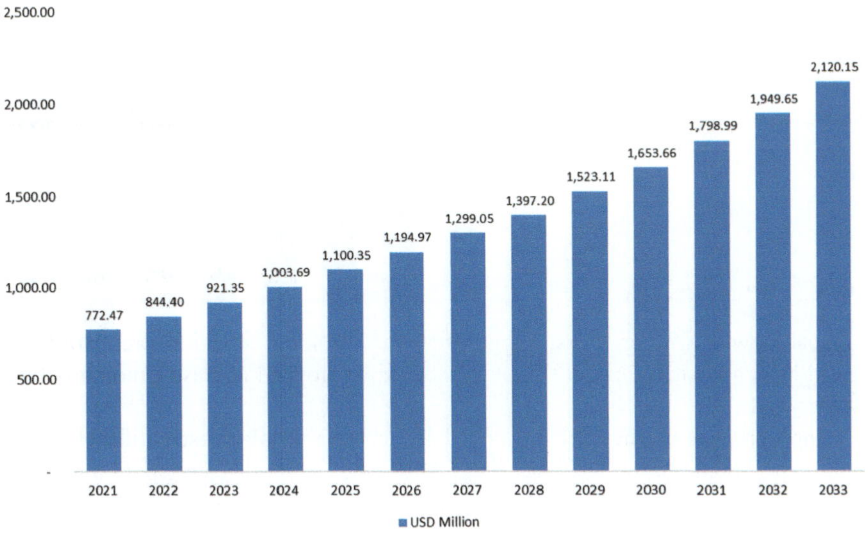

Fig. 8.2 Global Nitinol self-expanding stents market, by carotid Nitinol self-expanding stents 2021–2033 (USD Million)

Gastrointestinal (GI) Nitinol Self-Expanding Stents

Key Market Trends, Growth Factors, and Opportunities

Gastrointestinal (GI) Nitinol self-expanding stents are primarily used to manage malignant obstructions in the esophagus, duodenum, biliary tract, and colon. These stents provide a minimally invasive option to restore luminal patency, particularly for patients who are not surgical candidates due to advanced disease or comorbidities. Their Nitinol composition ensures high flexibility, radial strength, and resistance to external compression, making them especially effective in complex anatomical locations of the GI tract. Demand for these stents is rising as gastrointestinal cancers such as esophageal, colorectal, and pancreatic cancers show growing incidence worldwide. Moreover, the expanding geriatric population, which is more prone to GI malignancies and benign strictures, contributes to market growth. Innovations such as anti-migration designs, drug-eluting coatings, and covered versus uncovered stent variations are expanding therapeutic possibilities and addressing complications like tumor ingrowth and stent migration. Additionally, improvements in endoscopic techniques and the rising preference for palliative care interventions have enhanced the adoption of GI Nitinol self-expanding stents. Healthcare systems in emerging markets are also increasingly adopting these solutions due to improvements in cancer screening and diagnosis. Overall, this segment is expected to see steady demand growth, driven by oncology prevalence, technological advancements, and the increasing shift toward minimally invasive endoscopic interventions (Fig. 8.3).

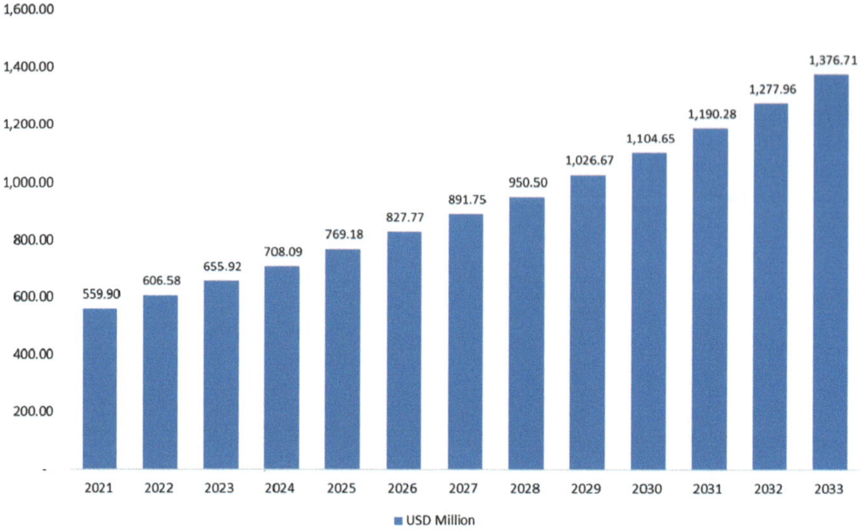

Fig. 8.3 Global Nitinol self-expanding stents market, by gastrointestinal (GI) Nitinol self-expanding stents 2021–2033 (USD Million)

Bronchial Nitinol Self-Expanding Stents

Key Market Trends, Growth Factors, and Opportunities

Bronchial Nitinol self-expanding stents are designed for use in the management of central airway obstructions caused by lung cancer, tracheobronchial stenosis, or benign airway strictures. These stents are particularly valuable for patients with advanced lung cancer, where airway compression significantly impairs breathing. Nitinol's flexibility and biocompatibility make these stents ideal for adapting to the dynamic respiratory environment, ensuring they maintain airway patency while minimizing tissue trauma. Unlike silicone stents, Nitinol stents are self-expanding, allowing for easier placement using bronchoscopy and reducing procedural complications. The segment is experiencing rising demand as global lung cancer incidence remains high and as awareness of minimally invasive pulmonary interventions increases. Innovation within the segment targets drug-coated and anti-granulation surface treatments to reduce restenosis and granulation tissue formation—a common challenge in airway stenting—plus designs that minimize migration while preserving mucociliary clearance. Interdisciplinary expansion of interventional pulmonology and thoracic endoscopy capabilities in tertiary centers is improving access and procedure volumes. Regions with high smoking prevalence and poor air quality are expected to be especially important growth markets. Although still smaller in absolute terms compared to cardiovascular and PAD segments, the pulmonary category's elevated CAGR reflects clinical unmet needs, active device R&D, and increasing clinician comfort with minimally invasive airway

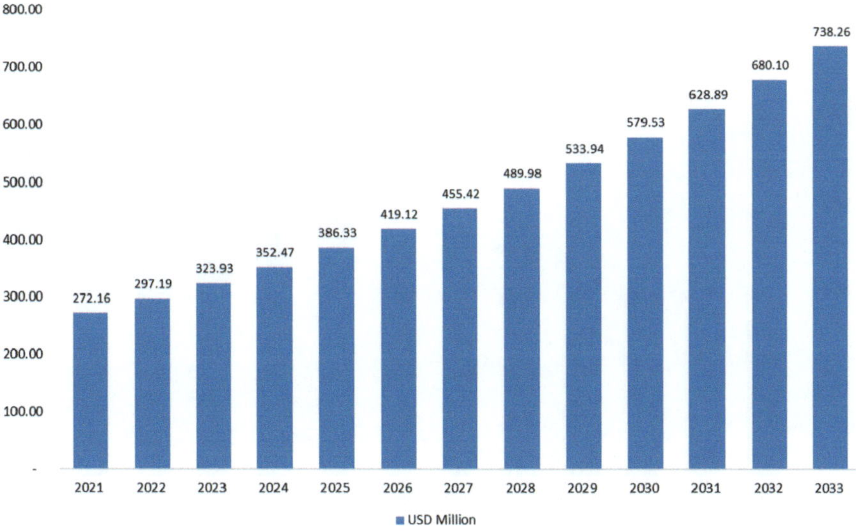

Fig. 8.4 Global Nitinol self-expanding stents market, by bronchial Nitinol self-expanding stents 2021–2033 (USD Million)

interventions. Furthermore, technological enhancements such as drug-coated bronchial stents, bioabsorbable designs, and hybrid silicone-Nitinol solutions are expected to improve patient outcomes and reduce complications like granulation tissue formation. Growth is also supported by advancements in interventional pulmonology and the availability of improved imaging-guided bronchoscopic placement techniques. Emerging markets are likely to contribute significantly as access to advanced respiratory care improves. As respiratory diseases, both malignant and benign, remain a global health concern, bronchial Nitinol self-expanding stents will continue to serve as a crucial solution in palliative and life-extending care (Fig. 8.4).

Drug-Eluting Nitinol Self-Expanding Stents

Key Market Trends, Growth Factors, and Opportunities

DES represent a transformative innovation in stent technology, combining the mechanical benefits of Nitinol with the therapeutic advantage of localized drug delivery. These stents are primarily used in peripheral artery disease (PAD), and increasingly in other vascular applications. By releasing antiproliferative drugs such as paclitaxel or sirolimus, they help prevent restenosis, a common complication in bare-metal stents caused by neointimal hyperplasia. The integration of self-expanding Nitinol ensures flexibility and durability, allowing for use in complex vascular anatomies, especially in tortuous or dynamically moving vessels like the superficial femoral artery. The demand for drug-eluting Nitinol stents is rising due to the high prevalence of cardiovascular diseases globally, coupled with clinical

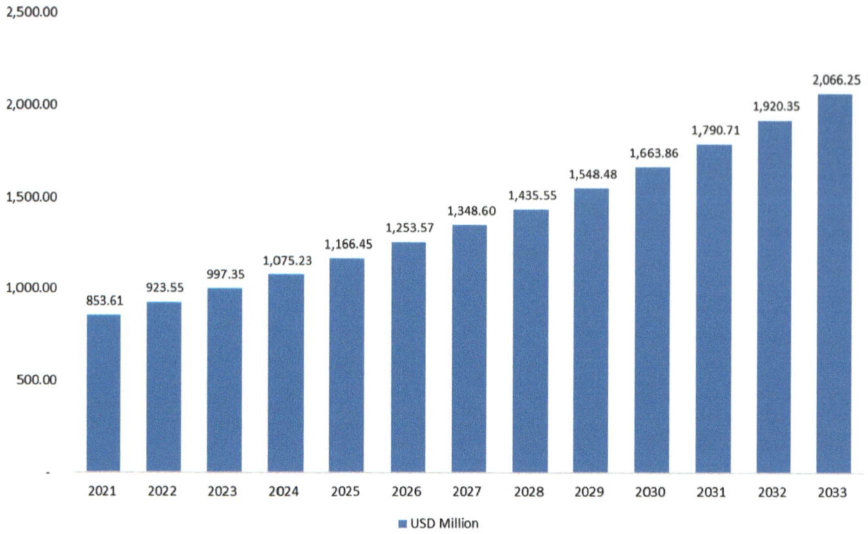

Fig. 8.5 Global Nitinol self-expanding stents market, by drug-eluting Nitinol stents 2021–2033 (USD Million)

evidence supporting superior long-term patency rates compared to conventional stents. Ongoing innovations are focused on biodegradable drug coatings, dual-drug release systems, and optimized polymer technologies that enhance biocompatibility and reduce late thrombosis risks. Additionally, health systems increasingly prioritize value-based care, making stents that reduce re-intervention rates highly attractive. Growth opportunities are especially strong in developed regions with high cardiovascular disease burdens, but adoption is also expanding in emerging economies due to improvements in healthcare infrastructure. With cardiovascular diseases continuing as a leading cause of mortality worldwide, the drug-eluting Nitinol self-expanding stents market is poised for strong growth (Fig. 8.5).

Nitinol Self-Expanding Stent-Grafts

Key Market Trends, Growth Factors, and Opportunities

Stent-grafts are a specialized category of Nitinol-based self-expanding stents designed primarily for use in endovascular aneurysm repair, such as thoracic or abdominal aortic aneurysms, peripheral arterial aneurysms, or arterial rupture/perforation with internal bleeding. These devices combine a metallic Nitinol scaffold with a fabric graft (commonly ePTFE or Dacron), creating a hybrid solution that reinforces blood vessels while excluding aneurysmal sacs or injured segment of a vessel. Their adoption has surged as endovascular treatments are increasingly preferred over open surgical repair due to their minimally invasive nature, reduced recovery times, and lower perioperative risks. Stent-grafts are widely used in

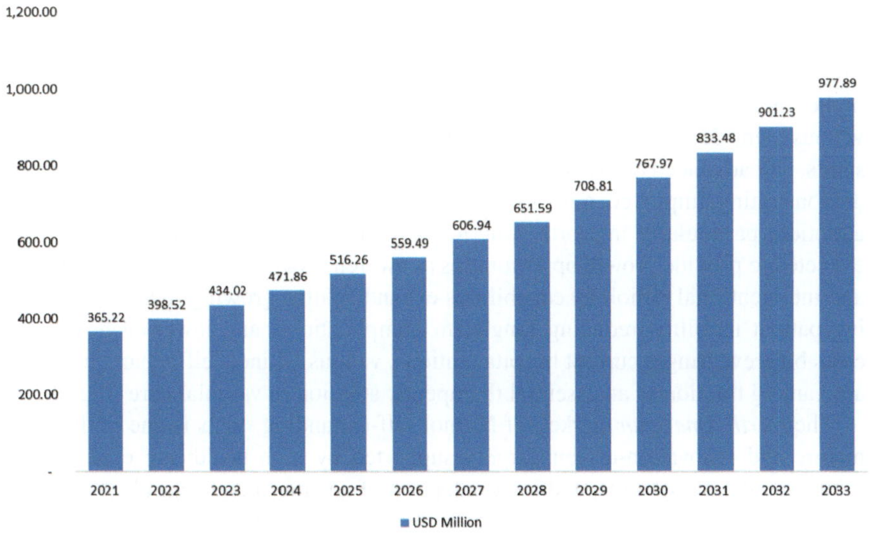

Fig. 8.6 Global Nitinol self-expanding stents market, by stent-grafts 2021–2033 (USD Million)

abdominal aortic aneurysms (AAA) and thoracic aortic aneurysms (TAA), conditions with growing prevalence among the aging global population. The flexibility of Nitinol allows these stent-grafts to adapt to the complex curves of the vessels while maintaining long-term patency. Technological advancements have led to fenestrated and branched stent-grafts, expanding their applicability to anatomically challenging cases. The market is also witnessing rising demand due to increased screening for aortic aneurysms, improvements in imaging diagnostics, and better access to endovascular surgical capabilities in both developed and emerging regions. However, durability concerns, re-intervention rates, and high procedural costs remain challenges. Nonetheless, with expanding patient awareness, increasing adoption of minimally invasive vascular repair, and innovation in next-generation devices, the stent-graft segment is set for sustained growth (Fig. 8.6).

Venous Nitinol Self-Expanding Stents

Key Market Trends, Growth Factors, and Opportunities

Venous Nitinol self-expanding stents are specifically designed to manage chronic venous obstructions, deep vein thrombosis (DVT) complications, and post-thrombotic syndrome. Unlike arterial stents, venous stents require unique design features such as high radial strength, crush resistance, and long lengths to accommodate the distinct anatomy and low-pressure environment of venous systems. Nitinol's self-expanding properties make it highly suitable for these requirements, ensuring flexibility and long-term patency. The demand for venous stents is rising due to increased diagnosis of chronic venous insufficiency, which causes significant morbidity and impacts quality of life. Additionally, risk factors such as sedentary lifestyles, obesity, prolonged immobilization, and aging populations contribute to higher incidences of venous disease globally. Recent innovations include dedicated venous stent designs (as opposed to adapted arterial stents), drug-eluting venous stents, and advanced delivery systems that simplify implantation. Clinical evidence demonstrating improved outcomes with these specialized stents has accelerated adoption, particularly in North America and Europe. Emerging markets are also expected to provide growth opportunities as awareness of venous diseases increases and interventional radiology capabilities expand. With a growing focus on improving patient mobility, reducing long-term complications, and lowering healthcare costs by preventing recurrent hospitalizations, venous Nitinol self-expanding stents are gaining traction as an essential therapeutic solution in vascular care (Fig. 8.7).

The *North American* market for Nitinol self-expanding stents is one of the most mature and innovation-driven, largely supported by high healthcare expenditure, robust regulatory systems, and rapid adoption of advanced endovascular therapies. The United States dominates the region due to the high prevalence of peripheral artery disease (PAD), carotid artery stenosis, and gastrointestinal obstructions, conditions that are increasingly managed with minimally invasive procedures. Favorable reimbursement frameworks from Medicare and private insurers further encourage the use of Nitinol-based stents across hospitals and specialty clinics. The region also benefits from strong R&D activity, with key players such as Boston Scientific, Abbott, and Medtronic actively investing in drug-eluting Nitinol stents and coated variants to reduce restenosis rates. Additionally, the aging population, coupled with lifestyle-related risk factors like obesity and diabetes, fuels demand for vascular and

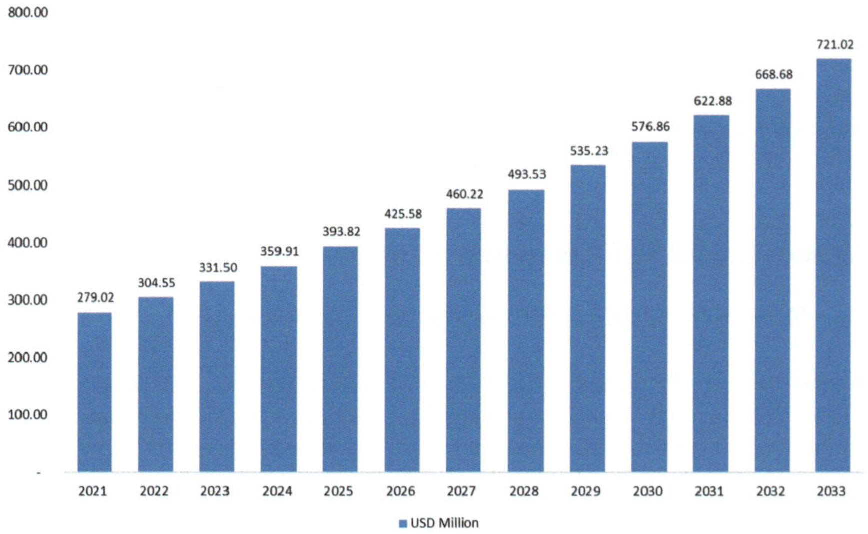

Fig. 8.7 Global Nitinol self-expanding stents market, by venous self-expanding stents 2021–2033 (USD Million)

venous stents. Canada is witnessing steady growth as well, supported by government healthcare coverage and a rising focus on interventional cardiology. Market growth is also driven by the presence of advanced ambulatory surgical centers (ASCs), which increasingly adopt self-expanding stents due to shorter recovery times and cost-effectiveness compared to inpatient hospital procedures. Looking forward, technological innovation in stent-grafts, integration of biodegradable coatings, and AI-assisted imaging for stent deployment are expected to enhance clinical outcomes, further expanding market penetration. However, challenges such as stringent FDA approval requirements may delay commercialization of next-generation devices, though overall demand in North America will remain strong over the forecast period (Table 8.2).

Europe represents a significant market for Nitinol self-expanding stents, driven by the region's aging population, well-established healthcare infrastructure, and strong demand for minimally invasive therapies across both vascular and non-vascular applications. Countries such as Germany, France, the UK, and Italy lead adoption, with Germany particularly strong due to its advanced cardiovascular treatment facilities and reimbursement systems that support stent implantation procedures. The European Medicines Agency (EMA) and CE marking requirements provide a clear but stringent regulatory pathway, which has encouraged innovation in coated stents, drug-eluting variants, and stent-grafts tailored to complex vascular anatomies. Rising incidence of chronic diseases such as atherosclerosis, gastrointestinal cancers, and pulmonary complications has also accelerated clinical usage. In recent years, Eastern European countries including Poland and Hungary have started showing higher demand, largely due to increasing investments in public healthcare modernization and greater accessibility to advanced interventional devices. The region's stent market is also being shaped by ongoing collaborations between research institutions and medical device manufacturers, particularly in biodegradable and hybrid stent technologies. Furthermore, governments are encouraging early detection and treatment of vascular diseases through screening programs, indirectly driving demand for self-expanding stents. However, price sensitivity in some markets, combined with budget constraints in public hospitals, may limit premium adoption of coated and drug-eluting Nitinol stents. Still, the European market is projected to maintain steady growth, supported by clinical preference for Nitinol's flexibility and shape memory, which enhances patient outcomes in tortuous anatomies compared to stainless steel alternatives (Table 8.3).

The *Asia-Pacific* (APAC) market for Nitinol self-expanding stents is witnessing the fastest growth globally, supported by rising healthcare expenditure, growing awareness of endovascular therapies, and a surge in chronic disease prevalence across populous nations. China and India are at the forefront, accounting for a large patient base suffering from cardiovascular and gastrointestinal disorders, driven by changing lifestyles, urbanization, and high smoking rates. Japan, with its highly advanced healthcare system, represents another significant contributor, particularly in the adoption of coated Nitinol stents and drug-eluting technologies. The presence of local manufacturers in China and South Korea has improved affordability and accessibility, enabling broader adoption across tier-2 and tier-3 cities. Government

Table 8.2 North America Nitinol self-expanding stents market by country USD million 2025–2033

Country	2025	2026	2027	2028	2029	2030	2031	2032	2033	CAGR (%)
US	2354.88	2538.74	2732.2	2890.42	3107.17	3337.52	3608.55	3895.68	4200.21	7.5
Canada	265.69	298.79	336.56	371.57	414.63	460.87	484.20	510.24	538.81	9.2
Total	2620.58	2837.53	3068.8	3261.98	3521.80	3798.39	4092.75	4405.92	4739.01	7.7

Table 8.3 Europe Nitinol self-expanding stents market by country, USD Million 2025–2033

Country	2025	2026	2027	2028	2029	2030	2031	2032	2033	CAGR (%)
Germany	322.91	351.76	382.98	416.77	462.70	502.85	556.85	604.45	667.86	9.5
France	240.11	257.73	276.50	296.50	324.36	347.35	379.0	405.51	441.40	7.9
UK	324.35	350.89	379.41	410.05	452.11	487.95	536.64	578.50	634.80	8.8
Italy	114.09	121.54	129.40	137.71	149.50	158.88	172.06	182.64	197.34	7.1
Spain	94.45	102.05	110.22	118.97	131.02	141.24	155.15	167.05	183.09	8.6
Benelux	134.96	145.72	157.27	169.64	186.67	201.09	220.72	237.48	260.09	8.5
ROE	359.96	382.93	407.01	432.24	468.13	496.11	535.52	566.39	609.51	6.8
Total	1590.83	1712.62	1842.79	1981.88	2174.50	2335.47	2555.98	2741.93	2994.1	8.2

initiatives to expand healthcare coverage, particularly under China's Healthy China 2030 strategy and India's Ayushman Bharat program, are further expanding access to advanced interventional procedures. Moreover, medical tourism in countries like Thailand, Malaysia, and Singapore is boosting demand for Nitinol self-expanding stents, particularly for gastrointestinal and bronchial indications. Technological collaborations between Western device companies and Asian manufacturers are driving innovation in cost-efficient stent designs tailored for diverse anatomies. However, regulatory variability across countries and lack of reimbursement in developing economies pose challenges. Despite this, the APAC region is poised for robust growth as it combines a large patient pool, rising procedural volumes, and ongoing adoption of advanced stent technologies across both hospital and ambulatory care settings (Table 8.4).

Latin America's market for Nitinol self-expanding stents is expanding steadily, primarily driven by increasing cardiovascular disease prevalence, rising obesity and diabetes rates, and growing access to interventional procedures in countries such as Brazil, Mexico, and Argentina. Brazil leads the market due to its advanced network of private hospitals and expanding public healthcare programs, which are gradually incorporating advanced vascular and gastrointestinal stent procedures. Mexico follows closely, driven by cross-border healthcare dynamics and rising investment in specialty clinics and ambulatory surgical centers. The affordability of Nitinol stents compared to surgical interventions is a key factor fueling their demand in the region. Multinational companies are also expanding their presence in Latin America, partnering with local distributors and healthcare providers to strengthen market penetration. Awareness campaigns and physician training programs by global medtech firms are enhancing adoption of advanced coated and drug-eluting stents. However, challenges remain, including limited reimbursement coverage in some countries, reliance on imports due to limited local manufacturing, and economic volatility affecting healthcare budgets. Despite these barriers, the region is expected to witness long-term growth as governments focus on reducing the burden of chronic vascular and gastrointestinal diseases. Stent-grafts and venous Nitinol stents are expected to gain traction in the coming years, particularly as clinical outcomes demonstrate improved long-term patency rates. Latin America's growing middle-class population and demand for minimally invasive solutions further reinforce the positive growth outlook for Nitinol self-expanding stents (Table 8.5).

The *Middle East* and *Africa* (MEA) market for Nitinol self-expanding stents is still in the early stages of adoption but presents significant growth potential, particularly in Gulf Cooperation Council (GCC) countries such as Saudi Arabia, the UAE, and Qatar. These nations are investing heavily in modernizing healthcare infrastructure and expanding access to advanced interventional cardiology and gastroenterology services. The high prevalence of cardiovascular diseases, diabetes, and obesity in the Middle East is a major driver of stent demand, with Nitinol's flexibility and self-expanding properties making it a preferred choice in complex anatomies. In Africa, South Africa remains a key hub for advanced medical procedures, while other nations are gradually improving access through public-private partnerships and medical tourism initiatives. International medical device companies are

Table 8.4 Asia Pacific Nitinol self-expanding stents market share by country, USD Million 2025–2033

Country	2025	2026	2027	2028	2029	2030	2031	2032	2033	CAGR (%)
China	423.33	455.26	493.74	529.94	573.32	624.64	673.95	731.98	793.79	8.2
India	388.54	426.44	471.99	517.01	570.84	634.73	698.92	774.72	857.40	10.4
Japan	169.78	183.19	199.34	214.67	233.02	254.73	275.76	300.50	326.96	8.5
SE Asia	193.05	210.88	232.30	253.25	278.30	307.98	337.52	372.35	410.13	9.9
Australia	43.52	46.71	50.55	54.15	58.46	63.57	68.45	74.19	80.30	8.0
Korea	66.51	71.74	78.03	84.00	91.15	99.61	107.79	117.42	127.71	8.5
ROAP	110.87	118.61	127.80	136.12	145.95	157.38	167.82	179.86	192.16	7.1
Total	1395.59	1512.82	1653.75	1789.15	1951.04	2142.64	2330.20	2551.02	2788.4	9.0

Table 8.5 Latin American Nitinol self-expanding stents market by country, USD Million 2025–2033

Country	2025	2026	2027	2028	2029	2030	2031	2032	2033	CAGR (%)
Brazil	148.31	161.87	175.74	189.91	204.40	219.19	234.28	249.69	265.40	7.5
Mexico	112.73	122.15	131.70	141.35	151.13	161.02	171.04	181.17	191.43	6.8
ROLA	292.47	313.95	335.30	356.50	377.58	398.52	419.32	440.00	460.54	5.8
Total	553.51	597.98	642.73	687.77	733.10	778.72	824.64	870.86	917.37	6.5

expanding their footprint in the region by collaborating with local distributors and establishing training centers to build physician expertise in endovascular therapies. However, affordability and lack of reimbursement remain major barriers, particularly in lower-income African countries where healthcare systems are still underdeveloped. Limited local manufacturing capacity also results in dependence on imports, raising overall treatment costs. Despite these challenges, growing investments in tertiary care hospitals, coupled with government initiatives to combat noncommunicable diseases, are expected to accelerate adoption. In the near future, coated Nitinol stents and drug-eluting stents are likely to see stronger uptake in GCC countries, while basic self-expanding Nitinol stents will dominate demand in African markets due to cost considerations. Overall, MEA represents a high-potential but unevenly developed market for Nitinol self-expanding stents (Table 8.6).

Globally, self-expanding stents remain a steady, mature market that grows in the mid-single digits. Recent industry trackers peg the overall self-expanding stents segment at roughly USD 3.6–3.8 billion in 2024–2025 with ~3–5% CAGR through 2030, and Nitinol continues to dominate this category thanks to its superelasticity and fatigue resistance.

Within that, venous stenting is the fastest-rising subsegment. Multiple dedicated iliofemoral venous systems gained US PMA in recent years (Vici, Abre, Zilver Vena, and, most recently, Philips Duo in 2024), which expands indications, competition, and physician familiarity. Forecasts now place the global venous stent market around USD 1.1–1.27 billion in 2024 with ~8–8.5% CAGR into the early to mid-2030s—above arterial growth.

Peripheral arterial Nitinol stents are seeing renewed momentum in drug-eluting platforms as the 2023 FDA update concluded that paclitaxel-coated devices for PAD are unlikely to increase mortality. That clarification stabilized clinical confidence and reimbursement narratives after years of uncertainty, and it supports continued investment in polymer-based and polymer-free paclitaxel stents.

On performance, contemporary drug-eluting Nitinol stents such as Eluvia and Zilver PTX continue to report competitive patency and reintervention profiles in randomized trials and pooled analyses, which is gradually tilting practice toward DES for long, complex femoropopliteal disease while drug-coated balloons retain share in shorter, less complex lesions. (Manufacturers report ~85–90% primary patency at one year in mixed-lesion cohorts and durable two- to five-year outcomes; independent commentaries and head-to-head data suggest no consistent mortality or safety penalty.)

Bare-metal Nitinol is not standing still. Biomechanics-centric designs (e.g., helical-centerline stents intended to encourage swirling flow and lower fracture risk) are accumulating supportive registry and RCT signals, creating a niche where "smart geometry" BMS can rival DES in select anatomies—another reason overall Nitinol volumes should remain resilient even as DCBs proliferate.

Manufacturing innovation is a quiet but important driver. Additive manufacturing of Nitinol is moving from research to pre-commercial feasibility, enabling fine control of strut architectures, graded porosity, and potentially patient-specific geometries—all with preserved superelastic behavior. While regulatory and cost hurdles

Table 8.6 MEA Nitinol self-expanding stents market by country, USD Million 2025–2033

Country	2025	2026	2027	2028	2029	2030	2031	2032	2033	CAGR (%)
Saudi Arabia	79.09	82.62	87.05	90.73	95.33	100.88	105.68	111.44	117.33	5.1
South Africa	23.76	25.18	26.93	28.49	30.38	32.64	34.71	37.17	39.74	6.6
Rest of MEA	176.20	186.22	198.53	209.39	222.67	238.50	252.91	270.03	287.84	6.3
Total	279.05	294.03	312.50	328.61	348.38	372.02	393.30	418.65	444.91	6.0

remain, this toolbox is likely to spill into limited-release products and custom devices first (e.g., complex airway or biliary), then into vascular once process controls are fully validated.

Regulation will shape the market cadence. In Europe, MDR has raised evidence and documentation burdens, lengthened timelines, and increased costs—factors that can thin product lines and slow launches, especially for smaller firms. Conversely, China is streamlining pathways and local production rules, which should accelerate both multinational and domestic entries in high-end cardiovascular devices, widening the addressable market for Nitinol implants.

Here is the best view of who holds the Nitinol-stent market today and how the share likely breaks down. The figures below are synthesis across the largest Nitinol stent segments (peripheral arterial, venous, and GI/tracheo-bronchial) using recent market reports and product landscapes. Those sources consistently identify Boston Scientific, Medtronic, Cook Medical, BD/Bard, Terumo, and Cordis as the core global manufacturers, with Biotronik and several endoscopy-focused firms (e.g., Micro-Tech) contributing meaningful regional share.

On a global basis (2024–2025) (Fig. 8.8), Boston Scientific holds around one -quarter of the market, buoyed by a broad Nitinol portfolio across peripheral (e.g., Eluvia/INNOVA), venous (VICI), and GI (WallFlex) plus ongoing portfolio expansion; Medtronic near one-fifth on strength in peripheral (EverFlex/Protégé) and leadership in dedicated venous stents (Abre); Cook Medical in low-teens anchored by Zilver (including Zilver PTX DES) and venous (Zilver Vena); BD/Bard

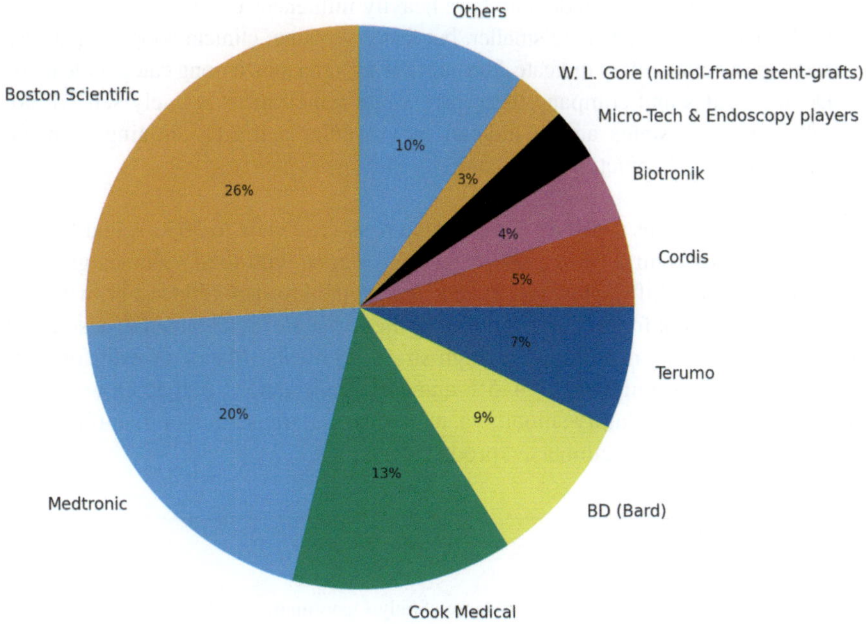

Fig. 8.8 Estimated global market share of Nitinol stent manufacturers 2024/2025.

Table 8.7 Global Nitinol self-expanding stents market share and products 2024/2025

Company	Market share (%)	Key products/segments
Boston Scientific	26	Peripheral stents, Eluvia DES
Medtronic	20	EverFlex/Protégé, Abre
Cook Medical	13	GI stents, Zilver, (venous, pulmonary)
Becton Dickinson (BD)	9	LifeStent/LifeStar
Terumo	7	Misago, Roadsaver Carotid stent
Cordis	5	SMART, PRECISE Pro Rx
Biotronik	4	Pulsar/Astron
Micro-Tech and other endoscopy players	3	GI Endoscopy stents
W.L. Gore	3.0	Nitinol-frame stent-grafts
Others	10	

mid-single digits to ~10% via LifeStent/LifeStar; Terumo mid-single digits (Misago and other peripheral lines); Cordis mid-single digits (SMART); Biotronik a few percentage (Pulsar/Astron); several endoscopy-centric manufacturers (e.g., Micro-Tech) adding a few percentage, and a long tail of region-specific players. Evidence points to Abre and Zilver Vena as among the most adopted dedicated venous stents, supporting Medtronic and Cook positions in that fast-growing niche (Table 8.7).

- Peripheral vascular stents are the largest Nitinol-stent segment and grow ~7% CAGR through 2030; leadership here heavily influences the overall picture.
- Dedicated venous stents are smaller, but faster-growing; clinical adoption patterns and expert commentary indicate Abre and Zilver Vena rank among category leaders.
- Device guides and company lists corroborate which firms actively sell Nitinol self-expanding stents across indications (vascular and GI), aligning with the "major players" depicted in the chart.

Taking these forces together, a reasonable base-case view to 2030 is that Nitinol will maintain its central role in self-expanding stents, with total volumes growing modestly and mix shifting toward (1) dedicated venous systems (fastest growth), (2) drug-eluting Nitinol for complex femoropopliteal disease, and (3) niche, design-led bare-metal solutions in tortuous or high-strain segments. Macro growth for self-expanding stents should track ~4–5% annually, with venous outpacing at ~8%+, and upside tied to regulatory smoothing and successful translation of manufacturing advances into scalable, reimbursed products.

Reference

1. Global Nitinol Self-Expanding Stents Market: Study, Opportunities, and Forecast (2025–2033). Straits Research; 2025.

Index

I. Rabkin, D. J. Rabkin, *Bloodline of Nitinol Stents*,
https://doi.org/10.1007/978-3-032-25697-3

GPSR Compliance

The European Union's (EU) General Product Safety Regulation (GPSR) is a set of rules that requires consumer products to be safe and our obligations to ensure this.

If you have any concerns about our products, you can contact us on ProductSafety@springernature.com

In case Publisher is established outside the EU, the EU authorized representative is:

Springer Nature Customer Service Center GmbH
Europaplatz 3
69115 Heidelberg, Germany

Batch number: 10726135

Printed by Printforce, the Netherlands